ENPC
Provider Manual

Community Nurse • Emergency Nurse • School Nurse •

Critical Care Nurse • Home Health Nurse • Trauma Nurse •

Office Nurse • Prehospital Nurse * Perioperative Nurse •

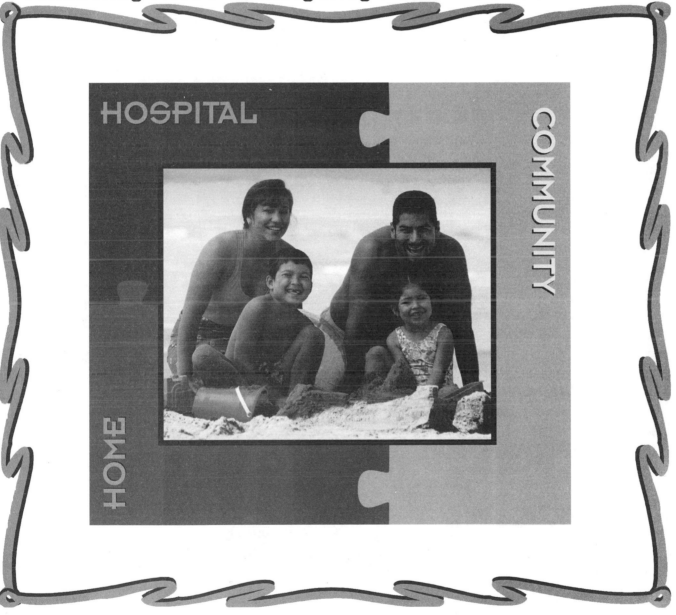

HOSPITAL

COMMUNITY

HOME

Medical-Surgical Nurse • Flight Nurse • Urgent Care Nurse •

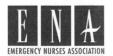

EMERGENCY NURSES ASSOCIATION

SECOND EDITION

Copyright © 1998
Emergency Nurses Association

ISBN 0-935890-34-3

The official Emergency Nursing Pediatric Course of the Emergency Nurses Association of New South Wales Inc. (Australia).

The official Emergency Nursing Pediatric Course of the National Emergency Nurses Association, Inc. of Canada.

Table of Contents

Tables

Figures

Appendixes

Skill Stations

Acknowledgments

The Emergency Nurses Association (ENA) would like to extend its appreciation to the 1997-1998 Emergency Nursing Pediatric Course Task Force for the development and implementation of the Emergency Nursing Pediatric Course (ENPC).

EDITORS

Nancy Eckle, RN, MSN, CEN, CNS
Program Manager, Emergency Services
Children's Hospital
Columbus, OH

Kathy Haley, RN, BSN, CEN
Trauma Coordinator, Trauma Program
Children's Hospital
Columbus, OH

Pam Baker, RN, BSN, CCRN, CEN
Director: Trauma, Pediatrics, and EMS
Emergency Nurses Association
Park Ridge, IL

1998 ENPC TASK FORCE

Kathy Haley, RN, BSN, CEN
Trauma Coordinator, Trauma Program
Children's Hospital
Columbus, OH

Nancy Eckle, RN, MSN, CEN, CNS
Program Manager, Emergency Services
Children's Hospital
Columbus, OH

Harriet Hawkins, RN, CCRN
Neonatal/Pediatric Transport Nurse
Transport Team
Children's Memorial Hospital
Chicago, IL

Reneé Semonin-Holleran, RN, PhD, CEN,
    CCRN, CFRN
Chief Flight Nurse/Clinical Nurse Specialist,
    Emergency Nursing
University of Cincinnati Medical Center
Cincinnati, OH

Beth Nachtsheim, RN, MS, PCCNP
Pediatric Critical Care Nurse Practitioner
Pediatric Intensive Care
Rush Presbyterian-St. luke's Medical Center
Rush University
Chicago, IL

1992 ENPC TASK FORCE

Lisa Bernardo, RN, MSN, PhD
Clinical Nurse Specialist
Children's Hospital of Pittsburgh
Pittsburgh, PA

Jan Fredrickson, RN, MSN, CPNP
Lecturer Maternal Child Health/Primary
    Ambulatory Care
UCLA School of Nursing
Pediatric Critical Care Clinical Specialist
Northridge Hospital Medical Center
Simi Valley, CA

Janice Rogers, RN, MS, CS
Pediatric Nurse Practitioner
Emergency Department
University of Rochester Medical Center
Rochester, NY

Reneé Semonin-Holleran, RN, PhD, CEN,
    CCRN, CFRN
Chief Flight Nurse/Clinical Nurse Specialist
Emergency Nursing
University of Cincinnati Medical Center
Cincinnati, OH

Treesa Soud, RN, BSN
Pediatric Emergency Nurse Consultant
Pediatric Emergency Services
Baptist Medical Center
Jacksonville, FL

Donna Thomas, RN, MSN, CEN
Director
Emergency Department
Primary Children's Medical Center
Salt Lake City, UT

CONTRIBUTING AUTHORS

Ray Bennett, RN, BSN, CEN, MICN
Emergency Department
Cooper Hospital
University Medical Center
Camden, NJ

Camillia S. Brandt, RN, MSN
Staff Nurse
Emergency Department
Cook Children's Medical Center
Fort Worth, TX

Tracey Bray, RN, MCN, Cert Paediatric
    Oncology
Senior Nurse Manager
Emergency Department
Sydney Children's Hospital
New South Wales, Australia

Patrick Callaway, RN, BSN, CEN
Care Coordinator
Emergency Department
Methodist/Children's Hospital
Omaha, NE

Cathy Carrico, RN, MS, CEN, FNP
Nurse Practitioner
Emergency Department
Children's Hospital
Omaha, NE

R. Warren Crow, Jr., RN, BSN, MICN
Director
Mobile Critical Care
Moses H. Cone Health System
Greensboro, NC

Neil Ead, RN, MSN, CCRN
Pediatric Nurse Practitioner
Hasbro Children's Hospital
Department of Pediatric Surgery
Providence, RI

Anne Morrison, RN, BN(Hon), Paed ICU Cert
Clinical Nurse Consultant
Paediatric ICU
New Children's Hospital
New South Wales, Australia

Sally Snow, RN, BSN, CEN
Pediatric Trauma Nurse Coordinator
Trauma Services
Cook Children's Medical Center
Fort Worth, TX

ORIGINAL CONTRIBUTING AUTHORS

Laurel Campbell, RN, MSN, CEN
Consultant Pediatric Clinical Nurse
Specialist
Adjunct Assistant Professor
Montana State University
Bozeman, MT

Neil Ead, RN, MSN, CEN, CCRN
Pediatric Nurse Practitioner
Hasbro Children's Hospital
Department of Pediatric Surgery
Providence, RI

Nancy Eckle, RN, MSN, CEN, CNS
Program Manager, Emergency Services
Children's Hospital
Columbus, OH

Sandra Jo Hammer, RN, MSN, MPH
Nurse Consultant II
State of California Department of Health
    Services
Adolescent Family Program
Sacramento, CA

Harriet Hawkins, RN, CCRN
Neonatal/Pediatric Transport Nurse
Transport Team
Children's Memorial Hospital
Chicago, IL

Susan J. Kelley, RN, PhD, FAAN
Associate Professor School of Nursing
Boston College
Boston, MA

Linda Manley, RN, BSN, CEN, CCRN
EMS Coordinator, Emergency Services
Flight Nurse/SkyMed
Children's Hospital
Columbus, OH

Melissa Taylor, RN, BSN
Nurse Manager
Emergency Services
Baptist Medical Center
Jacksonville, FL

CONTENT REVIEWERS

Mary E. Barkey, MA, CCLS
Child Life Clinical Specialist
Rainbow Babies and Children's Hospital
Cleveland, OH

Ray Bennett, RN, BSN, CEN, MICN
Emergency Department
Cooper Hospital
University Medical Center
Camden, NJ

Cathy Carrico, RN, MS, CEN, FNP
Nurse Practitioner
Emergency Department
Children's Hospital
Omaha, NE

Liz Cloughessy, RN, A&E Cert Executive
Emergency Nurses Association of New South
    Wales
and
Clinical Manager
Department of Emergency Medicine
Westmead Hospital
New South Wales, Australia

Carla Coffey, RN
Trauma Nurse Clinician
Children's Hospital
Columbus, OH

Neil Ead, RN, MSN, CCRN
Pediatric Nurse Practitioner
Hasbro Children's Hospital
Department of Pediatric Surgery
Providence, RI

Jane Ervin, RN, BSN
Clinical Leader
Emergency Department
Children's Hospital
Columbus, OH

Mary Fecht-Gramley, RN, PhD, CEN
Educational Coordinator to Trauma Services
Loyola University Health Center
Maywood, IL

Peggy Hamlin, RN, MSN, CRNP, CEN
Clinical Nurse Practitioner
University of South Alabama Physicians
Ob/Gyn Department
Mobile, AL

Mary Hayes, RN, MSN, CEN
Nursing Unit Director
Emergency Department
Catholic Medical Center – Mary Immaculate
    Hospital
Jamaica, NY

Jacqueline Jardine, RN
Nursing Director
Emergency Department
Arkansas Children's Hospital
Little Rock, AR

Mark Laubacker, RN, BSN, CSPI
Poison Information Specialist
Central Ohio Poison Center
Children's Hospital
Columbus, OH

Beth Malehorn, RN, BSN
RN Care Manager
Children's Hospital
Columbus, OH

Elizabeth Nicholson, MSSW, LISW
Director
Care House
Dayton, OH

Shawn Pruchnicki, RPH, EMT-P, CSPI
Poison Information Specialist
Central Ohio Poison Center
Children's Hospital
Columbus, OH

Cherie Revere, RN, MSN, CEN, CRNP
Clinical Nurse Specialist
Emergency Department
University of South Alabama
Medical Center
Mobile, AL

Andrea Self, RN, CEN
RN Care Manager
Emergency Department
Children's Hospital
Columbus, OH

Katherine H. Shaner, RN, BSN, CEN
RN Care Manager
Emergency Department
Children's Hospital
Columbus, OH
and
Transport Nurse
MedKids, MedFlight of Ohio
Columbus, OH

Sally Snow, RN, BSN, CEN
Pediatric Trauma Nurse Coordinator
Trauma Services
Cook Children's Medical Center
Fort Worth, TX

Barbara Kurfis Stephens, RN, MAN, CCRN
Clinical Nurse Specialist
Health Hill Hospital for Children
Cleveland, OH

STAFF SUPPORT

Pam Baker, RN, BSN, CCRN, CEN
Director: Trauma, Pediatrics, and EMS
Emergency Nurses Association
Park Ridge, IL

Sharon Tarnoff
Group Director, Association Resource
Development and Promotion
Emergency Nurses Association
Park Ridge, IL

Karen Charewicz
Administrative Assistant: Trauma, Pediatrics,
    and EMS
Emergency Nurses Association
Park Ridge, IL

MEDICAL ILLUSTRATOR

Leonard Morgan
Leonard Morgan Medical Art
Bolingbrook, IL

Preface

Trauma is the leading cause of death in children. However, acute illness is also a source of unnecessary pediatric death. Among all children who are patients in an emergency department (33% of all ED visits nationwide), fewer than 5% present with a true medical or surgical emergency. While national attention has recently focused on the standardization of trauma care, less effort has been made to standardize emergency pediatric care. To lessen the morbidity and mortality of children, emergency nurses must be knowledgeable about preventive strategies for injury and disease, as well as triage assessment and categories, nursing assessment, and the appropriate interventions for children requiring emergency care.

In response to requests by the ENA's membership for a greater focus on the pediatric patient, the ENA Pediatric Committee was formed in 1991. One of the charges of this new committee was to assess the need for a pediatric emergency nursing course. A needs assessment done at the 1991 ENA Scientific Assembly overwhelmingly supported the need for such a course.

The Emergency Nursing Pediatric Course (ENPC) Task Force was formed in 1991 to develop ENPC, and again in 1998 to revise the course. Since 1993, over 30,000 nurses have attended ENPC throughout the world. The focus of the ENPC is to teach nurses the various aspects of pediatric emergency nursing care, including, but not limited to, pediatric trauma. The ultimate goal of ENPC is to improve the care of the pediatric patient in the emergency care setting and to increase the skill and confidence of emergency nurses who care for children worldwide. The curriculum was written by nurses skilled in the care of the pediatric patient, both in general and pediatric emergency departments. The course is intended to increase the cognitive and technical skills necessary to care for children in the emergency care setting.

The ENPC Task Force would like to extend a special appreciation to Nancy Eckle, Pam Baker, and Kathy Haley for serving as editors for the ENPC project. ENA would also like to recognize Harriet Hawkins for obtaining and contributing many of the picture slides for the course. The dedication of these individuals to this project and the advancement of pediatric emergency nursing is unsurpassed.

The ENPC represents a dream of many people and has received the overwhelming support of the ENA, NENA and ENA New South Wales. It also represents many hours of work and collaboration and, most importantly, responds to the needs of each organization's membership. We are proud of the ENA's commitment and leadership, as well as the many nurses involved in this project.

Emergency Nursing Pediatric Course

SAMPLE QUESTIONS

1. An 8-month-old infant with pneumonia has severe intercostal and substernal retractions, weak muscle tone, lethargy, and gray skin color. The infant's condition does not improve after bag-valve-mask ventilation. The next step in treatment is most likely to be:

   A. Administration of epinephrine.

   B. Supplemental warming measures.

   C. Rapid sequence induction.

   D. Administration of albuterol.

   Reference: Chapter 5, Respiratory Distress and Failure.

2. An infant with hypernatremic dehydration suddenly loses consciousness and exhibits rigid posturing and fine tremors. The nurse should first:

   A. Open the patient's airway.

   B. Obtain intraosseous access.

   C. Begin chest compressions.

   D. Administer intravenous diazepam.

   Reference: Chapter 11, Medical Emergencies.

3. A 9-month-old infant is crying loudly throughout the nursing assessment, and the caregiver is becoming distraught. The nurse should ask the caregiver to:

   A. Read a story to the infant.

   B. Offer the infant a pacifier.

   C. Return when the infant is consoled.

   D. Ignore the infant's behavior.

   Reference: Chapter 3, The Pediatric Patient.

4. Which infant would be triaged as nonurgent?

   A. A 9-month-old with a 5% deep partial-thickness burn to the right hand who is crying.

   B. A 3-month-old with a history of premature birth and a respiratory rate of 40 breaths/minute and labored.

   C. A 6-month-old with a history of ear infections and a temperature of 38°C (101.4°F) who is active and alert.

   D. A 12-month-old who fell down a flight of stairs, vomited once, and is crying and fussy.

   Reference: Chapter 4, Initial Assessment and Triage.

5. An experienced nurse is precepting a new graduate nurse during the resuscitation of a child. When the child is pronounced dead, the new graduate nurse bursts into tears. The preceptor's most appropriate response would be:

   A. "Let's stop and talk about what you are feeling."

   B. "Unfortunately, this happens frequently in the emergency department."

   C. "We can talk about your feelings later after work."

   D. "Pull yourself together. We don't have time for this."

   Reference: Chapter 13, Crisis Intervention.

6. An unresponsive 2-year-old child was found by his mother with a bottle labeled "Elavil 50 mg" by his side. Which piece of information is important to obtain from his mother?

   A. The size of the medication bottle.

   B. The expiration date of the medication.

   C. The number of pills left in the bottle.

   D. The person for whom the medication was prescribed.

   Reference: Chapter 12, Toxicologic Emergencies.

7. Which combination of medications is best to have prepared for a pediatric resuscitation?

   A. Dopamine and sodium bicarbonate.

   B. Epinephrine and glucose.

   C. Naloxone and lidocaine.

   D. Pentothal and vecuronium.

   Reference: Chapter 7, Cardiovascular Emergencies.

8. During an intubation attempt, the child's heart rate drops to 40 beats/minute. Which intervention is initiated?

   A. Ask the physician to stop the intubation attempt and perform bag-valve-mask ventilation.

   B. Apply cricoid pressure and establish intravenous access.

   C. Inform the physician of the heart rate and ask the physician to intubate faster.

   D. Administer blow-by oxygen and begin chest compressions.

   Reference: Chapter 7, Cardiovascular Emergencies.

9. A nurse providing crisis intervention to the family of a seriously ill child can best keep the family informed of the child's condition by:

   A. Placing them a secluded room.

   B. Referring to their child as "the patient."

   C. Telling the family how they should feel.

   D. Appointing one staff member to communicate with them.

   Reference: Chapter 13, Crisis Intervention.

10. A 20-day-old infant has a 1-week history of not eating well. The infant has a weak cry and is jittery. Which laboratory test is indicated immediately?

    A. Arterial blood gas.

    B. Finger-stick glucose.

    C. Complete blood count with differential.

    D. Toxicology screen.

    Reference: Chapter 10, The Neonate.

11. A 6-week-old infant is pale, has marked substernal retractions, expiratory grunting and poor muscle tone. The emergency nurse should first:

    A. Obtain intravenous access.

    B. Apply a pulse oximeter.

    C. Prepare for chest x-ray.

    D. Administer 100% oxygen.

    Reference: Chapter 5, Respiratory Distress and Failure.

12. A 16-month-old child was an unrestrained front-seat passenger in a motor vehicle crash. The chest x-ray reveals multiple rib fractures. These findings suggest what type of injury?

    A. Minor surface injury.

    B. Significant underlying injury.

    C. Significant surface injury.

    D. Minor underlying injury.

    Reference: Chapter 6, Pediatric Trauma.

13. Which intervention should be performed next if tactile stimulation, positioning, drying and blow-by oxygen administration do not increase a newborn's heart rate?

    A. Chest compressions.

    B. Umbilical vein cannulation.

    C. Endotracheal intubation.

    D. Bag-valve-mask ventilation.

    Reference: Chapter 10, The Neonate.

14. The best method to open the airway in an injured child is:

    A. Placing the head and neck in hyperextension.

    B. Using the jaw thrust maneuver.

    C. Placing the head and neck in flexion.

    D. Using the head tilt maneuver.

    Reference: Chapter 4, Initial Assessment and Triage.

15. Which piece of information is most important to know prior to transferring a patient to another facility?

    A. Documentation of the family's health insurance coverage.

    B. Pertinent family health history.

    C. Confirmation of acceptance from the receiving hospital.

    D. Confirmation of a medical diagnosis.

    Reference: Chapter 14, Stabilization and Transport.

16. A 10-kg child has deep partial-thickness burns over 35% of the total body surface area. Which evaluation parameter indicates that fluid resuscitation is adequate?

    A. Heart rate of 160 beats/minute.

    B. Respiratory rate of 34 breaths/minute.

    C. Blood pressure of 80/60 mm Hg.

    D. Urine output of 22 ml/hour.

    Reference: Chapter 8, Burns.

17. A 4-year-old child with a history of the flu has a heart rate of 80 beats/minute, respirations of 16 breaths/minute, and capillary refill of more than 3 seconds. The proper sequence for nursing interventions would be to first:

    A. Position the airway, administer 100% oxygen, obtain venous access, and administer 20 ml/kg of an isotonic solution.

    B. Administer 100% oxygen, obtain venous access, administer 0.1 mg/kg of epinephrine 1:10,000, and prepare for endotracheal intubation.

    C. Position the airway, provide bag-valve-mask ventilation, provide synchronized cardioversion, and provide supplemental warmth.

    D. Administer 100% oxygen, prepare for a venous cutdown, administer 20 ml/kg of an isotonic solution, and obtain a chest x-ray.

    Reference: Chapter 7, Cardiovascular Emergencies.

18. A 10-year-old child who was struck by a car has a distended, tense abdomen. The child's heart rate is 144 beats/minute, respirations 24 breaths/minute, and blood pressure 120/80 mm Hg. Capillary refill is more than 3 seconds and skin is pale and cool. The patient's signs and symptoms suggest:

    A. Obstructive shock.

    B. Distributive shock.

    C. Hypovolemic shock.

    D. Cardiogenic shock.

    Reference: Chapter 6, Pediatric Trauma.

19. Activated charcoal is effective in the absorption of which agent?

    A. Acetaminophen.

    B. Hydrocarbons.

    C. Iron.

    D. Caustics.

    Reference: Chapter 12, Toxicologic Emergencies.

20. A 7-year-old female sustains a minor head injury and did not lose consciousness. She does not respond to commands and groans in response to questions. Which action will quickly determine if her behavior indicates a serious head injury?

A. Review her medical record for pre-existing developmental problems.

B. Obtain a head computerized tomography scan.

C. Conduct a developmental screening test.

D. Ask the parents if her behavior is unusual.

Reference: Chapter 6, Pediatric Trauma.

21. A 3-year-old is transported by prehospital personnel after being struck by a car. The parents are en route. The child is screaming and uncooperative. Which is the best approach while conducting the secondary survey?

A. Hold the child to comfort him.

B. Wait for the parent's arrival.

C. Observe for behavioral pain cues.

D. Use a doll to demonstrate the examination.

Reference: Chapter 3, The Pediatric Patient.

22. A school-aged child is about to receive stitches. To evaluate his understanding of the procedure, you tell him:

A. "Young people your age have questions about getting stitches. What are your questions?"

B. "Don't cry while you are getting the stitches. Be brave like a man."

C. "You will probably receive 10 stitches. Do you have any questions before we restrain you?"

D. "Does your cut hurt? Would you like your mommy to hold you?"

Reference: Chapter 3, The Pediatric Patient.

23. An 8-month-old child presents with purpura, irritability, and a rectal temperature of 39.4°C (102.9°F). An intervention of high priority is:

A. Encouraging the caregiver to hold and comfort the child.

B. Monitoring for signs and symptoms of increased cranial pressure (ICP).

C. Collecting urine for toxicology screen.

D. Encouraging oral fluids and food.

Reference: Chapter 11, Medical Emergencies.

24. Which ocular finding is associated with child maltreatment?

A. Glaucoma.

B. Conjunctivitis.

C. Iritis.

D. Retinal hemorrhage.

Reference: Chapter 9, Child Maltreatment.

25. Which intervention must be initiated in the child with a hemopneumothorax prior to transfer?

A. Nasogastric tube insertion.

B. Endotracheal tube insertion.

C. Chest tube insertion.

D. Central line insertion.

Reference: Chapter 14, Stabilization and Transport.

ENPC Sample Questions

ANSWER KEY

1.	C	10.	B	18.	C
2.	A	11.	D	19.	A
3.	B	12.	B	20.	D
4.	C	13.	D	21.	C
5.	A	14.	B	22.	A
6.	C	15.	C	23.	B
7.	B	16.	D	24.	D
8.	A	17.	A	25.	C
9.	D				

Overall Course Objectives

On completion of this course, the learner should be able to:

- Describe the characteristics of life-threatening illness and injury in children.

- Identify the anatomic and physiologic characteristics of children as a basis for signs and symptoms.

- Identify the most frequent causes of illness or injury in children.

- Describe the assessment of children with illness or injury.

- Identify the appropriate nursing diagnoses and expected outcomes based on the assessment findings.

- Plan the specific interventions needed to manage the child with illness or injury.

- Evaluate the effectiveness of nursing interventions related to patient outcomes.

- Identify health promotion strategies related to the pediatric population.

Psychomotor Skill Station Objectives

On completion of this course, the learner should be able to:

- Demonstrate a standardized, systematic, and organized approach to assessment, planning, intervention, and evaluation.

- Perform a primary and secondary assessment.

- State patient problem based on assessment data.

- Identify an appropriate plan of care.

- Set priorities for nursing interventions based on assessment data.

- Implement appropriate interventions.

- Evaluate patient response to nursing interventions.

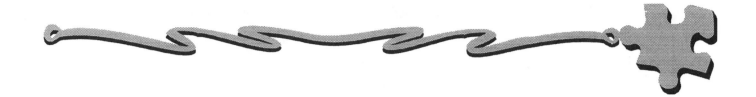

CHAPTER 1

The Emergency Nursing Pediatric Course

OBJECTIVES

On completion of this lecture, the learner should be able to:

- ✦ Describe the development of pediatric emergency care as a unique discipline.

- ✦ Identify three nursing roles in pediatric emergency care.

- ✦ Describe the purpose and structure of the Emergency Nursing Pediatric Course (ENPC).

INTRODUCTION

All infants, children, and adolescents must have access to emergency care executed by health care providers knowledgeable in the care of pediatric emergency conditions.[1] Although children younger than 18 years of age account for approximately 30% of all emergency department (ED) visits, many health care providers have difficulty developing and maintaining critical pediatric skills.[2] The majority of ED visits by children are for nonemergent problems; however, every emergency department has the potential to receive a child in need of lifesaving intervention. All emergency health care providers must be prepared to provide immediate emergency care and appropriate referral for definitive pediatric care.[1-3] Over the last two decades, an increasing level of commitment to the improvement of emergency care for children has been demonstrated by[1,3]:

- • The creation of pediatric committees by nursing and medical organizations.

- • The emergence of pediatric emergency medicine and nursing as recognized subspecialties of pediatric care and a corresponding increase in nurses and physicians specializing in pediatric emergency care.

- • The establishment of professional organizations that provide a forum for pediatric emergency practitioners.

- • The development and dissemination of national educational programs on pediatric emergency care and resuscitation.

- The funding of pediatric emergency medicine residencies and fellowship programs.

- The availability of board certification in pediatric emergency medicine, offered jointly by the American Board of Pediatrics and the American Board of Emergency Medicine.

- Significant increases in the publication of pediatric emergency care textbooks in nursing and medicine, research, and clinical articles.

- The ongoing funding of the Emergency Medical Services for Children (EMSC) grant program.

The scope of emergency nursing practice encompasses nursing assessment, intervention, and evaluation of patients of all ages and all acuity levels. The Emergency Nurses Association (ENA), the Emergency Nurses Association of New South Wales, and the National Emergency Nurses Association of Canada support the development of standards to ensure adequate and safe emergency care for children with injuries and illnesses. In response to the needs of children and emergency nurses, ENA developed the ENPC in 1991. The ENPC provides nurses and other health care providers with a standardized, internationally disseminated pediatric educational program to enhance their knowledge, skill, and expertise in the care of children.

ENA has continued to respond to the needs of children by: 1) monitoring and proposing legislation, 2) identifying issues related to pediatric emergency care, 3) collaborating with other organizations to enhance the emergency care of children, and 4) developing educational resources for emergency nurses who care for children. This chapter describes the role of the emergency nurse in pediatric emergency care and the structure of the ENPC.

ROLES OF THE EMERGENCY NURSE IN PEDIATRIC EMERGENCY CARE

The evolution of pediatric emergency care as a separate and recognized discipline has been a catalyst for improvement in the emergency care of infants, children, and adolescents. Nurses perform a pivotal role in all phases of pediatric emergency care.

Physiologic baselines and responses to illness or injury in the child differs from the adult. Anatomic and physiologic characteristics as well as emotional, psychosocial, and cognitive responses differ among age groups. These factors are compounded by the fact that children represent a smaller percentage of the total population seen in emergency care settings. Generally, emergency nurses have a lower experience level in providing care for children, especially pediatric patients with life-threatening illness or injury.

To lessen the morbidity and mortality of children, the emergency nurse must be able to quickly recognize and intervene for the pediatric patient in crisis. Essential knowledge for the emergency nurse includes growth and development, pediatric triage and acuity level identification, pediatric assessment and intervention techniques, common pediatric disease and injury processes, and prevention strategies as they relate to the infant, child, and adolescent.[1] Core-level and continuing education are necessary for the development and maintenance of competence in pediatric emergency care.

Nurses who provide emergency care to children must assure that policies and procedures, specific to the pediatric patient, are developed to guide and maintain consistency in the delivery of emergency care.[1] Additionally, supplies and equipment in a wide array of sizes must be available and functional to provide emergency interventions for children from birth to adolescence.

Providing Family-Centered Care

Pediatric emergency care requires assessment and intervention to meet the physiologic, psychosocial, and emotional needs of children and their families. Strategies to integrate psychosocial care into practice must include the adoption of a *family-centered care philosophy*. An interdisciplinary approach that supports and integrates the *family* into the emergency care process is vital for both the child and family.[1]

The child's normal behavior and routines are best described by the child's *caregiver*. Parents or caregivers may be unclear of their role in the child's care in the emergency care setting. It is important to assess the caregiver's comfort level with the treatment process and encourage the caregiver's participation in care. The primary role of the caregiver during assessment and interventions is to provide support and comfort measures to the child. Anxious caregivers may increase the child's fears and resistance. It is important to listen to the concerns of the caregiver and communicate in terms he or she can understand. Providing caregivers and family members the option to be with their child throughout emergency treatment, stabilization, or resuscitation is an ethically based practice grounded in the philosophy of family-centered care.[1]

The key elements of family-centered care include[4]:

- Recognizing that the family is the constant in a child's life.

- Facilitating family and professional collaboration at all levels of hospital, home, and community care.

- Recognizing and honoring diversity, strengths, and individuality within and across all families; this includes ethnic, racial, spiritual, social, economic, educational, and geographic diversity.

- Recognizing and respecting different methods of coping, and implementing policies and programs to meet the diverse needs of families.

- Recognizing the range of strengths, concerns, emotions, and expectations of families and children.

Promoting Prevention of Injury and Illness

Because of the episodic nature of emergency care, a single patient encounter may be the only opportunity the nurse has to affect the health practices of a family. Therefore, nurses must be cognizant of their role in the prevention of childhood illness and injury. Early identification of children at risk is an important element in the primary prevention of illness, injury, and child maltreatment. Evaluation of risk factors and the formulation of practical intervention strategies are actions that may enhance or influence family health practices. Each encounter with a child and family provides an opportunity for education, counseling, and anticipatory guidance.[1]

Emergency nurses also have the opportunity to participate in public endeavors directed at injury and/or illness prevention. The activities may include involvement in: 1) public and professional education, 2) legislative efforts for injury control and prevention, 3) legislative efforts for regionalization of pediatric emergency care services, 4) child advocacy, and 5) injury or illness prevention initiatives.[1] ENA and EN CARE injury prevention programs include EN CARE Learning to CARE, TAKE CARE, and Dare to CARE programs; injury prevention workgroups; grant and training programs, Master Lock Gun Safety Campaign; Polaroid – Family Violence Campaign; Global Med-Net which is an emergency information database program; and multiple injury prevention resources and professional services.

Participating in Programs to Enhance Emergency Medical Services for Children

In 1984, Congress adopted legislation authorizing the establishment of the Emergency Medical Services for Children (EMSC) grant program. The purpose of this ongoing grant program is to reduce pediatric morbidity and mortality by expanding access to and improving the quality of emergency medical services for children. The EMSC program is operated jointly by the Maternal and Child Health Bureau (MCHB) and the Health Resource and Services Administration (HRSA) of the US Department of Health and Human Services in collaboration with the National Highway Traffic Safety Administration (NHTSA).[5] With current funding of $12.5 million, EMSC provides grants to support the development and implementation of projects related to pediatric emergency care across the country. The development of educational materials, training programs, pediatric protocols, and pediatric emergency care systems has been funded through EMSC. Through the collaboration of physicians, nurses, and prehospital providers, EMSC grants have provided education and training for providers in all phases of emergency care. Information and assistance to those interested in issues related to emergency medical services for children are available through the EMSC resource center.[2,5]

THE EMERGENCY NURSING PEDIATRIC COURSE (ENPC)

Course Description

The ENPC is a 16-hour course designed to provide the learner with cognitive knowledge and psychomotor skills. The nursing process is used to standardize the approach to pediatric emergency care and is reflected in the content and approach of the chapters and psychomotor skill stations. Participants receive 18.6 continuing education credit hours (CECH) for attending the course.

Lectures and psychomotor skill stations are presented by ENPC Instructors and ENPC Instructor Candidates. The lecture content is organized to provide the learner with substantive knowledge for use in the psychomotor skill stations. Evaluation of the learner includes 1) a written multiple choice examination designed to assess his or her acquisition of content presented in the manual and during the lectures, and 2) performance at psychomotor skill stations designed to evaluate the acquisition of important skills. To successfully complete the ENPC, the learner must achieve a minimum of 80% on the written examination and demonstrate 70% of all steps in each skill station.

If the written examination score is between 70 and 80%, a learner may repeat the written examination one time only if he or she is successful in all psychomotor skill stations. A learner may repeat one psychomotor skill station as long as he or she successfully completes the multiple choice examination the first time.

Purpose

The purpose of the ENPC is to present core-level knowledge and psychomotor skills associated with implementing the nursing process in the care of children from birth through adolescence. The psychomotor skill stations facilitate initial integration of psychomotor abilities in a setting that simulates pediatric patient situations. It is the intent of ENPC to enhance the nurse's ability to rapidly and accurately assess the pediatric patient's responses to the illness or injury event. It is anticipated that the use of the knowledge and skills learned in the ENPC will ultimately contribute to a decrease in the morbidity and mortality associated with pediatric emergencies.

Course Participants

Nurses and other health care providers practicing in clinical areas other than an emergency care setting may desire to take ENPC. It is assumed that the course participant has an understanding of emergency care terminology and is familiar with standard emergency equipment. The course content and psychomotor skill stations provide valuable information and skill practice within a supportive learning environment.

Only registered nurses are eligible for evaluation and verification in the ENPC. Other health care providers are not eligible for evaluation or verification in the ENPC; however, they may attend a course and receive a certificate of attendance and/or continuing education contact hours if approved by their professional accrediting body.

THE NURSING PROCESS AND ORGANIZATION OF THE ENPC MANUAL

The nursing process serves as a basis for the standardized approach to initial pediatric care. The *Standards of Clinical Nursing Practice*, developed by the American Nurses Association,[6] the *Standards of Emergency Nursing Practice*, developed by the Emergency Nurses Association,[7] and the *Standards of Pediatric Clinical Nursing Practice*, developed by the Society of Pediatric Nurses and the American Nurses Association,[8] are the standards that describe the implementation of the nursing process. The nursing process describes and organizes the essential phases of nursing care, including assessment, nursing diagnoses, outcome identification, planning and implementation, and evaluation. Following the sequential phases of the nursing process provides the foundation for a structured approach to nursing care activities and clinical decision making.[6]

To enhance learning, each ENPC chapter follows a consistent format and includes the six components of the nursing process. The ENPC manual design reinforces and supplements lectures and psychomotor skill station content. Chapter format includes the following:

- Objectives: Behavioral and learning objectives are stated at the beginning of each chapter. The objectives identify the key lecture content and areas for evaluation.

- Introduction: Within this section, information regarding epidemiology and pediatric-specific information on the topic are presented.

- Anatomic, Physiologic, and Developmental Characteristics as a Basis for Signs and Symptoms: A brief review of relevant anatomic, physiologic, and developmental concepts are presented to enhance understanding of the illness or injury process for the topics covered in the chapter. The section presents specific information on the unique characteristics of infants and children.

- Definitions and Causes: Definition of the disorder and common etiology are described in selected chapters.

- Nursing Care of the Child: The nursing process is used to organize the nursing care principles. The phases of the nursing process are presented as follows:

  - Assessment – Appropriate history and physical assessment principles are described. A mnemonic for the assessment of the pediatric patient describes and organizes the assessment components. This mnemonic approach to assessment and intervention is consistent throughout the text. Pertinent historical data and expected physical findings (signs and symptoms) specific to the patient problem or emergency condition are noted in each chapter.

♦ The assessment content is organized, where appropriate, using the assessment skills of inspection, auscultation, and palpation.

♦ In the diagnostic procedures section, appropriate laboratory, radiographic, and monitoring procedures are listed.

- Nursing Diagnoses and Outcome Identification – Nursing diagnoses, developed by the North American Nursing Diagnosis Association, are used to categorize the patient's responses to the illness or injury event. The nursing diagnoses provide a foundation for the identification of interventions and determining expected patient outcomes. Interventions and expected outcomes associated with each nursing diagnosis are listed in a table format.

- Triage and Acuity Decisions – The assessment findings and patient condition allow categorization into three levels of acuity: Emergent, urgent, and nonurgent.

- Planning and Implementation – In the planning and implementation section, interventions are listed in a descending order of priority. This classification of interventions stresses the need to set priorities for pediatric patient care based on the correction of life-threatening conditions first.

- Evaluation and Ongoing Assessment – A description of desired patient responses and ongoing assessments are listed. Based on achievement or lack of achievement of expected outcomes, nursing interventions can be adjusted to meet the changing needs of the patient.

● Selected Emergencies: This section presents a variety of specific disease processes or injury types associated with a particular body system or type of emergency condition. A brief description of the selected emergency is followed by a discussion of specific or additional signs and symptoms that may be present. Only interventions that vary from those presented earlier in the chapter are described.

● Health Promotion: This section provides an overview of injury and illness prevention strategies and related anticipated guidance topics.

● Pediatric Considerations Supplement: Select chapters are followed by information on selected procedures and interventions relevant to chapter content.

Psychomotor Skill Stations: Additional information is also presented in each skill station. Preparation for the course includes reading and becoming familiar with the skill station content. Each psychomotor skill station uses the following format:

● Equipment needed for the station.

● Station preparation.

● Introductory information.

● Principles of the station assessment.

● Intervention techniques taught in the station, steps in the skill performance, and summary.

Case scenarios are utilized to provide the participant with an opportunity to assimilate knowledge and psychomotor skills into the care of the pediatric patient.

Appendixes: Supplemental and reference information is presented in the appendixes. Relevant appendixes are referred to in the associated chapter text.

Glossary: Definitions of terms and phrases used in the ENPC manual. Words and phrases defined in the glossary are identified the first time they appear by italics in the text.

SUMMARY

The provision of competent emergency care for children must become an inherent part of the emergency care system. The community, hospital, and home environments are integral in the provision of emergency care to children and their families. Nurses practicing in a variety of environments encounter children with emergent conditions that require prompt recognition and intervention. The delivery of quality nursing care to the pediatric patient requires specialized knowledge, training, equipment, and planning. The ENPC provides comprehensive pediatric emergency care information and describes definitive interventions. Although the level of intervention described may not be applicable in all settings (school, private office, clinic, home, prehospital environment), the principles of pediatric emergency nursing care and the nursing process cross all care environments.

Competent emergency nursing care for children is essential for the reduction of pediatric morbidity and mortality. Each of the organizations that disseminate ENPC believes that the knowledge and psychomotor skills identified in the ENPC will assist the professional nurse to systematically assess the pediatric patient and provide appropriate interventions.

HOSPITAL-BASED NURSING
- Emergency Nurse
- Critical Care Nurse
- Transport/Flight Nurse
- Pediatric Nurse
- Perioperative Nurse
- Postoperative/Postanesthesia Care Nurse
- Medical/Surgical Nurse
- Rehabilitation Nurse

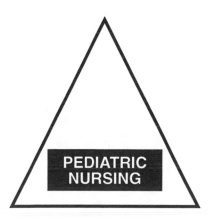

PEDIATRIC
NURSING

HOME-BASED NURSING
- Home Health Nurse
- Public Health Nurse
- Rehabilitation Nurse

COMMUNITY-BASED NURSING
- School Nurse
- Office Nurse
- Public Health Nurse
- Prehospital/EMS Nurse
- Extended Care Facility Nurse
- Poison Information Specialist Nurse

REFERENCES

1. Emergency Nurses Association. *Emergency Nursing: Pediatric Emergency Care Policy Statement*. Park Ridge, Ill: Author; 1995.

2. Institute of Medicine, Division of Health Care Services, National Research Council. Emergency medical systems origin and operations. *Emergency Medical Services for Children*. Washington, DC: National Academy Press; 1993:66-107.

3. Institute of Medicine, Division of Health Care Services, National Research Council. Risking our children's health: A need for emergency care. *Emergency Medical Services for Children*. Washington, DC: National Academy Press; 1993:38-65.

4. Shelton TL, Stepanek JS. Key elements of family-centered care. *Family-Centered Care for Children Needing Specialized Health Care and Developmental Services*. Bethesda, Md: Association for the Care of Children's Health; 1994:vii.

5. Weintraub B. Emergency medical services for children. *J Emerg Nurs*. 1997;23:274-275.

6. American Nurses Association. *Standards of Clinical Practice*. Kansas City, Mo: Author; 1991:3.

7. Emergency Nurses Association. *Standards of Emergency Nursing Practice*. 3rd ed. St. Louis, Mo: Mosby-Year Book; 1995.

8. Society of Pediatric Nurses and American Nurses Association. *Statement on the Scope and Standards of Pediatric Clinical Nursing Practice*. Washington, DC: American Nurses Publishing; 1996.

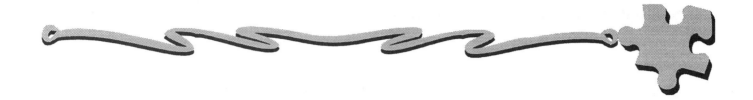

CHAPTER 2

Epidemiology

OBJECTIVES

On completion of this lecture, the learner should be able to:

+ Identify characteristics of pediatric patients seen in the emergency department.

+ Describe the characteristics of life-threatening illness in children.

+ Discuss the impact of pediatric injuries on child morbidity and mortality.

+ State topics for injury prevention teaching based on the child's age.

INTRODUCTION

The needs of children were generally overlooked during the development of emergency medical services. It was not until the mid-1970s that the prehospital and hospital-based emergency care needs of children began to be addressed.[1] The unique attributes of pediatric emergencies are influenced by the growing anatomy, immature physiology, and variable developmental achievements of children.[2] These factors affect the types of illnesses and injuries sustained as well as the typical clinical presentation. This chapter describes the characteristics of the pediatric population and the epidemiology of pediatric emergencies.

CHARACTERISTICS OF THE PEDIATRIC POPULATION

The characteristics of the pediatric population treated in the emergency care setting are being influenced by changes in health care systems, access to pediatric tertiary care, advances in health care practices, and socioeconomic and community conditions. A combination of these factors and social circumstances may influence the caregiver's utilization of the emergency department for episodic care.[3]

Access to Pediatric Health Care Services

- Not all communities have pediatric hospitals or pediatric specialty services. Children may have to be transferred to a pediatric tertiary care or pediatric trauma center for definitive care.

- Many children's hospitals and large metropolitan hospitals maintain facilities and personnel to treat the most complex, rare, and life-threatening pediatric emergencies. The presence of a pediatric center impacts the pediatric census in general emergency departments in the same service area. Consequently, personnel in general emergency departments may have significantly less exposure to children with serious illnesses or injuries.

- There has been enormous growth in enrollment in managed care plans and health maintenance organizations (HMOs) in the United States. Such plans typically include cost-containment and utilization-management features. Many plans include gatekeeping functions by the primary care provider that may require emergency care referral or authorization. Additionally, a child may be enrolled in a plan that does not include the pediatric hospital or the area hospital with a pediatric emergency department or pediatric services.

- Currently, information provided to enrollees concerning the definition of emergency conditions is often vague and adult based without reference to emergency conditions in children.[4] Primary care providers or HMOs may advise parents to take their children to the emergency department in cases of emergency; however, conditions perceived as an emergency by the caregiver may not be considered an emergency by the health plan (caregiver refers to parents, guardians, or any individual responsible for the child). In addition, the caregiver may delay seeking appropriate emergency care to obtain authorization. Managed care can potentially result in underutilization of appropriate services and a reduced quality of care.[5] State and federal legislative efforts are underway to standardize the definition of emergency conditions utilizing the *prudent layperson definition.*

Continued Use of the Emergency Department as a Primary Source of Episodic Health Care

- Children who lack access to primary and well-child health care are more likely to utilize emergency care services. The emergency department is often the easiest and least restricted entry into the health care delivery system, especially for those who are uninsured. Recent data indicate that 21% of American children live in poverty, and hundreds of thousands are homeless.[6,7] Families with children constitute the fastest growing group of the homeless, accounting for up to 43% of the homeless population.[7] These children often do not have an established relationship with a primary care provider.[7]

- Because of decreased funding, many primary clinics have decreased their hours of access. For some caregivers, the emergency department may offer the only easily recognizable and accessible alternative for health care.[8]

- Restrictions or limitations in the operating hours of primary care provider's offices and clinics often force caregivers to seek treatment at other sites. Lack of available care and actual or perceived inaccessibility of primary care providers have also been identified as factors in the use of the emergency department for nonurgent problems.[9,10]

Referral Patterns of Primary Care Providers

- Many physicians are reluctant to handle pediatric patients with complex problems, especially in the office or clinic setting. Therefore, children are referred to an emergency department for evaluation and treatment.[11] Unlike offices or clinics, an emergency department provides 24-hour availability of diagnostic facilities and access to experienced physicians and nurses.

- Primary care physicians with limited knowledge of pediatrics or who lack familiarity with the child may be reluctant to assess signs and symptoms by telephone, particularly in view of the potential liability.[12] Therefore, the caregiver and child may be referred to an emergency department.

- In the United States, a combination of full office schedules, lack of open appointments, and a problem that is felt to be medically urgent by the primary care provider or *gatekeeper* may influence decisions regarding referrals or approvals of nonurgent ED visits.[10]

Higher Survival Rates and a Greater Number of Children with Chronic Illness

- Because of technology and the advancements in health care, children who have diseases that have historically been fatal in childhood or adolescence are now living well into adulthood. Acute exacerbations, however, often require rapid, expert emergency care and hospitalization.

- Many children afflicted with complicated medical problems are dependent on medical technology such as oxygen, home ventilators, and long-term central venous access devices. These children are often at greater risk for the development of emergent conditions such as respiratory failure and sepsis.

Violence Against Children

- Violence against children occurs in both the family and community environments. Inflicted injury has had a significant impact on pediatric morbidity and mortality, as well as the types of injuries pediatric patients sustain.

- The United States leads the world in pediatric homicide and suicides.

- All forms of child maltreatment have risen significantly. Currently almost 3 million cases of suspected child maltreatment are reported annually in the United States; of these, approximately 1 million cases are substantiated.[13] Despite improved recognition and reporting of child maltreatment, a significant number of cases remain unreported.

- Physical assault has been recognized as the leading cause of homicide in infants and toddlers.[14] In older children and adolescents, an argument or criminal activity is often the precipitating factor in a violent death or homicide in which the perpetrators are peers, acquaintances, or gang members.[14]

- Exposure to violence in the community and through the media, in combination with other social experiences, can increase the risk for involvement with violence. Access to firearms, substance abuse, and involvement in antisocial or violent groups are factors that increase a child's risk for entanglement in violent situations.[15]

- Gang activity and influences are increasingly evident in inner city, suburban, and rural areas. Violence affiliated with gang activity is extremely volatile and is often associated with illegal drugs, "turf wars," and weapons. As a result, children are increasingly the victims of penetrating trauma, as either a participant in or an innocent bystander to gang activities.

Nonimmunized and Underimmunized Children

Although immunization rates for children younger than 3 years of age have improved in some regions, a significant percentage of young children are not fully immunized. Approximately 67.5% of children younger than 3 years of age were reported to be up-to-date on their immunizations in 1994, a significant improvement over 1991's rate of 37%.[16] However, regional outbreaks of rubella, rubeola, pertussis and other preventable illnesses have been directly related to inadequate immunization. Children who contract one of these highly communicable diseases may develop emergent complications or present in the emergency department for acute care in response to the illness.

Infrequent Use of Prehospital Emergency Medical Services

Fewer than 10% of requests for emergency medical services are for children.[17] Caregivers often choose to transport their critically or seriously ill or injured child to an emergency department by private vehicle rather than waiting for emergency medical services to respond. Consequently, emergent pediatric patients routinely present to the emergency department without benefit of prehospital care.

EPIDEMIOLOGY OF PEDIATRIC EMERGENCIES

The exact epidemiology of pediatric emergencies is not known.[2] Determining the precise incidence and prevalence of pediatric emergency illness and injury is complicated by a number of factors:

- Age definitions for "pediatrics" are not standardized. The American Academy of Pediatrics defines *pediatrics* as a continuum from birth through adolescence, or 0 to 21 years of age.

- ED data are not consistently reported by age category.

- Qualitative and quantitative data that accurately document indicators, such as delayed or missed diagnosis, are difficult to obtain.

- Statistics regarding children with emergencies are seriously limited.

- The number of children with emergency conditions who are treated by primary care providers and in urgent care facilities is unknown.[2,18]

- There is no nationally standardized reporting system for pediatric emergencies.[2]

In 1993, approximately 4,500 hospitals reported providing emergency services.[13] Of the 96 million ED visits in 1995, 40% (more than 38 million) were made by persons 24 years of age or younger.[16] Children younger than 15 years of age represented a total of 23 million visits (24%).[16] It is estimated that more than 60,000 children seek emergency care for injuries or illnesses every day in the United States.[19]

Because of the limited number of pediatric emergency departments, the majority of children seeking emergency care are treated in general emergency departments.[2] Therefore, all emergency health care providers must be familiar with the signs and symptoms of a life-threatening illness or injury as well as subtle signs of a deteriorating condition in children. Recognition of such conditions can be difficult for those who lack pediatric training and experience.[17] Accurate assessment is essential to rapidly providing the child with the appropriate interventions and stabilization.

PEDIATRIC ILLNESS

The frequency of pediatric illness varies significantly according to the age, season, and time of day. Usage of emergency departments by pediatric patients tends to be higher during evening hours and in the winter months.[20] Caregivers often use emergency departments because an illness develops or the child becomes sicker during times when primary care availability is most limited.[21] No published data have substantiated significant misuse of emergency departments for "well-child care." In general, caregivers use emergency departments because they are worried about their child's health and are poorly supported by primary health care.[1,22]

Determining the actual incidence of illness-related pediatric emergencies is very difficult. No illness-related diagnosis sets have been defined. Only aggregate data for pediatric deaths and hospital discharges are readily available for broad categories of pediatric illness.[17] More detailed epidemiologic data may be available through institutional statistics or published research studies. Wheezing-related illnesses, fever, respiratory distress, abdominal pain, seizures, and gastroenteritis are among the most common complaints of children presenting to emergency departments.[2,23]

Although fewer children die from acute illness than from injury, illness accounts for many more hospitalizations. Approximately two thirds of all ED visits by children are the result of illness.[24] Severe, life-threatening illness is still relatively infrequent compared to the incidence of all acute illness in children. Only about 5% of children who present to the emergency department have a life-threatening condition.[18] Most critically ill children are younger than 6 years of age and present with respiratory or central nervous system emergencies.[18,25] The following, alone or in combination, are among the characteristics of life-threatening illness in children.

- Involve initial subtle signs of illness that progress to a condition that requires emergent intervention.

- Have relatively rapid onset with precipitous deterioration.

- Frequently involve the respiratory system or central nervous system.

- Require rapid intervention.

- Necessitates care at a tertiary pediatric center.

Pediatric Hospitalizations Resulting from Illness

In 1994, there were more than 30 million hospitalizations; of these, more than 2 million (7%) occurred in children younger than 15 years of age. The top three primary diagnoses for these children included: 1) acute respiratory infection, 2) pneumonia, all types, and 3) bronchitis and asthma. Respiratory system illnesses accounted for 38% of the admissions in children younger than 15 years of age.[2,13,19] Other common admission diagnoses included seizures, abdominal pain, and poisoning.[2,22]

Pediatric Deaths Resulting from Illness

The number of children who die before reaching 1 year of age is reflected in the infant mortality rate. In 1996, there were 28,100 deaths in children younger than 1 year of age, or 7.2 infant deaths per 1,000 live births.[26] Birth-related conditions and congenital anomalies account for the majority of deaths in the neonatal period. Sudden infant death syndrome is the second leading cause of death in infancy and the primary cause of infant death outside of the neonatal period, accounting for approximately 5,000 infant deaths annually.[2,13,27] Other leading causes of illness-related pediatric death include heart disease, pneumonia, septicemia, stroke, meningitis, infection with the human immunodeficiency virus, and cancer.[27] After 1 year of age, however, injury becomes the leading cause of death in the pediatric population.[2,27]

PEDIATRIC TRAUMA

Trauma has a greater impact on pediatric morbidity and mortality than any other disease. Injury accounts for approximately 40% of ED visits by children.[21,27] In 1994, 44% of injury-related ED visits (17 million) were made by persons 24 years of age or younger. Children younger than 15 years of age accounted for more than 9 million of those visits.[13] Everyday 39,000 children sustain injuries that require medical attention in emergency departments, physicians' offices, or other heath care facilities.[28] Treatment for injury is the second leading cause of hospitalization in children 14 years of age and younger.[28]

In Australia, the highest incidence of deaths from drowning occur in the childhood years. Suicide and transport deaths begin during adolescence. Males 15 to 24 years of age accounted for 22% of all transport deaths. In this same age range, females accounted for 9% of deaths. There were 129 deaths of children under 15 years of age related to road incidents, usually as motor vehicle passengers or pedestrians.[29]

The most prevalent pediatric injuries include minor trauma, such as sprains, lacerations, contusions, fractures, and mild head injury.[2,21,29] However, children are also at risk for disabling and life-threatening injuries. Common causes of injury in children include:

- Falls.
- Motor vehicle crashes.
- Being struck by a motor vehicle (pedestrians and bicyclists).
- Bicycle crashes and collisions.
- Drowning.
- Thermal sources.
- Poisoning.

- Sports and recreational activities.

- Suffocation or choking.

- Penetrating events such as gunshots, stabbing, cutting, piercing.

- Child maltreatment.

As in the adult population, boys have a higher rate of injury-related ED visits than girls.[24,25] The prevalence of specific injury events and injuries sustained also varies among age groups. These variations are related to the differences in cognitive, perceptual, motor, and language abilities among age groups as well as physical development.[28] The variation in developmental maturity, in combination with the child's proximity to high-risk surroundings or high-risk behaviors, can increase his or her risk for some injury events.

Falls are the leading cause of unintentional injury for children. Children 14 years of age or younger account for 33% of all fall-related ED visits.[28] More than 2.5 million children are treated in emergency departments annually for falls. Because of their developmental level, motor skills, and curiosity, children younger than 10 years of age are at greatest risk for injury from a fall.[28]

Motor vehicle-related injury is a leading cause of unintentional injury and death among children and adolescents.[27] Children are at risk for injury as occupants in motor vehicles as well as pedestrians and bicyclists. Annually, more than 300,000 children are injured in motor vehicle-related crashes, the vast majority as passengers.[28]

Fires, flames, and scalds continue to be a factor in pediatric deaths. In 1997, approximately 920 U.S. children 1 to 24 years of age died as a result of fire. During 1995 in Australia, one third of all deaths due to a house fire were children younger than 15 years of age. Approximately 16% of deaths from fire were children 0 to 4 years of age.

In addition to age and developmental abilities, the child's environment and typical activities are factors affecting the child's risk for injury. Annually, a significant number of pediatric injuries and deaths involve nursery furnishings, toys, recreational equipment, and playground apparatus.[16,28,30] Sports and occupational injuries are also evident in the pediatric population, with the greatest number occurring in the adolescent age group.[30]

In 1994, there were 2.9 million reports of suspected child maltreatment.[13] It has been estimated that as many as 10% of injuries in children younger than 5 years of age are due to child maltreatment.[32] Children 4 years of age and younger are at greatest risk for inflicted injury.

The rate of suicide of Australian males 15 to 24 years of age has remained consistent since the 1980s. There were approximately 25.2 deaths per 100,000 population reported in 1995 due to suicide. Overall, the death rate in males from suicide was 4 times the death rate in females.[29]

Pediatric Disability Resulting from Injury

In 1993, more than 50,000 children younger than 14 years of age were permanently disabled from unintentional injuries.[28] The National Pediatric Trauma Registry (NPTR) database includes injury information on more than 42,000 children, from birth to 19 years of age, admitted to the hospital for acute injury. Of those children surviving an injury, 32% suffered either short-term or long-term disability. Children 5 to 9 years of age demonstrated the greatest proportion of disability among the various age groups.[33]

Falls were the most frequent cause of disabling injury in children from birth to 9 years of age. The NPTR reported that child maltreatment accounted for 23% of the injuries resulting in disability in children younger than 1 year of age, second only to falls for this age group.[33] In 1990, 18,000 children sustained inflicted injury that resulted in permanent disability.[34] In children 5 to 19 years of age, 50 to 57% of disabling injuries were attributed to motor vehicle crashes and other traffic-related injuries (e.g., pedestrian struck by a vehicle).[33]

Pediatric Deaths Resulting from Injury

Trauma is the leading cause of death in children older than 1 year of age, accounting for almost one half of all pediatric deaths annually. Motor vehicle crashes are the leading cause of unintentional injury deaths in children of all age groups. In children younger than 12 years of age, motor vehicle crashes cause about one of every three injury-related deaths.[28] Children younger than 4 years of age and adolescents are at highest risk for unintentional injury-related death.[27]

Child maltreatment is the leading cause of intentional death in children 4 years of age or younger.[34] In the United Sates, fatal child maltreatment occurs at a rate of 5.4 of every 100,000 children 4 years of age or younger. Approximately 2,000 children die as a result of inflicted injury each year, more than five children per day.[34] Severe head trauma is the primary cause of death from child abuse.[34,35] In 1995, 16 Australian children 0 to 4 years of age and seven children 5 to 9 years of age died from homicide or child maltreatment.

Cost of Pediatric Injury

For every pediatric injury-related death, there are 45 children who require hospitalization and 1,300 ED visits related to an injury. Annually, one child in four will be injured seriously enough to require medical attention, and an estimated 300,000 children will require hospitalization for those injuries. The health care costs for these children exceed $11 billion in medical costs alone. The annual lifetime cost of all injuries to children exceeds $250 billion when medical costs, future earnings, and quality of life are considered.[36]

Measures to prevent and control childhood injuries have a positive impact in reducing the incidence and cost of injury and injury-related deaths. However, injury continues to plague the pediatric population. In a study conducted by the Centers for Disease Control, 41% of the bicycle-related head injury deaths, and 76% of bicycle-related head injuries, occurred among children younger than 15 years of age. Researchers estimated that if all bicyclists had worn helmets during the 5-year study period, one death could have been prevented every day, and one head injury could have been prevented every 4 minutes.[37]

HEALTH PROMOTION

Most childhood injuries are preventable. Therefore, it is essential to include prevention information in ED care. The following are examples of prevention measures that an emergency nurse can provide:

Safety Teaching/Injury Prevention

- Develop and provide caregivers with age-appropriate printed instruction sheets that address anticipatory guidance topics for each age group.

- Include teaching on safety and injury prevention as a part of discharge from the emergency department and every health care setting for every pediatric patient.

- Provide caregivers with information concerning resources in their community for safety programs, safety restraint seats, and helmets. Explore and develop systems for hospital distribution of helmets and child restraint seats.

- Provide safety and educational displays, video programs, and brochures (e.g., "Give the Gift of Safety" by ENA, National Safe Kids, EN CARE) in waiting lobbies[38] (see Appendix A for Injury Prevention Resources).

- Demonstrate different methods of medication administration to caregivers to prevent drug administration error.

Health Promotion/Community Involvement

- Provide prevention lectures for school and community organizations (i.e., Trauma Nurses Talk Tough, Farm Safety for Kids, EN CARE programs).

- Assist caregivers in locating local Women, Infants and Children (WIC) offices.

- Evaluate the immunization status of all pediatric patients treated in the emergency department. Provide education and referral for all patients who are not fully immunized:

  - Explore and develop systems to administer vaccines, in addition to tetanus toxoid, in the emergency department.

  - Participate in community- or hospital-based immunization initiatives or programs.

- Participate in ED tours for schoolchildren and youth groups.

- Encourage and promote public education (e.g., for caregivers, grandparents, baby-sitters) in pediatric basic life support and first aid.

SUMMARY

This chapter describes the interaction between the hospital, community, and home environments in relation to the incidence of pediatric illness and injury. Epidemiology provides a foundation for understanding the health care needs of children and their families. Health promotion and injury prevention are driven by these identified needs.

REFERENCES

1. Haller JA, Shorter N, Miller D, Colombani P, Hall J, Buck J. Organization and function of a regional trauma center. Does system management improve outcomes? *J Trauma*. 1983;23:691-696.

2. Dieckmann RA. Epidemiology of pediatric emergency care. In: Dieckmann RA, Fiser DH, Selbst SM, eds. *Illustrated Textbook of Pediatric Emergency and Critical Care Procedures*. St. Louis, Mo: Mosby-Year Book; 1997:3-6.

3. Grossman M, Dieckmann RA. *Pediatric Emergency Medicine: A Clinician's Reference*. Philadelphia, Pa: JB Lippincott; 1991.

4. Uva JL. HMOs and the barrier to access for the pediatric population requiring emergency medical services. *Pediatr Emerg Care*. 1996;12:189-200.

5. American Academy of Pediatric. Guiding principles for managed care arrangements for the health care of infants, children, adolescents and young adults. *Pediatrics*. 1995;95:613-615.

6. Annie E. Casey Foundation. *Kids Count Data Book*. Baltimore, Md: Author; 1997.

7. American Academy of Pediatrics. Health needs of homeless children and families. *Pediatrics*. 1996;98:789-791.

8. Mayefsky JH, El-Shinaway Y, Kelleher P. Families who seek care for the common cold in the pediatric emergency department. *J Pediatr*. 1991;119:933-934.

9. Padgett DK, Brodsky B. Psychosocial factors influencing non-urgent use of the emergency room: a review of the literature and recommendations for research and improved service delivery. *Soc Sci Med*. 1992; 35: 1189-1197.

10. Kini NM, Strait RT. Nonurgent use of the pediatric emergency department during the day. *Pediatr Emerg Care*. 1998;14:19-21.

11. Altieri M, Bellet J, Scott H. Preparedness for pediatric emergencies encountered in the practitioner's office. *Pediatrics*. 1990;85:710-714.

12. Troutmann J, Weight J, Shifrin D. Pediatric telephone advice: Seattle hotline experience. *Pediatrics*. 1991;88:814-816.

13. Statistical Abstracts of the United States, 1996. 116th ed. *The National Data Book*. Washington, DC: US Bureau of the Census; 1996.

14. Christoffel KK. Violent death and injury in US children and adolescents. *Am J Dis Child*. 1990;144:697-706.

15. American Psychological Association. *Violence & Youth: Psychology's Response, Report of the APA Commission on Violence and Youth*. Washington, DC: Author; 1993.

16. Statistical Abstracts of the United States, 1996. 117th ed. *The National Data Book*. Washington, DC: US Bureau of the Census; 1997.

17. Institute of Medicine, Division of Health Care Services, National Research Council. Risking our children's health: A need for emergency care. *Emergency Medical Services for Children*. Washington, DC: National Academy Press; 1993:38-65.

18. Ludwig S, Selbst SM. A child oriented emergency medical services system. *Curr Probl Pediatr*. 1990;20:15-18.

19. American Academy of Pediatrics. Access to emergency medical care. *Pediatrics*. 1992;90:14.

20. Krauss B, Harakal T, Fleisher GR. The spectrum of frequency of illness presenting to a pediatric emergency department. *Pediatr Emerg Care*. 1991;7:67-71.

21. Pachter L, Ludwig S, Groves A. Night people: utilization of a pediatric emergency department during the night. *Pediatr Emerg Care*. 1991;7:12-14.

22. Weir R, Rideout E, Crook J. Pediatric use of the emergency department. *J Pediatr Health Care.* 1989;3:204-210.

23. Nelson DS, Walsh K, Fleisher G. Spectrum and frequency of pediatric illness presenting to a general community hospital emergency department. *Pediatrics.* 1992;90:5-10.

24. Emergency Nurses Association. *Emergency Nursing: Pediatric Emergency Care Policy Statement.* Park Ridge, Ill: Author; 1995.

25. Kissoon N, Walia M. The critically ill child in the pediatric emergency department. *Ann Emerg Med.* 1989;18:30-33.

26. *Monthly Vital Statistics Report.* US Department of Health and Human Services, National Center for Health Statistics. 1996;45:1-19.

27. National Safety Council. *Accident Facts.* 1998 ed. Itasca, Ill: Author; 1998.

28. National Safe Kids Campaign. *Fact Sheets: Childhood Injury, Falls, Motor Vehicle Occupant Injury.* Washington, DC: Author; March 1996.

29. Bordeaux S, Harrison J. Injury mortality Australia, 1995. *Australian Injury Prevention Bulletin.* 1998; 17.

30. Gallagher SS, Finison K, Guyer B, Goodenough S. The incidence of injuries among 87,000 Massachusetts children and adolescents: results of the 1980-1981 statewide childhood injury prevention surveillance system. *Am J Public Health.* 1984;74:1340-1347.

31. Children's Safety Network. *A Data Book of Child and Adolescent Injury.* Washington, DC: National Center for Education in Maternal Child Health; 1991.

32. Johnson CF, Showers J. *Diagnosis and Management of Physical Abuse of Children: A Self-Instructional Program.* Columbus, Ohio: Children's Hospital; 1987.

33. National Pediatric Trauma Registry. *Children and Adolescents with Disability Due to Traumatic Injury: A Data Book.* Boston, Mass: Department of Physical Medicine and Rehabilitation, New England Medical Center; 1996.

34. US Advisory Board on Child Abuse and Neglect. *A Nation's Shame: Fatal Child Abuse and Neglect in the United States.* Washington, DC: US Department of Health and Human Services; 1995.

35. Kelley SJ. Child abuse and neglect. In: Kelley SJ, ed. *Pediatric Emergency Nursing.* 2nd ed. Norwalk, Conn: Appleton & Lange; 1994:87-107.

36. Children's Safety Network. *Childhood Injury: Cost and Prevention Facts.* Washington, DC: CSN Economics and Insurance Resource Center; March, 1996.

37. Sacks JJ, Holmgreen P, Smith S, Sosin DM. Bicycle-associated head injuries and deaths in the United States from 1984 to 1988: How many are preventable? *JAMA.* 1991;266:3016-3018.

38. Ellerby P, Ward P. Development of a pediatric injury prevention program for emergency departments. *J Emerg Nurs.* 1989;15:224-228.

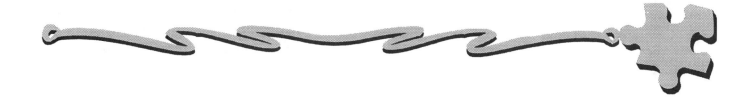

The Pediatric Patient

OBJECTIVES

On completion of this lecture, the learner should be able to:

✦ Discuss how pediatric developmental stages affect the child's reaction to illness, injury, pain, and death.

✦ Delineate the specific nursing interventions for the pediatric patient based on developmental stages.

✦ Identify basic anatomic and physiologic differences between adult and pediatric patients.

INTRODUCTION

Caring for ill or injured children can be an exciting challenge for some health care providers, while others approach the care of children with uneasiness. Understanding how children are different from adults often lessens the mystification associated with pediatric care. With this knowledge, the emergency nurse may feel more comfortable when caring for an ill or injured child.

Children are not small adults! Children vary in size, thought processes, physical and emotional maturity, and their ability to interact socially. The purpose of this chapter is to highlight pediatric developmental changes, identify pain responses, and describe specific approaches to the child.

REACTIONS TO ILLNESS AND INJURY

Unexpected health-related emergencies can be stressful events for children and their families. Although physical stabilization is usually the primary concern of the emergency health care provider, psychological stress should not be overlooked.[1] Physical deterioration associated with responses to psychological stress may be avoided by using simple techniques directed toward decreasing a child's anxiety.

The child's physiologic response to illness and injury is determined by many factors, including developmental level, culture, previous experiences and developed coping strategies, availability of support systems, and the nature of the present situation. Psychosocial and cognitive maturation will also affect the child's ability to understand illness and injury, treatments, procedures, hospitalizations, and the meaning of death.

The pediatric patient may regress developmentally during or after a stressful situation. A child may cope with a stressful situation by temporarily retreating to a "safer" developmental level. Typically, the child manifests this regression through a loss of the most recently acquired developmental milestone.[2] Family members must be made aware of the possibility of a temporary regression in the child's behavior and be assured that this is not an unusual response in children.

APPROACH TO CARE OF PEDIATRIC PATIENTS

All facets of development proceed as an individualized sequence of orderly changes in the child's physical, psychosocial, and cognitive abilities. Ages at which developmental milestones are accomplished may vary. To minimize stress and maximize a positive patient outcome, the emergency team must provide interventions based on the knowledge of specific developmental stages. The optimal approach to the ill or injured child is determined by age, acuity of illness or injury, and developmental stage.

The following are general guidelines that are used during care for all pediatric age groups. Pertinent developmental and physiologic characteristics, additional communication guidelines, and age-specific responses to pain are delineated throughout the chapter. Appendix B provides more detailed information on growth and development. Appendix C presents considerations in choosing language when caring for the child. Appendix D provides information on physiologic and anatomic characteristics.

Approaching Diversity

The approach to the pediatric patient also includes considerations of family and cultural diversity. Family structure in today's society is variable. Divorce, single parents, parents in the workforce, and children in day care settings impact family function and lifestyles. Cultural traditions and values also influence family function, health care practices, and the family and child's response to an illness or injury. Culture, religion, and ethnicity affect health care practices in a variety of ways. Health-related cultural perceptions and the perceived meaning of illness affect approaches to treatment and help-seeking behaviors.[3] Appendix E lists some cultural considerations of Southeast Asian folk healing practices.

Because of the diversity of society, the emergency care provider is often confronted not only by an ill or injured child, but also with a range of diverse beliefs related to health and healing practices. The process of performing a cultural assessment is an approach the ED team can utilize to facilitate understanding of the family's lifestyle, beliefs, and decision-making processes. When caring for children and families from various cultural origins, health care providers should identify health care patterns and beliefs that may be a factor in treatment interventions or discharge preparation.[4]

The information obtained from the cultural assessment is essential in the provision of culturally competent care. Assessment of the views and beliefs of the child and family facilitates treatment and discharge planning, incorporation of cultural practices, and negotiating culturally acceptable modifications.[5] If the family's approach or practices may be harmful to the child, the emergency team can address these issues and provide the family with information concerning the implications of those customs. The detail and depth of the cultural assessment will be dependent on the situation and the needs of the child and family. Table 1 provides a practice model for assisting emergency care providers in their approach to diversity.[3]

Table 1

DIVERSITY PRACTICE MODEL[3]	
Definition	**Application to Assessment**
Assumptions: The act of taking for granted or supposing that a thought or idea is true.	What are my assumptions and what are they based on? • Assumptions are often based on limited experience, bias, or generalizing.
Beliefs and behaviors: Beliefs are shared ideas about how a group operates. Behaviors are the ways a group conducts itself.	How do your assumptions compare to what you believe about certain groups? • All patients must be treated with the same respect and dignity, regardless of their diversity.
Communication: The two-way sharing of information that results in an understanding between the receiver and the sender.	• An early assessment must be made regarding the patient's ability to comprehend what is being said. • As communication begins, the body language of the emergency care provider must be one of acceptance and respect.
Diversity: The way in which people differ and the effect that differences have on the response to health care.	How does the patient's diversity affect his or her response to health or illness or the emergency care provider's response to the patient? • There is a wide variety of symptom management among diverse groups.
Education and ethics: Gaining knowledge about a diversity group and recognizing that ethical issues may be viewed differently by different diverse groups.	• The development of a cultural reference manual or collection of reference materials on cultural practices and health beliefs is indispensable to the emergency department. • Criteria for evaluation of staff competency must be developed with periodic evaluation.

The following are a series of questions that may assist the emergency nurse in identifying religious and cultural beliefs related to a child's illness and the family's usual health care routines, including folk healing practices.[4-6] When asking questions regarding what may be a sensitive subject, the emergency care provider must be nonjudgmental.

- Why do you think your child has this problem? The family may believe illness is caused by Karma, evil or offended spirits, or have demonic origins.

- Why did it start when it did?

- In your home country, whom would you see about this problem, and who would treat the child? The family may see a healer or a family elder. What kind of treatment would be done and who would administer the treatment?

- How long do you think this illness or problem will last?

- What treatments have you or your healer tried at home or in the past?

- What results do you hope your child will receive from the treatments? What treatment do you think your child should receive?

- Do you plan to continue to use those treatments or are there treatments you will use along with those prescribed in the emergency department?

- Will your healer or others involved work with us to make your child well?

Sensitivity to the issues of culture and religion is essential in the emergency care of the child. It is impossible for the emergency care team to have knowledge of all types of diversity. Therefore, the use of a diversity model is an integral part of the nursing process.

General Safety

The health care setting may not always be a safe environment for the child. Children must always be supervised; therefore, caregivers need to be instructed on supervision of their children during hospital visits. Consider child safety and injury prevention when purchasing furniture, room decorations, and toys for waiting room lobbies and patient rooms.

Family Presence

The development of a family-supportive environment is an important piece of providing family-centered care. The family is a constant in the child's life and must be able to provide comfort and support to the child during emergency care. Family participation and involvement in the child's health care promotes collaborative relationships among the health care professional, the patient, and the family. Facilitating *family presence* during invasive procedures or resuscitation situations is a core component of family-centered care practices.[7]

The option to remain present during invasive or resuscitation procedures must be the choice of the caregiver based on predetermined policies. If the caregiver chooses to remain with his or her child, the health care team must ensure that the caregiver is: 1) provided clear explanations of the procedure and the child's expected responses, 2) provided instruction on strategies to use to facilitate the child's coping with the procedure, as appropriate, 3) assessed in relation to his or her support needs, 4) provided emotional support and ongoing explanations by designated staff during resuscitation measures, and 5) provided support by staff, as needed, during other invasive procedures. Refer to *Presenting the Option for Family Presence*, published by ENA for additional information. If the caregiver chooses not to stay with the child, health care providers must respect that decision and continue to provide appropriate support and explanations of the procedure and treatment plan.

General Approach for Communication, Assessment, and Health Promotion

- Establish cheerful, private, and decorated examination areas that are appropriate for pediatric patients. Decorations such as mobiles, ceiling stickers, cartoon pictures, and youthful music can provide useful and thoughtful age-appropriate distractions. See Appendix F for information on developing a distraction or coping kit.

- Allow the caregiver to remain with the child whenever possible.

- Provide privacy (essential).

- Observe the child's level of consciousness, activity level, interaction with environment and caregiver, position of comfort, skin color, respiratory rates and effort, and degree of discomfort before touching the child. An appropriate time to accomplish this assessment is during the initial history.

- Compare assessment findings with the caregiver's description of the child's normal behavior (e.g., eating and sleeping habits, activity level, level of consciousness).

- Address the child by his or her name. Ask the child or caregiver what name to use when addressing the child.

- Use a kind, firm, direct approach. Demonstration is useful.

- Be honest with the child and caregiver.

- Acknowledge positive behavior and praise the child after procedures. Rewards such as stickers, hugs, or handshakes are helpful.

- Assess for pain using age-appropriate assessment tools and guidelines. Pain is assessed by a composition of physiologic behavior and self-report indicators. Explore past pain experiences with the caregiver to identify the child's typical response to pain and methods that have previously provided comfort:

  - Pain is usually characterized by a global pattern of physiologic arousal that can result in increased heart rate, increased blood pressure, and increased respiratory rate and depth. However, if pain has persisted for several hours or days, these responses are often modified, and cardiovascular and respiratory measurement may be normal.

  - Provide pharmacologic agents, as ordered, and nonpharmacologic pain reduction measures, as indicated. Children of all ages are capable of experiencing pain. There are few, if any reasons, for underuse of appropriate analgesia in children.[8]

- Health promotion teaching must be tailored to the child's age and potential risks and needs associated with the child's current developmental level and upcoming developmental changes. Well-care, injury prevention, and illness prevention are components of health promotion. Health promotion education or instructions applicable to all age groups include:

  - The importance of establishing a relationship with a primary care provider for the child and providing referral or contact information to a primary care provider.

  - Immunization schedules and community resources for obtaining low-cost or no-cost immunizations.

  - Health risks associated with the child's exposure to secondhand smoke.

  - Hand washing and, as appropriate, limiting contacts to prevent the spread of viral and bacterial infections.

  - Injury prevention focused on risks associated with developmental level, including use of safety seats and seat belts, helmets, and other protective equipment.

  - Poison center information and telephone numbers for the local poison information center. Most poison information centers will provide emergency departments with telephone stickers or magnets.

  - Child maltreatment prevention and community domestic violence resources.

  - Parenting information and community resources for parenting education.

Infants (1 Month to 1 Year of Age)

PSYCHOSOCIAL DEVELOPMENT

- Infancy is a period of rapid physical and psychosocial growth and development. Infants are dependent on caregivers to meet their needs.

- Infants understand and experience the world through their bodies. Being held, cuddled, rocked, or comforted with familiar touch and smells soothes infants.

- Common fears, especially for older infants, include separation and stranger anxiety. The infants' relationship with the primary caregiver is crucial to promote a sense of well-being.

- Infants explore objects by sucking, chewing, and biting. The more mobile, older infant has an increased risk for injury by poisoning, foreign-body aspiration, falls, and drowning.

ANATOMIC AND PHYSIOLOGIC CHARACTERISTICS

- 50th percentile weight is 3.5 to 10 kg.

- Infants are obligate nose breathers for the first several months of life. Blocked or partially blocked nasal passages may cause respiratory distress.

- Infants breathe predominately using abdominal muscles. Any pressure on the diaphragm from above or below can impede respiratory effort.

- The metabolic rate in an infant is approximately two times the adult rate. This results in an increased need for oxygen and calories.

- The infant's circulating blood volume is 90 ml/kg. Volume losses that may be perceived as insignificant can cause circulatory compromise. Volume losses occur primarily due to inadequate intake, vomiting and diarrhea, increased insensible losses, or hemorrhage.

- Infants in the first few months of life have immature renal function. The kidneys cannot efficiently adjust to fluid changes. Normal urine output is 2 ml/kg/hour.

- In infants, the autonomic nervous system is not fully developed. The ability to control body temperature in response to environmental changes is limited.

- Although the central nervous system remains immature, by 6 to 8 weeks, newborns can fix on and follow objects placed in front of them.

- In the first month of life, primary reflexes such as *sucking, rooting, startle*, and *grasp* are present. Arm and leg recoil to a state of complete flexion is symmetric.

APPROACH

- Approach the infant slowly, gently, and calmly. Loud voices and rapid movements may frighten the infant.

- Assess the infant while he or she is held by the caregiver, whenever possible, to decrease separation anxiety.

- Provide comfort. Up to about 7 months of age, the infant can be comforted by strangers, as long as his or her basic needs are met.[9] Stranger anxiety varies among infants and is dependent on the variety of caregivers in the child's life and the infant's individual temperament.

- Vary the sequence of the assessment with the infant's activity level. If the infant is calm and quiet, obtain the respiratory rate and auscultate the lungs at the beginning of the assessment.[10]

- Complete the most distressing components of the examination last, such as touching. When the infant is being examined, using warmed hands and stethoscope is less distressing.

- Avoid insertion of intravenous lines into the infant's favored extremity whenever possible because he or she may want to suck the fingers, thumb, or hand.

- Explain to the caregivers that the infant will cry once the procedure is initiated. Unlike other age groups, young infants make no link between approaching stimulus and pain.

PAIN ASSESSMENT AND COMFORT MEASURES

- Although there is no physiologic response unique to pain, physiologic measures of heart rate, blood pressure, and respiratory rate are a useful component in the pain assessment of infants. Other physical ailments and interventions can also effect these physiologic responses.

- Young infants, unlike older children, are unable to anticipate pain.

- Young infants respond to pain in a generalized manner. This includes generalized thrashing of arms, legs, and torso, rigidity, and exaggerated reflex withdrawal. Young infants will close their eyes tightly when experiencing pain. Specific behaviors such as vocalizations, like crying or groaning, closing eyes tightly, and inability to be consoled are useful assessment clues to estimate an infant's pain intensity. Caregivers can assist with the interpretation of cries and other sounds.

- Older infants (6 months to 1 year of age) respond to pain similarly but have a more localized response with deliberate withdrawal of the affected area.

- Provide nonpharmacologic comfort measures in conjunction with pharmacologic pain management. Sensorimotor soothing techniques such as pacifiers, stroking the skin, rocking, swaddling, playing music, speaking in quiet, soothing tones, darkening the room, and minimizing noxious stimuli are effective measures. See Appendix G for nonpharmacologic guidelines for pain management.

HEALTH PROMOTION

- Encourage caregivers to lessen the risk for injury within the home by shortening window shade cords and covering electrical outlets.

- Provide age-appropriate injury prevention pamphlets such as those provided by Safe Kids, EN CARE, Emergency Nurses Association, and American Academy of Pediatrics.

- Instruct caregivers to transport infants safely in infant carriers and when traveling in motor vehicles and by aircraft. The safest place for placement of an infant car seat is in the rear seat. Provide air bag information, including the risk of injury associated with air bag deployment and car seats.

- Discourage caregivers from using shopping carts to carry infants while shopping. Serious injury and deaths have occurred to infants from falling out of a shopping cart.

- Discourage caregivers from using movable baby walkers for their older infants. Walker use increases mobility and height, placing infants at risk for serious injury resulting from falls and the ability to reach potentially dangerous items on tables and counters.

- Provide poison center information and encourage caregivers to remove poisoning hazards before the infant becomes mobile!

- Infants explore with their mouth, which places them at greater risk for foreign-body airway obstruction. Encourage caregivers to keep small objects from infants. Provide a "choke tube." The choke tube is a commercially available safety measure that is intended to simulate the size of a child's airway in relationship to the safe size of an object for a small child. If the device is unavailable in your area, an empty toilet tissue roll can be used in the same manner.

Toddlers (1 to 2 Years of Age)

PSYCHOSOCIAL DEVELOPMENTAL

- Toddlers are in a stage of rapid physical and psychological growth and development. By about 18 months of age, the toddler is able to run, grasp, and manipulate objects, feed himself or herself, play with toys, and communicate with others.

- Toddlers may have erratic eating patterns compared to infants and older children.

- Toddlers are curious and have improved mobility but have no sense of danger.

- Cognitively, toddlers' thinking is concrete. They have increased ability to solve problems by trial and error.

- Toddlers are able to communicate verbally. Their negativism and insistence express an increasing need for autonomy, or doing things for themselves.

- Common fears include separation from the caregiver and loss of control. They delight in the ability to control themselves and others. The toddler tends to cling to a caregiver when apprehensive.

- Toddlers' experiences are still strongly sensory based: Seeing is believing.

ANATOMIC AND PHYSIOLOGIC CHARACTERISTICS

- *50th percentile weight* is 10 to 12 kg.

- A *Babinski's reflex* is normally present until the toddler starts walking. After 2 years of age, the child should have a *plantar reflex*.

- The toddler continues to use abdominal muscles for breathing.

- The toddler has improved thermoregulatory ability but may still develop *cold stress* when critically ill or injured and exposed for extended periods of time.

APPROACH

- Approach the toddler gradually. Keep physical contact minimal until the toddler is acquainted with you. Use a quiet, soothing voice.

- Incorporate play while assessing the toddler (e.g., "Show me your belly button"). If the child becomes upset or apprehensive, complete the assessment as expeditiously as possible.

- Encourage the caregiver to hold and comfort the child during the assessment and interventions.

- Introduce and use equipment gradually. Allow the child to handle minor equipment such as a stethoscope.

- Provide the toddler with limited choices, such as, "Do you want me to listen to your belly (chest) or your back first?" This provides the toddler with a sense of control.

- Prepare the child immediately before a procedure, using simple, concrete terms. Throughout the procedure, provide reassurance.

- Tell the child when the assessment or procedure is completed.

PAIN ASSESSMENT AND COMFORT MEASURES

- Assess for pain by evaluating behavioral and physiologic responses. The verbal toddler can state that he or she has pain but is generally incapable of describing its intensity and location. Normal behavioral responses to inflicted pain may include biting, hitting, and kicking; therefore, plan for adequate immobilization.

- Unusual behaviors such as whining, quietness, or listlessness may indicate discomfort or pain.

- Decreased movement or avoiding use of an extremity could indicate pain.[6]

- Promote the use of comforting objects, such as favorite blankets, familiar toys, and pillows.

- Provide distraction measures. For example, bubble blowing is popular among children 1 year of age and older. Ask the toddler to blow a bubble while you cleanse the intravenous site. In addition to providing a distraction, it also promotes regular breathing to help relieve pain and fear.

- Facilitate the caregiver's participation in care. Incorporate the caregiver in comfort and distraction measures during and after procedures.

- Stroking the toddler's arm, hand, or forehead in a light, rhythmic fashion can provide temporary comfort and distraction measures.

- Provide stickers, awards, and praise.

HEALTH PROMOTION

- The toddler has become more mobile, requiring closer supervision. Encourage caregivers to minimize home hazards for injury. For example, place hazardous household products and medications in a secure location and eliminate clutter around stairways to lessen the risk of stairway falls.

- Safety restraint devices are required. Instruct caregivers that appropriate car seats vary by model of car and child's size. References for caregivers include the car manual, car seat packaging information, and local car seat experts. Review information regarding injury risk with air bag deployment and safety seats.

Preschoolers (3 to 5 Years of Age)

PSYCHOSOCIAL DEVELOPMENT

- Preschoolers are magical and illogical thinkers. They often confuse coincidence with causation, have difficulty distinguishing fantasy from reality, and have many misconceptions about illness, injury, and body functions (e.g., if they have a cut, their "insides" will leak out).

- Preschoolers do not have a well-developed concept of time.

- Preschoolers often have an imaginary playmate.

- Preschoolers often take words and phrases literally (see Appendix C).

- Common fears include body mutilation, especially genitalia, loss of control, death, darkness, and being left alone.

ANATOMIC AND PHYSIOLOGIC CHARACTERISTICS

- 50th percentile weight is 14 to 18 kg.
- Normal urine output is 1 ml/kg/hour.
- The preschooler continues to use abdominal muscles for breathing.

APPROACH

- Allow the child to handle equipment, or similar play equipment, such as a stethoscope.
- Immediately before the procedure, prepare the child by using simple, concrete terms. Explain in terms of the sensory experience (e.g., hearing, feeling, seeing). Delays in starting the procedure soon after preparing the child can lead to increased anxiety.
- Set limits on behavior, but offer choices whenever possible to enhance feelings of control.
- Enlist the child's help (e.g., tell the child to hold still, but give him or her permission to cry). Do not link "good" behavior with stoic behavior.
- Assess the child's level of understanding and correct erroneous or unclear ideas as adult vocabulary may be misleading.
- Consider age-related language in explaining procedures to the child (see Appendix C).
- Use games to gain cooperation.
- Use dressings (e.g., adhesive bandages) freely to promote the preschooler's feelings of body integrity.

PAIN ASSESSMENT AND COMFORT MEASURES

- Verbal statements are the most important factors in assessing pain.[11,12] Pain assessment tools such as the Oucher Scale may be useful for children who are 3 years of age and older (see Appendix H). Young children may prefer to use face scales.
- Ask preschool children to describe their illness or injury, such as "Point to where it hurts." Their precision of indicating the site of pain is present but increases with age. Preschoolers vocabulary for pain is limited to a few simple words such as "bad," "boo-boo," and "ouch."[12]
- Preschoolers' motor responses to pain may include thrashing of the arms and legs, guarding, restlessness, and reluctance to move. Their expressive responses to pain include crying, screaming, and verbalizing pain (e.g., verbal reprimands, such as "I hate you," clinging to support person, pleading).
- Preschoolers have gained the ability to anticipate pain.
- Preschoolers do not always understand why they are experiencing pain, what has caused the pain, and how long it will last.

- Nonpharmacologic methods for pain management include use of distraction techniques such as pop-up books, activity books, watching videos, blowing bubbles to control breathing, kaleido-scopes, and discussion of favorite television shows. Additional distraction and comforting measures include imagery, music, toys, and warmed blankets. Pharmacologic pain management is enhanced when combined with nonpharmacologic methods.

- Provide reassuring comments. Assure the child that the pain is not associated with punishment.

HEALTH PROMOTION

- Safety restraint devices are still required for most children in this age group. Children learn by example, and children in this age group will begin noticing if caregivers are not using safety restraints.

- Riding toys are beginning to be used. Remind caregivers that safety helmets must be correctly fitted and worn.

- Instruct caregivers to place beds away from windows because this age group is at risk of falls from windows.

School-aged Children (6 to 10 Years of Age)

PSYCHOSOCIAL DEVELOPMENT

- School-aged children are developing a sense of accomplishment and mastery of new skills. Successes contribute to positive self-esteem and a sense of control.

- Although the ability for logical thought processes is beginning, misinterpretation of words and phrases is common.

- Their concept of time is improved; awareness of possible long-term consequences of illness is present.

- By 9 years of age, children can understand simple explanations about their anatomy and body functions.

- Older school-aged children tend to hide their thoughts and feelings.

- Common fears include separation from friends, loss of control, and physical disability. Risk-taking behavior is emerging.

- School-aged children develop a general knowledge of medical intervention, often based on media reports, television shows, and nightmarish fantasies.[9]

- They are more likely to want to be involved in their care.

ANATOMIC AND PHYSIOLOGIC CHARACTERISTICS

- 50th percentile weight is 20 to 32 kg.

- By about 8 years of age, the child's respiratory anatomy and physiology approximates that of an adult. The child's circulatory blood volume is 80 ml/kg.

APPROACH

- Provide the older school-aged child with the choice of having the caregiver present during assessment.

- Explain procedures simply and request return feedback. The school-aged child may be reluctant to ask questions or to admit not knowing something that the child perceives he or she is expected to know.

- Provide privacy. Privacy needs are changing (e.g., some children may not want caregivers in the room when they undress).

- Be honest, explain procedures, and describe how the child can be involved in his or her own care (e.g., holding tape, adhesive bandages).

- Reassure the child that he or she did nothing wrong. The procedure, illness, or injury discomfort is not punishment and is unrelated to his or her actions.

PAIN ASSESSMENT AND COMFORT MEASURES

- Use age-appropriate pain assessment scale tools. By 7 or 8 years of age, many children can use a numeric scale.[11] Children in this age group can describe the intensity and location of their pain in greater detail.

- Assess for physical, behavioral, and emotional responses to pain. Motor responses include clenched fists, body stiffness, and facial grimaces. The child may exhibit bargaining behavior. Physiologic responses to pain include tachycardia and tachypnea.

- They may deny their pain because they fear receiving a "shot."

- Comfort measures include distraction techniques, such as music, imagery, watching videotapes, and discussion of favorite sports team or a music group. Bubble blowing is still effective until about 10 years of age.[11]

HEALTH PROMOTION

- Remind the caregiver and the patient that bicycle helmets must be worn. Helmets must be replaced every 3 years or sooner, depending on the child's head growth, or if cracks or chips develop in the helmet material, or sustain damage in a significant crash.

- Remind the caregiver and patient that safety pads for the knees, elbows, and wrists must be worn when the child is in-line skating or skateboarding.

- Caregivers need to assure the child's proper use of seat belts. The safest place in a motor vehicle for all children younger than 12 years of age is the rear seat with proper restraint. Provide information regarding injury risks associated with air bag deployment.

- Provide safety information on the avoidance of strangers and "saying no" to the use of alcohol and drugs.

- Provide information to caregivers on methods to prevent foreign body aspiration.

Early and Middle Adolescents (11 to 18 Years of Age)

PSYCHOSOCIAL DEVELOPMENT

- Adolescence is a period of experimentation and risk-taking activity.

- Adolescents are acutely aware of their body appearance. Anything that differentiates them from their peers is perceived as a major tragedy.

- Psychosomatic complaints are common.

- Adolescents' quest for independence from their families often leads to family dissension.

- Peers are important for psychological support and social developments. Sexual interests are common.

- Adolescents may experience mood swings, depression, eating disorders, suicidal ideation, and violent behavior. The differential diagnosis of an emerging mental health disorder versus normal adolescent responses should be considered.

- Common fears include changes in appearance, dependency, and loss of control.

- Beliefs may be influenced by peer group based on concerns with acceptance and rejection.

- Adolescents may regress to earlier stages of development for comfort.[10]

- Adolescents move from concrete to formal operational cognitive development. However, they still lack the conceptual thinking skills of the adult. They need concrete explanations.[13]

ANATOMIC AND PHYSIOLOGIC CHARACTERISTICS

- Weights range from 36 kg to adult weight.

- Adolescence is characterized by rapid growth and heightened emotions, usually associated with hormonal changes.[12]

- Puberty begins with an average onset age of 12½ years for females, and 15½ years for males. The average age of menarche is 12½ to 13 years. *Tanner staging* is a method used to assess pubertal development.[13]

APPROACH

- Introduce yourself to the patient and family.

- Sit down and converse with the adolescent. Avoid interruptions and distractions.

- Be honest and nonjudgmental. Do not talk down to him or her or use jargon or slang. Use terms the adolescent can understand.

- Encourage the adolescent to ask questions and participate in his or her own health care. Address his or her concerns as well as those of the parents.

- Be attentive to nonverbal cues.

- Respect privacy and confidentiality, unless the information divulged is harmful to the adolescent or others (e.g., suicidal ideation). Questions concerning sexual activity, including date of last menstrual period, must be included. However, these questions should be asked in private without caregivers in the room.

- Include a screening for health risks when obtaining the history. The HEADSS method may be used to identify the adolescent at risk.[14]

    - H = Home: Who lives at home? How does everyone get along?

    - E = Education: What school and grade do you attend? How are your grades? Do you have a job after school?

    - E = Eating: Review eating behaviors, meal frequency, and content.

    - A = Activities: What activities are you involved in both in and out of school, weekends, after school, and evenings?

    - A = Affect: What is the affect? Is there evidence of depression or anxiety?

    - D = Drugs: Ask about illicit drugs, inhalants, over-the-counter medications with abuse potential, alcohol, and smoking. Are peers involved in drugs?

    - S = Suicidal ideations and attempts: Have there been any attempts? Are there suicidal ideations currently?

    - S = Sexual history: Sexual practices, number of partners, use of contraception. Any sexually transmitted diseases? Has there been a history of sexual abuse?

- Provide older children and adolescents with concrete information about their illness or injury, normal body functions, and the plan of care, treatments, and diagnostic tests.

PAIN ASSESSMENT AND COMFORT MEASURES

- Adolescents tend to deny their pain, especially when in the presence of friends because they fear losing control.

- Adolescents are able to identify the site, type, onset, duration, and intensity of pain.

- Assess for pain using age-appropriate assessment tools. With clear instructions, adolescents can report their pain on a scale of 0 (no pain) to 10 (worst pain).

- Assess for pain responses that include mood swings, crying, and regressions to an earlier developmental stage. Adolescents tend to ignore or dismiss their pain and delay or refuse treatment in the presence of their peers. Common motor responses to pain include muscle tension and decreased activity.

- Comfort measures include imagery, music, controlled breathing, watching videotapes, and cutaneous stimulation.

HEALTH PROMOTION

- Promote recreational safety and the use of helmets and other appropriate safety equipment.

- Promote proper seat belt use.

- Provide counseling related to reducing the risk of sexually transmitted diseases, use of birth control methods, safe sexual practices, and responsible sexual behavior.

- Provide injury awareness and prevention literature about driving safely and the hazards of driving under the influence of drugs and alcohol. Use resources available through agencies such as the American Academy of Pediatrics, Emergency Nurses Association, EN CARE, and others.

- Promote and provide health guidance information on[15]:

  - Parenting.

  - Development.

  - Diet and physical activity.

  - Healthy lifestyles (includes sexual behavior and avoidance of tobacco, alcohol, and other drug use).

  - Injury prevention.

- Promote annual *preventive services* visit with the primary care provider for the adolescent.[15] The preventive services visit facilitates early recognition of potential and actual health problems and the early establishment of health promotion practices.

APPROACH TO SPECIAL NEEDS CHILDREN

The term *special needs* is widely used but poorly defined.[16,17] Commonly, the term is defined as any type of condition with the potential to interfere with normal growth and development. Prevalence rates do not exist.[16] Special needs children can include those with physical disabilities, developmental or learning disabilities, technological dependencies, and chronic illnesses. Technologically dependent children have a varied range of supports, which may include one or more of the following: Home ventilators, tracheostomy, gastric tube, supplemental oxygen, apnea monitor, pulse oximeter, long-term intravenous catheter, peritoneal dialysis, or continuous parenteral or enteral nutrition. Children with special needs related to chronic illnesses may include those with digestive allergies, diabetes, traumatic brain injury, epilepsy, frequent or severe headaches, and cerebral palsy. Asthma and congenital heart defect account for two thirds of all cases of chronic illness in children.[16]

Children with special needs are a growing component of the pediatric population. Multiple advances in highly specialized areas of medicine have enabled children with severe or complex medical problems to survive. Although the initial principles of emergency nursing do not differ for this group, many of these children require modification in certain areas of acute care management.

Advances in the treatment of children with special medical problems occur rapidly, and it is difficult for nurses to be familiar with the details of every congenital or acquired pediatric problem. In some emergency departments, a profile or informational card for certain disorders is used. These reference systems are unique to each institution's referral community and are designed to provide rapid information about new research and regional experts.[18] The American Academy of Pediatrics and the American College of Emergency

Physicians are developing a system to facilitate obtaining medical information about these children by adopting a form approved by both organizations. Primary care providers will be encouraged to use the Children with Special Health Care Needs Data Form for any of their patients with special needs. Schools, area hospitals, or any other facilities that may have a use for this information are encouraged to have access to the form. The form will include a brief explanation of the child's condition, medications, allergies, and any other pertinent information. It is anticipated that the program will begin in the Fall of 1999.

Special needs children may require frequent hospitalization. When caring for the special needs child, the emergency health care team must use age-specific guidelines, and:

- Listen to the caregiver. Obtain a careful history (e.g., How is the child's condition today in comparison to the "norm?") Identify the child's "chief complaint" and reason for the ED visit. Caregivers can often provide the emergency team with information concerning approaches that work best, typical routines, rituals, and typical responses and behaviors. Caregivers know the child best. Their assistance in interpreting responses and behaviors aids the emergency team in understanding and meeting the child's acute care needs. The presence of the caregiver may be comforting to the child.

- Approach the child with a developmental delay or decreased mental ability using a developmentally appropriate level rather than age-specific guidelines. Communicate with the child in a manner appropriate to his or her ability. Sometimes children with a chronic illness or technology dependency may not progress developmentally as rapidly as other children. However, the presence of a physical disability does not mean that a child is also cognitively impaired. Drawing, communication boards, or Braille material may be useful for communication.

- Focus on the child's developmental age rather than chronologic age or diagnosis. This emphasizes the child's abilities, not disabilities. Concentrating on what the child is able to do promotes self-esteem and a positive self-image.

- Use "special needs" informational resources. All pediatric patients with special needs must maintain some form of identification to alert health care providers of the "special need." Some children wear jewelry that contains medical information; others wear a jewelry-type identifier that alerts the medical staff to contact an agency that provides specific information about the child.

SUMMARY

This chapter has provided an overview of the biophysical, psychosocial, and intellectual differences among pediatric age groups. Key pieces include diversity, family presence, and health promotion. It is essential that nurses use the appropriate techniques to approach and assess the child based on his or her age and/or developmental level. By using these techniques and promoting the use of pharmacologic and non-pharmacologic distraction therapies, the child's and caregiver's fear and anxiety can be reduced. This leads to a more cooperative and collaborative care environment. On this foundation, further knowledge of pediatric assessment and nursing care can be established.

REFERENCES

1. Lewandowski L. Psychosocial aspects of pediatric critical care. In: Hazinski MF, ed. *Nursing Care of the Critically Ill Child*. 2nd ed. St. Louis, Mo: Mosby-Year Book; 1992:19-77.

2. Wong D. Impact of hospitalization on the child and family. In: Wong D, ed. *Pediatric Nursing*. 5th ed. St. Louis, Mo: Mosby-Year Book; 1997:608-672.

3. Emergency Nurses Association. *Approaching Diversity: An Interactive Journey*. Park Ridge, Ill: Author; 1998.

4. Tripp-Reimer T, Brink PJ, Saunders JM. Cultural assessment: content and process. *Nurs Outlook*. 1984;32:78-82.

5. Kelley BR. Cultural diversity in clinical practice. In: Fox JE, ed. *Primary Health Care of Children*. St. Louis, Mo: Mosby-Year Book; 1997:32-40.

6. Tripp-Reimer T, Afifi LA. Cross-cultural perspectives on patient teaching. *Nurs Clin North Am*. 1989;25:613-619.

7. Emergency Nurses Association. *Presenting the Option for Family Presence*. Park Ridge, Ill: Author; 1995.

8. Callahan J. Pharmacologic agents. In: Dieckmann RA, Fiser D, Selbst SM, eds. *Illustrated Textbook of Pediatric Emergency and Critical Care Procedures*. St. Louis, Mo: Mosby-Year Book; 1997:53-71.

9. McKenze I, Gaukroger P, Ragg P, Brown T, eds. *Manual of Acute Pain Management in Children*. New York, NY: Churchill Livingstone; 1997.

10. Engel J. Preparation for examination. In: Engel J, ed. *Pocket Guide to Pediatric Assessment*. 3rd ed. St. Louis, Mo: Mosby-Year Book; 1997:46-51.

11. Kuttner L, ed. *A Child in Pain*. Point Roberts, Wash: Hartley & Marks Publishers; 1996.

12. Betz C, Sowden L. Pain in children. In: Betz C, Sowden L, eds. *Pediatric Nursing Reference*. 3rd ed. St. Louis, Mo: Mosby-Year Book; 1996:596-601.

13. Strasburger VC, Brown RT. Growth and development. In: Strasburger VC, Brown RT, eds. *Adolescent Medicine: A Practical Guide*. 2nd ed. Philadelphia, Pa: Lippincott-Raven; 1998:1-22.

14. Emergency Nurses Association. *Caring for the Adolescent in the Emergency Department*. Park Ridge, Ill: Author; 1999.

15. American Medical Association. *Guidelines for Adolescent Preventive Services*. Chicago, Ill: Author; 1996.

16. Wong D. Impact of chronic illness, disability, or death on the child and family. In: Wong D, ed. *Pediatric Nursing*. 5th ed. St. Louis, Mo: Mosby-Year Book; 1997:524-543.

17. Gay JC, Muldoon JH, Neff JM, Wing LJ. Profiling the health service needs of populations: Description and uses of the NACHRI classification of congenital and chronic health conditions. *Pediatr Ann*. 1997;26:655-663.

18. Sacchetti A, Geradi M, Barkin R, Santamaria J, Cantor R, Weinburg J, Gausche M. Emergency data set for children with special needs. *Ann Emerg Med*. 1996;28:324-327.

Pediatric Considerations:
Pain Management and Medication Administration

HELPING CHILDREN COPE WITH STRESSFUL AND PAINFUL PROCEDURES

Children experience pain as a result of illness, injury, and routine emergency care procedures. Although pain is a common experience for children, management of acute pain in children is often inadequate.[1,2] The pain experience is a composite of physiologic and psychologic variables.[3] Factors that may influence children's pain experience include underlying medical conditions; experience with previous painful events; cultural, family, or environmental influences; developmental level; the part of the body involved; preparation for the procedure; type of medication administered; and use of nonpharmacologic interventions. Unfortunately, misconceptions about pediatric pain often prevent caregivers and professionals from appropriately treating children's pain. Table 2 discusses facts and fallacies about children and pain.

Pediatric pain management involves recognition and anticipation of painful events as well as a spectrum of interventions to relieve and prevent pain. Interventions include both nonpharmacologic and pharmacologic methods. Age-specific pain assessment information and nonpharmacologic interventions were discussed in Chapter 3 and Appendixes F, G, and H. Approaches to procedural pain management are described in the following section.

NONPHARMACOLOGIC INTERVENTIONS

Preparing Children and Their Families for Procedures

Developmentally appropriate preparation for a procedure is essential in gaining the cooperation of the child, decreasing the child's and the caregiver's anxiety, and helping the child cope with the procedure. When preparing the child and family for procedures:

- Consider the child's developmental level when determining the preparation approach and timing.

- Explain the procedure to the child and family in a manner that is developmentally appropriate for the child. Use age-appropriate and developmentally appropriate words and techniques and consider cultural variances (see Appendix C).

Table 2

FALLACIES AND FACTS ABOUT CHILDREN AND PAIN	
Fallacy	**Fact**
Infants do not feel pain.	Infants demonstrate behavioral, especially facial, physiologic, and hormonal indicators of pain. Fetuses have the neural mechanisms to transmit noxious stimuli by 20 weeks of gestation.
Children tolerate pain better than adults.	Children's tolerance for pain actually increases with age. Younger children tend to rate procedure-related pain higher than older children.
Children cannot tell you where they hurt.	By 4 years of age, children can accurately point to the body area or mark the painful site on a drawing; children as young as 3 years of age can use pain scales, such as the faces scale.
Children always tell the truth about pain.	Children may not admit to having pain to avoid an injection. Because of constant pain, they may not realize how much they are hurting. Children may believe that others know how they are feeling and not ask for analgesia.
Children become accustomed to pain or painful procedures.	Children often demonstrate increased behavioral signs of discomfort with repeated painful procedures.
Behavioral manifestations reflect pain intensity.	Children's developmental level, coping abilities, and temperament, such as activity level and intensity of reaction to pain, influence pain behavior. Children with more active, resisting behaviors may rate pain lower than children with passive, accepting behaviors.
Parents do not want to be involved in their child's pain control.	Parents do want to be involved. They know their child best and can help in assessing pain and pain relief measures. Since they may not have seen their child in severe pain, they may need guidance in interpreting pain responses.
Narcotics are more dangerous for children than for adults.	Narcotics (opioids) are no more dangerous for children than they are for adults. Addiction to opioids used to treat pain is extremely rare in children. Reports of respiratory depression in children are also uncommon. By 3 to 6 months of age, healthy infants can metabolize opioids similarly to older children.

Adapted from Wong DL. Family-centered care of the child during illness and hospitalization. In: Wong DL, Hockenberry-Eaton M, Winkelstein ML, Ahmann E, DiVito-Thomas PA, eds. *Whaley and Wong's Nursing Care of Infants and Children.* 6th ed. St. Louis, Mo: Mosby-Year Book; 1999:1082. Used with permission.

- Include procedural and sensory information for the child and caregiver[4]:

  - Be realistic about the time required for a procedure. Five minutes easily stretches into 15 or 20 minutes.

  - Show the child the equipment and/or supplies that will be used. Allow the child to touch the equipment and supplies as appropriate, or have similar "play" equipment available for the child to explore.

  - Explain any alarms that may ring; let the caregiver and child hear what the alarm sounds like; explain why it may ring and what the staff's response will be to the alarm.

  - Provide the child with objective information about what they may feel, hear, smell, or taste. Do not introduce words such as *hurt* or *cry.*

- Consider the child's previous experiences. Prior painful and/or stressful health care encounters may influence the responses. Obtaining information concerning the child's previous experience with a procedure or painful event is useful in understanding his or her reaction, anxiety level, and perception of the current situation.

- Assess the child's understanding of the information and correct any misconceptions.

- Offer the caregiver the option of staying or leaving during the procedure. Not all caregivers are comfortable being present during invasive or painful procedures. Provide adequate explanations and support for the caregiver to make the decision:

  - Provide the caregiver with a clear explanation of his or her role during the procedure.

  - Respect and support the decision.

  - Adolescents may be uncomfortable having a caregiver present for some examinations and procedures. Ask if they prefer the caregiver to stay or leave.

- Prepare the caregiver to assume a comforting role during and after the procedure. When the caregiver understands the procedure, its sequence, and the child's potential responses, the caregiver is better able to comfort the child:

  - Encourage the caregiver to use comforting strategies typically used in the home environment.

  - Identify and discuss coping strategies that may be helpful for the child.

- Provide words of encouragement during and after the procedure to promote the child's self esteem.

Coping Skills

Strategies to reduce pain and distress in children undergoing painful procedures typically involve a combination of approaches. In combination with psychologic preparation, the use of specific coping strategies may assist in decreasing the child's anxiety, distress, and pain during a painful or stressful procedure. While providing preparation information, remain aware of the child's responses and assess his or her coping style. Consider teaching the child and caregiver a specific coping strategy to use during the procedure.

The use of distraction is an expedient coping technique because it requires little patient or caregiver preparation. The distraction techniques selected should be age-appropriate and developmentally appropriate. The caregiver's participation with the distraction technique should be encouraged. A coping kit with a variety of items that facilitate distraction for various age groups is a helpful tool in implementing this technique (see Appendix F). General distraction approaches include:

- Playing soothing music, children's stories, or songs during the procedure.[5]

- Playing a videotape for the child to view during the procedure.

- Using soap bubbles, glitter wands, or puppets to engage the child's attention.

- Asking the caregiver to read or tell the child a story during the procedure.

- Asking the child to sing a song or count aloud slowly. The child may be instructed to sing or count louder or faster if needed.[5]

Other distraction or coping techniques require teaching the child the strategy as well as providing an opportunity for the child to rehearse the technique. These techniques are most useful in older children and adolescents. Examples of these techniques include:

- Deep breathing: The child is coached in deep breathing, focusing on inhalation and exhalation phases of each breath to initiate a relaxed breathing pattern.[6]

- Blowing away the pain: The child is instructed to blow out the pain, imagining he or she is blowing out candles slowly and steadily. Having the child blow bubbles or a pinwheel also works with this technique.[7]

- Imagery: The child is talked through a pleasant or enjoyable situation or activity. Developing the scenario requires the nurse to ask questions of the child and/or caregiver about an imagined situation.[6]

- Positive self-talk: The child is coached in saying positive statements ("I can do it," I'm doing great."). Positive self-talk may also be combined with thought stopping to decrease anticipatory stress. The child stops thinking about the fearful or anxiety-provoking aspects of the procedure and substitutes a positive thought.[6,7]

Comfort Measures

Physical positioning and comfort measures are components of nonpharmacologic pain management. Basic interventions are used to minimize pain and/or to prevent the exacerbation of pain. These measures may be initiated in response to illness or injury or as part of a procedure. There may be variations in these interventions based on cultural factors. Comfort measures include:

- Applying splints or other immobilization techniques for suspected fractures or extremity injuries.

- Applying ice or cold packs to an injury site.

- Applying warm compresses.

- Elevating an injured extremity.

- Positioning the child in a comfortable position or support positioning with blankets or pillows.

- Covering wounds with a dressing to decrease airflow across the wound.

- Transporting the patient by wheelchair or stretcher to minimize movement associated with ambulation.

Positioning for Comfort During Procedures

The child should be positioned in a manner that is conducive to the procedure and comfortable for the child. One of the developmental milestones achieved in infancy is the ability to sit unsupported. After this milestone is achieved, attempts to force an infant or child to lie down are often met with resistance, crying, and struggling. As efforts to restrain a child in the supine position increase, so does the child's resistance and attempts to get up.[8] Lying down is a significant contribution to the child's stress during procedures. Stephen and Barkey[8] developed a nonaggressive approach to positioning children for invasive procedures.

A variety of invasive procedures commonly performed in the emergency care setting can be completed while the infant or child is in a sitting position. Placing children in a sitting position promotes a sense of control and decreases the stress of the event.[8] Positioning for comfort, coupled with preparation and other pain management techniques, improves the experience of an invasive procedure for the pediatric patient. The approach and methods advocated by Stephen and Barkey provide[8]:

- A secure, comforting, hugging hold for the child.

- Close physical contact between the child and the caregiver.

- An opportunity for the caregiver to participate in the child's care in a positive, comforting manner rather than a negative, restraining mode.

- Effective immobilization of the desired body area.

- A technique to complete the procedure using fewer people.

Examples of Stephen and Barkey's recommended positions[8] are illustrated in Figures 1, 2, and 3. Creative variations to the illustrated positions accommodate the performance of many procedures. The caregiver may be positioned on the stretcher to support and hold the child if sitting in a chair does not place the child at a height conducive to the procedure.

Points to Remember:

- Remove the child's shoes before starting procedures to avoid a painful kick.[4]

- When holding the legs, hold at the knees to stabilize the extremity.

- Utilize other staff members to assist with holding as needed.

- Instruct the caregiver in the holding procedure; ensure a secure hold before starting the procedure.

- Ensure that the caregiver is comfortable participating in holding the child during the procedure. If the caregiver is uncomfortable or unable to hold the child during the procedure, another staff member can hold the child using the techniques described. The caregiver may remain involved by providing comforting measures during and/or after the procedure.

The following figures demonstrate methods of holding a child for procedures.

Figure 1
SIDE-SITTING POSITION FOR INTRAVENOUS ACCESS

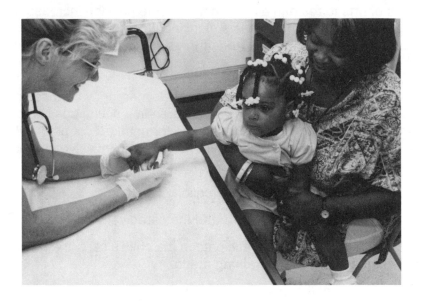

The child sits on the caregiver's lap, facing to the side. From the opposite side of the stretcher, the health care provider can then stabilize the arm for an intravenous access or phlebotomy.

Figure 2
CHEST TO CHEST WITH STANDING CAREGIVER FOR INJECTION

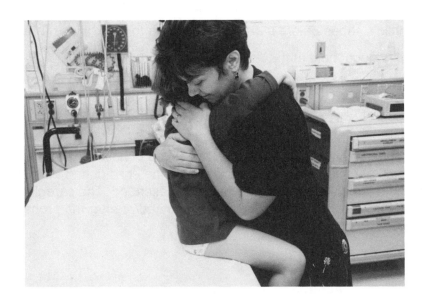

The child is positioned sitting on the stretcher or examination table with the caregiver standing in front of the child. The chest-to-chest position allows the caregiver to hug the child and secure the upper extremities, as illustrated in the figure. The health care provider controls the leg for the injection.

Figure 3
CHEST TO CHEST WITH SITTING CAREGIVER FOR INTRAVENOUS ACCESS

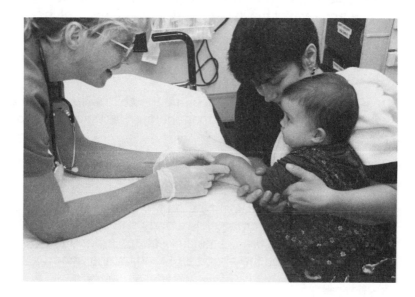

The child straddles the caregiver's lap, sitting chest to chest. The caregiver can hug the child and assist in securing the upper extremities, as pictured. The child's arm can be stabilized on the stretcher for intravenous access or phlebotomy. This position can also be used effectively for obtaining intravenous access in the foot of a younger child by having a staff member secure the lower extremity.

Use of Physically Restrictive Devices During Procedures

The least restrictive methods of controlling the child's movement should be used. Preparation for the procedure and the use of pain management techniques decrease the need for restrictive devices. When assessing the need for a physically restrictive device, evaluate the following:

- The child's developmental level and coping abilities.
- The procedure to be performed.
- The risk of harm to the patient if movement occurs.
- Any previous history of child maltreatment that may affect the child's response to being restrained.

Distraction and other pain management techniques are essential components when restrictive devices are used. The following approach should be used when restrictive devices are needed:

- Explain the need for restricting the child's movement and the method to be used to the child and caregiver.
- Consider the length of the procedure, the child's age, and the child's coping abilities when choosing a securing method.
- Use the least restrictive method or device.
- If the child must not touch the sterile field or move his or her arms and/or hands:
  - Have the child place his or her hands under the buttocks so that the child is sitting or lying on his or her hands. This will remind the child not to reach into the field.

- Place the child's arms in a pillowcase, pulling the pillowcase up to the child's shoulders. Position the child's arms at his or her side with the pillowcase across the back, so the child lies on the pillowcase. The child's weight on the pillowcase will keep the child's arms in the pillowcase and restrict movement. The head of the stretcher can be raised so the patient can be in a reclined or sitting position, or can lie flat. The pillowcase can be described as Superman's, Superwoman's, or Batman's cape.

- A child-restraint board can assist in controlling the child's movements:

  - To avoid stress and to lessen the chance that the child will struggle, always use distraction and other appropriate pain management techniques in conjunction with this method of physical immobilization.

  - Prepare the restraint board by opening the Velcro® straps on the board and placing a triangular sheet over the board (see Figure 4).

  - Place the child so that he or she is supine on the board with the arms at each side. Bring the right corner of the sheet over the child's body and tuck it under the child's left arm; repeat on the other side.[4] Secure the Velcro® straps around the child. If the child is resisting the placement, open the straps and readjust the sheet.

Figure 4

TECHNIQUE FOR USING A CHILD-RESTRAINT BOARD

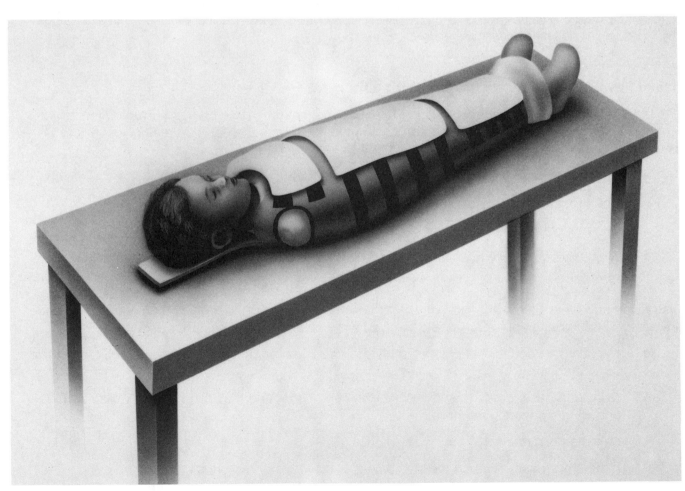

CHAPTER 3 PEDIATRIC CONSIDERATIONS

- Keep the caregiver in the child's line of vision whenever possible.

- Encourage the caregiver to talk to the child.

- If possible, keep one of the child's hands free so that the caregiver can hold the child's hand. There are typically three cloth straps or sections of the device; it may not be necessary to secure all the straps to control the child's movement.

- Allow the child as much control as possible.

- Monitor the child for potential vomiting and be prepared to intervene to prevent aspiration while the child is immobilized with this device.

PHARMACOLOGIC INTERVENTIONS

A spectrum of pharmacologic agents are used for pediatric pain management, including anesthetics, analgesics, and sedatives. Historically, analgesics and sedatives have been underused in the pediatric population.[9] Inadequate pain control is often related to misconceptions about pain in children, unrecognized pain, fear of side effects of medications, and lack of familiarity with medications and pediatric dosages rather than to true contraindications.[1,9]

Anesthetics

Anesthetics include a variety of agents. Local anesthetics are commonly used in wound closures and procedures that require an incision or sharp puncture of the skin (e.g., intravenous insertion, chest tube insertion, lumbar puncture). Anesthetic injections in the skin or an open wound are generally painful. Approaches used to reduce the pain associated with administration of local anesthetics or to eliminate the injection include the following:

- Buffering lidocaine hydrochloride with sodium bicarbonate to decrease the pain of the injection.[5] Buffered lidocaine hydrochloride is prepared with 1 part sodium bicarbonate to 10 parts lidocaine hydrochloride 1%.

- Applying topical and transdermal anesthetics:

  - Tetracaine hydrochloride, adrenaline, and cocaine hydrochloride solution (TAC solution)[5] or lidocaine hydrochloride, epinephrine hydrochloride, and tetracaine hydrochloride in a gel base, (LET gel, also known as TAL and XAP) are applied topically to lacerations:

    - Because of the effects of these medication combinations, they cannot be used on end organs, on or near mucous membranes, or on burns.

    - Anesthesia is attained in 20 to 30 minutes.

  - A eutectic mixture of prilocaine and lidocaine hydrochloride in a cream base (EMLA) is applied topically to intact skin, then covered by an occlusive dressing. Anesthesia is attained in approximately 60 minutes (see Appendix I for guidelines on using EMLA).

  - Transdermal administration of lidocaine with epinephrine by iontophoresis is another method of providing dermal anesthesia to intact skin[10]:

    - A battery-powered device (e.g., IOMED Numby Stuf) Is used to deliver a current through a special drug-delivery electrode, resulting in dermal anesthesia up to 10 mm in depth.

    - Anesthesia is achieved in approximately 10 minutes.

Other anesthetics that may be used in the emergency care setting require specialized equipment, training, and/or protocols. Nitrous oxide inhalation, which is a 50:50 mix of oxygen and nitrogen, or ketamine, are used in some emergency departments.[11]

Analgesics

Analgesics that may be given include nonnarcotic and narcotic medications:

- The following are characteristics of nonnarcotic analgesics:
    - Pain relief occurs at the site of injury or the peripheral nervous system.[5]
    - They are effective for acute or chronic pain and pain from trauma, surgery, or arthritis.[5]
    - They provide a ceiling effect on analgesia.
    - The category includes acetaminophen, ibuprofen, acetylsalicylic acid, and ketorolac tromethamine.
- The following are characteristics of narcotic analgesics:
    - They may be given by mouth, intramuscularly, subcutaneously, or intravenously.
    - The intravenous route provides rapid delivery and ability to titrate medication accurately.[1]
    - Side effects may include respiratory depression, sedation, hypotension, nausea, vomiting, chest wall rigidity (fentanyl citrate), or laryngospasm (fentanyl citrate).
    - The category includes morphine sulfate, fentanyl citrate, meperidine hydrochloride, codeine sulfate, and hydrocodone bitartrate.

Sedatives and Hypnotics

Sedatives and hypnotics provide no analgesia but are useful for reducing anxiety and providing sedation for painless procedures (e.g., computerized tomography scans and magnetic resonance imaging). These medications are frequently used in combination with analgesics for painful procedures:

- The following are characteristics of benzodiazepines (e.g., diazepam, lorazepam, and midazolam hydrochloride):
    - They may be given by mouth, rectally, intranasally, sublingually, intramuscularly, or intravenously.
    - The intravenous route allows for titration of medication.
    - Side effects include respiratory depression, a burning sensation with intranasal midazolam hydrochloride, and paradoxical inconsolability with midazolam hydrochloride.
    - The duration varies with the medication.
- Pentobarbital sodium is a sedative frequently used for painless procedures:
    - Side effects include respiratory depression and hyperactivity.
    - The duration is 2 to 3 hours when it is given intravenously.

Sedation and Analgesia for Painful Procedures

Sedation encompasses a continuum from mild sedation through noninteractive sedation, or arousal with moderate to intense stimuli. Conscious sedation is a state in which the patient maintains a patent airway, adequate cardiorespiratory function, and the ability to purposefully respond to verbal commands or tactile stimulation. In some institutions, specific policies have been developed delineating the care of patients based on various levels of sedation rather than using the broader category of conscious sedation. Levels of sedation are defined by the patient's level of responsiveness. In some states, the Nurse Practice Act dictates the level of practitioner required to monitor patients at some levels of sedation (e.g., anesthesiologist or certified registered nurse anesthetist).

In the emergency care setting, pediatric patients often require sedation and analgesia for painful procedures (e.g., fracture reduction). It is important to remember that patients may move rapidly from one level of sedation to another; vigilant monitoring and assessment are required to provide safe sedation. The following procedures and interventions are recommended when sedation and analgesics are given in the emergency care setting:

- Before the procedure is started, the following should be completed[12]:
  - The physician must obtain a presedation history:
    - Airway abnormalities (e.g., snoring, sleep apnea).
    - Chronic illness or conditions.
    - Previous adverse reactions to sedation, analgesia, or anesthesia.
    - Allergies.
    - Current medications.
    - Time of last oral intake, including solids or liquids.
  - The physician must complete a focused physical examination.
  - The physician must obtain informed consent as appropriate and per institution policy.
- Appropriate equipment must be available at bedside[12]:
  - Oxygen source and delivery method (oxygen mask, cannula).
  - *Bag-valve-mask device* and appropriate-sized face mask.
  - Suction apparatus and tonsil tip suction.
  - Intubation equipment and endotracheal tubes appropriate for the child's size.
  - Emergency medications and reversal agents.
  - Cardiac monitor.
  - Pulse oximeter.
  - Noninvasive blood pressure device.
  - End-expiratory CO_2 monitor (optional).

- Personnel requirements include:
  - An RN whose only role is to monitor the patient.
  - Practitioners capable of basic life support and airway management.
  - Person to assist with the procedure.
  - Person performing the procedure.
- Prior to the procedure the nurse should[6]:
  - Obtain intravenous access.
  - Place the patient on monitors, as listed above.
  - Obtain and document baseline vital signs and O_2 saturation.
- During the procedure, the nurse should[6]:
  - Prepare analgesic and sedative medications for administration (see Table 3).
  - Document all medications and doses administered.
  - Monitor and record vital signs every 5 to 10 minutes, including heart rate, respiratory rate, blood pressure, and oxygen saturation.
  - Monitor and document sedation level and level of consciousness.
  - Observe and document airway patency, respiratory pattern, and chest excursion.
  - Continue monitoring the patient until he or she returns to presedation level and discharge criteria are met.
- Discharge criteria should be standardized; before discharge, the patient[12]:
  - Must exhibit stable cardiovascular and respiratory status and vital signs that are returning to baseline levels.
  - Must be able to talk, sit up unaided, control his or her head and extremities, and follow commands; must be alert and oriented for age; must have returned to presedation state.
  - Must be able to maintain hydration status.

Important Points to Remember:

- When the noxious stimulus is decreased (e.g., fracture reduction is completed) an increased level of sedation may occur.
- Infants metabolize medications, especially narcotics, differently than do older children. Delayed reactions and delays in respiratory depression may occur. Infants require extended monitoring to ensure that they have returned to the presedation level.
- There is no ideal drug dosage or drug combination. Continuous monitoring of the patient and the ability to intervene are critical to safe sedation practices.
- Nonpharmacologic methods of pain management and coping are important adjuncts in managing pain in the pediatric patient.

Table 3

MEDICATIONS FOR CONSCIOUS SEDATION
Opioids*
• Morphine sulfate, 0.05 to 0.10 mg/kg intravenously over 1 to 2 minutes, given 5 minutes before procedure.   • Fentanyl citrate, 1 to 2 mcg/kg (0.001 to 0.002 mg/kg) intravenously 3 minutes before procedure.**   • Meperidine hydrochloride (if morphine sulfate or fentanyl citrate is not available), 0.5 to 1.0 mg/kg intravenously over 1 to 2 minutes, given 2 to 5 minutes before procedure, or 1.5 mg/kg orally, 45 to 60 minutes before procedure.
Sedatives*
• Diazepam, 0.2 to 0.3 mg/kg, maximum to 10 mg, orally, 45 to 60 minutes before procedure.   • Midazolam hydrochloride, 0.2 to 0.4 mg/kg, maximum to 15 mg intravenously. If given orally, administer 30 to 45 minutes before procedure. If given intravenously, administer 0.05 mg/kg 3 minutes before procedure.   • Pentobarbital sodium, 1 to 3 mg/kg intravenous bolus, to a maximum of 100 mg or until the child is asleep.   • Chloral hydrate, 20 to 75 mg/kg, to a maximum of 100 mg/kg or 2.0 grams, orally or rectally, 60 minutes before procedure.
*   Provide analgesia and sedation.   **   Not recommended for children who weigh less than 15 kg. Lozenge should be sucked, not chewed and swallowed. If chewed, the drug is less effective because part of it is metabolized by the liver before entering the bloodstream. Swallowing the drug rapidly does not increase risk of respiratory depression during first 15 to 30 minutes, which is the period of greatest risk for decreased respiration.   *** Provide sedation but no analgesia.

Adapted from Zeltzer LK. Report of the subcommittee on the management of pain associated with procedures in children with cancer. *Pediatrics.* 86;1990:826-831; and Cote CJ. Sedation for the pediatric patient. *Pediatr Clin North Am.* 41;1994:31-58. Used with permission.

MEDICATION ADMINISTRATION

- Before any medications are administered, the patient's identification band should always be checked against the chart. The caregiver should also be asked to state the child's name to verify the child's identity. If old enough, the child may be asked to state his or her name.

- All dosages are calculated based on weight. Ensure that the patient's weight is recorded accurately in kilograms.

- Table 4 provides an overview of common routes of administration and tips to facilitate administration.

Positioning for an Injection

Consider using positioning-for-comfort techniques. Have the caregiver hold the child on his or her lap (chest to chest) and hug the child, or have the caregiver stand in front of the child who is sitting on the stretcher (chest to chest) and hug the child.

Table 4

	MEDICATION ADMINISTRATION
Route	**Considerations**
Ear	• In children younger than 3 years of age, pull the pinna down and back. • In children older than 3 years of age, lift the pinna up and back. • Have the child position his or her head to side or rest his or her head on the caregiver's shoulder.
Nasal	• Have the caregiver hold the child across his or her lap with the child's head down. Place the child's arm that is closest to the caregiver around the caregiver's back. Firmly hug the child's other arm and hand with the caregiver's arm; snuggle the head between the caregiver's body and arm.[13]
Eye	• Explain the procedure; tell the child the medication will feel cool. Prepare the child if the medication may sting. • Have the child lie on his or her back with the hands under the buttocks; alternatively, have the child sit on the caregiver's lap and have the caregiver hug the child to secure his or her arms. • Have the child look up, then retract the lower lid and instill the medication. • Provide distractions.
Oral	• Consider the child's age when determining the medication preparation (liquid, chewable, sprinkles). • Use an oral syringe or calibrated cup to ensure correct dosage. • To prevent aspiration, administer oral medications while the child's head is raised or the child is in a sitting position. • For infants, liquid medication can be administered through a nipple, followed with 5 ml of sterile water.[14] • When administering medication with an oral syringe, place the syringe between the gum and cheek. Administer slowly, no more than 0.5 ml of medication at a time.[14] • Do not administer chewable tablets to children without teeth. Give children who do receive chewable tablets something to drink afterward. • Do not crush enteric-coated caplets or tablets. • Do not open capsules if medication is sustained release; check with the pharmacy before opening any capsules for administration.[14] • Avoid mixing medications with formula because the infant may refuse the formula thereafter. • When mixing medications with food or fluids, use as little diluent as possible. Masking the taste with food or fluid is often helpful; however, if the quantity is large, the child may not finish the entire amount and the full dose will not be given.
Rectal	• Consult a pharmacist prior to cutting a suppository; the medication is not necessarily distributed evenly through the suppository (e.g., acetaminophen suppositories must be divided lengthwise not widthwise). • Place the child in knee-chest position on his or her side. • Lubricate the suppository with water-soluble lubricant prior to insertion.

Intramuscular Injections

- Position and secure the child before the injection.

- Consider the child's age, weight, and muscle mass, as well as medication volume and viscosity, when selecting an injection site (see Table 5 and Figure 5 for considerations and location of injection sites).[13,15]

- Consider use of dermal anesthetic or placing a wrapped ice cube on the site for approximately 1 minute prior to the injection.[13]

- The medication volume for injection per intramuscular site is limited: Infants – 0.5 to 1.0 ml; older children – 2.0 ml.

- After the medication is drawn into the syringe, change the needle before giving the injection. Insertion of the needle through a vial stopper dulls the tip of the needle, and residual medication on the needle may irritate tissue and/or muscle.

- For the immunocompromised child, cleanse the site with povidone iodine and alcohol.[14]

- After the injection, comfort the child and give him or her a reward (e.g., sticker, popsicle).

Table 5

PEDIATRIC INTRAMUSCULAR INJECTION SITES		
Site	**Recommended Age**	**Considerations**

Vastus lateralis	Infant. Preferred for children younger than 3 years of age.	- Largest muscle group in children younger than 3 years of age.
		- Can tolerate large injection volumes:
		  - Infants 0.5 to 1.0 ml.
		  - Older children up to 2.0 ml.
		- Area free of important nerves or blood vessels.
		- Use 22-gauge to 25-gauge 5/8-inch to 1-inch needle.

Ventrogluteal	Child. Consider for children older than 3 years of age.	- Can tolerate large injection volumes. - Area free of important nerves or blood vessels. - Easily accessible site. - Health care professionals often unfamiliar with site. - Injection volume up to 2.0 ml. - Use 20-gauge to 25-gauge 1-inch to 1.5-inch needle.
Dorsogluteal	Contraindicated in children younger than 3 years or in children who have not been walking longer than 1 year.	- Large muscle mass in older children. - Can tolerate large injection volumes. - Danger of injury to sciatic nerve. - Exposure of site may cause embarrassment in older children. - Injection volume up to 2.0 ml. - Use 20-gauge to 25-gauge 1-inch to 1.5-inch needle.
Deltoid	Infant.	- Small muscle mass. - Can tolerate only small injection volumes (0.5 to 1.0 ml). - Easily accessible site. - Rapid absorption rate. - Danger of radial nerve injury in young children. - Use 22-gauge to 25-gauge 1/2-inch to 1-inch needle.

Figure 5
INTRAMUSCULAR INJECTION SITES IN CHILDREN

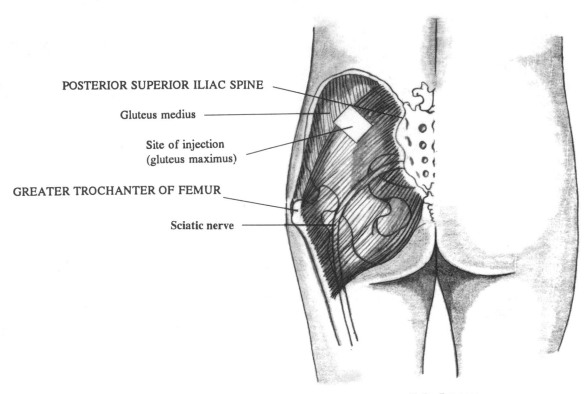

POSTERIOR SUPERIOR ILIAC SPINE

Gluteus medius

Site of injection
(gluteus maximus)

GREATER TROCHANTER OF FEMUR

Sciatic nerve

E.P. BRADY

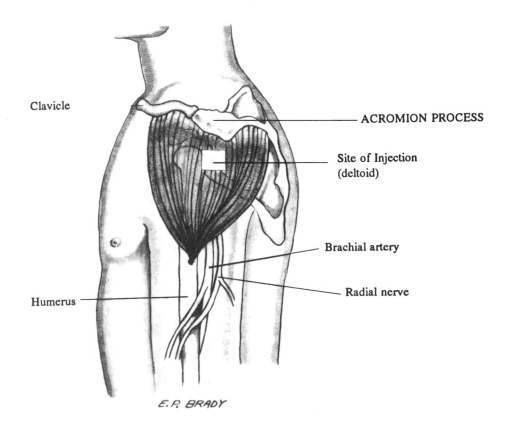

Clavicle

ACROMION PROCESS

Site of Injection
(deltoid)

Brachial artery

Radial nerve

Humerus

E.P. BRADY

Figure 5 (Continued)

INTRAMUSCULAR INJECTION SITES IN CHILDREN

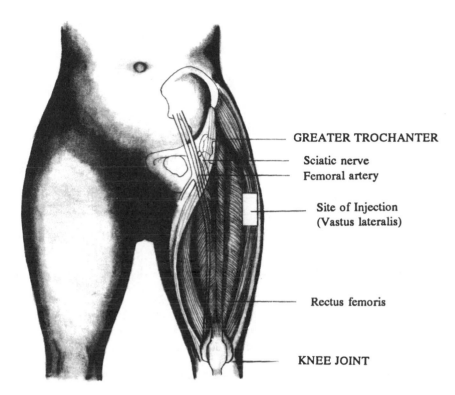

GREATER TROCHANTER

Sciatic nerve

Femoral artery

Site of Injection
(Vastus lateralis)

Rectus femoris

KNEE JOINT

F.P. BRADY

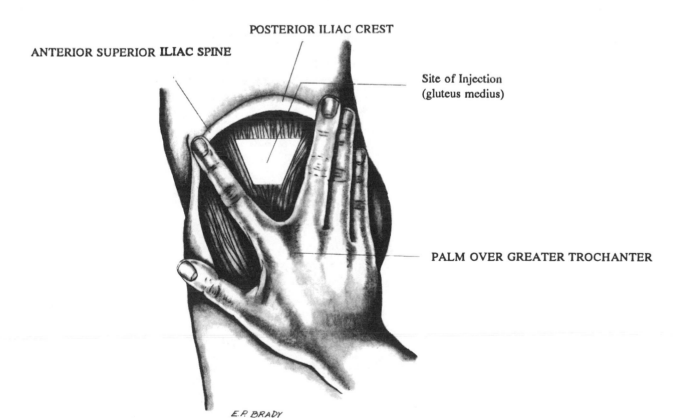

POSTERIOR ILIAC CREST

ANTERIOR SUPERIOR ILIAC SPINE

Site of Injection
(gluteus medius)

PALM OVER GREATER TROCHANTER

E.P. BRADY

Subcutaneous Medication Administration

- Sites include deltoid, anterior thigh, and anterior abdominal wall.

- Volume of medication administered is limited, 0.5 to 1.0 ml. Maximum of 1.0 ml in all age groups.

- Insert needle at a 90° angle.

- Needle size: Infant or thin child – 25-gauge, 1/2-inch; larger child – 25-gauge, 5/8-inch.[16]

Intravenous Medication Administration

- Administration time may vary. Drugs and fluids may be given by intravenous bolus, constant infusion, or intermittent infusion.

- A syringe pump or infusion pump is used to deliver continuous or intermittent medication infusions to ensure accurate and timely delivery of medications.

- Administer medications following guidelines for dilution and infusion of the specific drug. After drug administration, flush the intravenous tubing with normal saline fluid to clear any residual medication from the line. Syringe pumps with low-volume tubing are available to minimize the amount of flush solution needed.

- To administer an intravenous fluid bolus rapidly, a pressure bag may be applied to the intravenous solution bag with regular intravenous or large-bore intravenous tubing. However, a small catheter may impede gravity flow. When more rapid administration is needed, the following stopcock technique may be used:

  - Attach a 3-way stopcock between the T-connector and the intravenous tubing.

  - Attach a syringe to the stopcock; turn off the stopcock to the child (arrow toward the child).

  - Withdraw the syringe plunger, filling the syringe with intravenous solution.

  - When the desired amount is withdrawn, turn off the stopcock to the intravenous solution bag (arrow toward the bag) and push the solution from the syringe. Repeat this procedure until the desired fluid volume is administered.

  - If medications are administered through a stopcock, flush the stopcock with 3 to 5 ml of solution following the medication administration.

Endotracheal Administration

- In the absence of vascular access during resuscitation, the endotracheal route can be used to administer the following emergency drugs: lidocaine hydrochloride, epinephrine hydrochloride, atropine sulfate, naloxone.

- The recommended dose of epinephrine hydrochloride via the endotracheal tube during resuscitation is 10 times the intravenous or intraosseous dose.

- For a more rapid delivery, dilute the drug in 1 to 2 ml of normal saline and inject through a catheter inserted beyond the endotracheal tube tip. After the drug is administered, follow with several positive pressure ventilations.

Discharge Teaching for Caregivers Regarding Medication Administration

- Caregivers and children (when appropriate) should be given information about the drug name, route of administration, action, dosage, and potential side effects.

- Adequate discharge instructions promote compliance and the safe and accurate administration of medications at home. The following information should be included in the instructions:

  - Time medication should be given.

  - Duration of drug therapy.

  - Medication administration techniques, including methods of measuring suspensions.

REFERENCES

1. Selbst SM. Pain management in the emergency department. In: Schechter NL, Berde CB, Yaster M, eds. *Pain in Infants, Children, and Adolescents*. Baltimore, Md: Williams & Wilkins; 1993:505-518.

2. Schechter NL, Blankson V, Pachter LM, Sullivan CM. The ouchless place: No pain, children's gain. *Pediatrics*. 1997:99:890-894.

3. McKenzie IM. Developmental physiology and psychology. In: McKenzie IM, Gaukroger PB, Ragg PG, Brown TCK, eds. *Manual of Acute Pain Management in Children*. New York, NY: Churchill; 1997:7-10.

4. Bove MA. Positioning and securing children for procedures. In: Bernardo LM, Bove MA, eds. *Pediatric Emergency Nursing Procedures*. Boston, Mass: Jones & Bartlett; 1993:29-34.

5. McCaffey M, Wong DL. Nursing interventions for pain control in children. In: Schechter NL, Berde CB, Yaster M, eds. *Pain in Infants, Children and Adolescents*. Baltimore, Md: Williams & Wilkins; 1993:299-315.

6. Bernardo LM, Conway AE. Pain assessment and management. In: Soud TE, Roger JS, eds. *Manual of Pediatric Emergency Nursing*. St. Louis, Mo: Mosby-Year Book; 1998:686-711.

7. Kuttner L. *A Child in Pain*. Point Roberts, Wash: Hartley & Marks Publishers; 1996:90-132.

8. Stephen B, Barkey M. *Positioning for Comfort*. Mt. Royal, NJ: Association for the Care of Children's Health Hurt Alert Day Resource; March 1994.

9. Callahan JM. Pharmacologic agents. In: Dieckmann RA, Fiser DH, Selbst SM, eds. *Illustrated Textbook of Pediatric Emergency and Critical Care Procedures*. St. Louis, Mo: Mosby-Year Book; 1997:53-67.

10. Ashburn MS, Gauthire M, Loce G, Basta S, Gaylord B, Kessler K. Iontophoretic administration of 2% lidocaine HCL and 1:10,000 epinephrine in humans. *Clin J Pain*. 1997;13:22-26.

11. Froese N, Costarino AJ. Sedation and pain relief: Other agents. In: Dieckmann RA, Fiser DH, Selbst SM, eds. *Illustrated Textbook of Pediatric Emergency and Critical Care Procedures*. St. Louis, Mo: Mosby-Year Book; 1997:68-71.

12. American Academy of Pediatrics. Guidelines for monitoring and management of pediatric patients during and after sedation for diagnostic and therapeutic procedures. *Pediatrics*. 1992;89:1110-1115.

13. Wong D, Whaley L. *Clinical Manual of Pediatric Nursing*. 3rd ed. St. Louis, Mo: Mosby-Year Book; 1990.

14. O'Connor K. Medication administration. In: Bernardo LM, Bove MA, eds. *Pediatric Emergency Nursing Procedures*. Boston, Mass: Jones & Bartlett; 1993:207-240.

15. Newton M, Newton DW, Fudin J. Reviewing the big three injection routes. *Nursing*. 1992;22:34-42.

16. Scale N. *Manual of Pediatric Nursing Procedures*. Philadelphia, Pa: JB Lippincott; 1992.

ADDITIONAL RESOURCES FOR GUIDELINES ON CHILDREN'S PAIN

1. **Acute Pain Management: Operative or Medical Procedures and Trauma**
   Available at no charge from the Agency for Health Care Policy and Research Publications, PO Box 8527, Silver Spring, MD 20907; (800) 358-9295.

2. **Acute Pain Management in Infants, Children, and Adolescents; Operative and Medical Procedures**
   Available at no charge from the Agency for Health Care Policy and Research Publications, PO Box 8527, Silver Spring, MD 20907; (800) 358-9295.

3. **Management of Cancer Pain**
   Available at no charge from the Agency for Health Care Policy and Research Publications, PO Box 8527, Silver Spring, MD 20907; (800) 358-9295.

4. **Quick Reference Guide for Clinicians: Management of Cancer Pain: Adults**
   Available at no charge from the Agency for Health Care Policy and Research Publications, PO Box 8527, Silver Spring, MD 20907; (800) 358-9295.

5. **Principles of Analgesic Use in the Treatment of Acute Pain and Chronic Cancer Pain**
   Available from the American Pain Society, 4700 West Lake Ave., Glenview, IL 60025; (847) 375-4700.

6. **Management of Acute Pain: A Practical Guide**
   Available from the International Association for the Study of Pain (IASP), 909 NE 43rd St., Suite 306, Seattle, WA 98105; (206) 547-6409.

7. **Handbook of Cancer Pain Management**
   Available from the Wisconsin Cancer Pain Initiative, 3675 Medical Sciences Center, University of Wisconsin Medical School, 1300 University Ave., Madison, WI 53706; (608) 262-0078.

8. **Report of the Consensus Conference on the Management of Pain in Childhood Cancer**
   Published in *Pediatrics* 86(5, suppl):813-834; 1990; available from the American Academy of Pediatrics, PO Box 927, Elk Grove Village, IL 60009; (800) 433-9016.

9. **Guidelines for Standard of Care of Acute Painful Episodes in Patients with Sickle Cell Disease**
   Available from Samir K. Ballas, MD, Cardeza Foundation, 1015 Walnut St., Philadelphia, PA 19107.

10. **Clinical Reference Guide for Health Care Providers**
    Sickle Cell-Related Pain: Assessment and Management Conference Proceedings
    Available from the New England Regional Genetics Group (NERGG), PO Box 670, Mt. Desert, ME 04660; (207) 288-2704; Fax (207) 288-2705.

11. **American Nurses Association Position Statements on Promotion of Comfort and Relief of Pain in Dying Patients and on the Role of the Registered Nurse in the Management of Patients Receiving IV Conscious Sedation for Short-Term Therapeutic, Diagnostic, or Surgical Procedures**
    Published in *The American Nurse*, Feb. 1992, pp 7-8. Available from American Nurses Association Publications Distribution Center, PO Box 4100, Kearneysville, WV 25430; (800) 637-0323.

12. **Oncology Nursing Society Position Paper on Cancer Pain**
    By Spross JA, McGuire DB. Published in *Oncology Nursing Forum*, 1990; 17(5):753.

13. **Mayday Pain Resource Center**
    Available from City of Hope National Medical Center, Nursing Research and Education/Mayday Pain Resource Center, 1500 East Duarte Rd., Duarte, CA 91010; (818) 359-8111, ext. 3829; Fax (818) 301-8941.

14. **Whaley and Wong's Pediatric Pain Assessment and Management**
    Videotape available from Mosby, 11830 Westline Industrial Dr., St. Louis, MO 63146; (800) 426-4545.

ALSO AVAILABLE FOR FAMILIES

1. **Pain Control After Surgery: A Patient's Guide**
   Managing Cancer Pain: Patient Guide
   Available at no charge from the Agency for Health Care Policy and Research Publications, PO Box 8527, Silver Spring, MD 20907; (800) 358-9295.

2. **Children's Cancer Pain Can Be Relieved: A Guide for Parents and Families**
   Available from the Wisconsin Cancer Pain Initiative, 3675 Medical Sciences Center, University of Wisconsin Medical School, 1300 University Ave., Madison, WI 53706; (608) 262-0978.

3. **Pain Relief: How to Say No to Acute, Chronic, and Cancer Pain!**
   By Jane Cowles, 1993; available from MasterMedia Limited, 17 E. 89th St., New York, NY 10128; (212) 546-7650.

4. **Questions and Answers About Pain Control: A Guide for People with Cancer and Their Families**
   Available at no charge from the Office of Cancer Communications, Bldg. 31, Room 10A24, Bethesda, MD 20892; (800) 4-CANCER; and from local branches of the American Cancer Society; or call (800) ACS-2345.

5. **Sickle Cell-Related Pain: Assessment and Management – A Guide for Patients and Families**
   Available from the New England Regional Genetics Group (NERGG), PO Box 670, Mt. Desert, ME 04660; (207) 288-2704; Fax (207) 288-2705.

Information from Wong DL. Family-centered care of the child during illness and hospitalization. In: Wong DL, Hockenberry-Eaton M, Winkelstein ML, Ahmann E, DiVito-Thomas PA, eds. *Whaley and Wong's Nursing Care of Infants and Children*. 6th ed. St. Louis, Mo: Mosby-Year Book; 1999:1082.

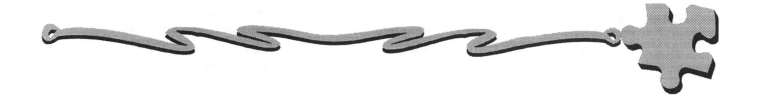

CHAPTER 4

Initial Assessment and Triage

OBJECTIVES

On completion of this lecture, the learner should be able to:

✦ Discuss the components of a pediatric primary assessment.

✦ Correlate life-threatening conditions with the specific component of the primary assessment.

✦ Describe interventions needed to manage life-threatening conditions found during the primary assessment.

✦ Identify the components of a pediatric secondary assessment.

✦ Identify the components of pediatric triage.

✦ Evaluate the effectiveness of nursing interventions as related to patient outcomes.

INTRODUCTION

Ill or injured children are often a source of anxiety for health care providers. Children may rapidly decompensate with few signs of impending arrest. Therefore, early identification of abnormal findings during the initial assessment is crucial for a positive patient outcome. The initial assessment of the pediatric patient involves a systematic process that recognizes life-threatening conditions, identifies injuries, and determines priorities of care based on the assessment findings.[1] The initial assessment is divided into two phases, primary and secondary.

Treatment priorities are determined by the initial and repeat assessments. *Triage,* which means to sort or choose, is a process used to determine the urgency of need for emergency care based on the assessment findings. The prioritization of patients is a continuous process and extends beyond the physical facilities of the triage area. Throughout the emergency care visit, children must be periodically reassessed to identify changes in condition and reset priorities of care.

In essence, triage and prioritization of care are integral components of the nursing process in all locations. The initial assessment is performed to collect enough information to make the initial triage decision. This chapter will identify the components of the initial assessment, interventions completed during the primary assessment, use of the Pediatric Assessment Triangle, components of pediatric triage, and the analysis of assessment data to formulate nursing diagnoses and determine an appropriate *triage decision*.

A Guide to Initial Assessment

The following mnemonic describes the components of the initial assessment of the pediatric patient. The materials presented in this chapter represent comprehensive primary and secondary assessments.

- Primary assessment:

    - A = Airway with simultaneous *cervical spine stabilization* for any child with suspected trauma.

    - B = Breathing.

    - C = Circulation.

    - D = Disability or neurologic status.

- Secondary assessment:

    - E = Exposure and environmental control to prevent heat loss.

    - F = Full set of vital signs, including weight, and family presence.

    - G = Give comfort measures.

    - H = Head-to-toe assessment and history.

    - I = Inspect posterior surfaces.

PRIMARY ASSESSMENT

An observational assessment is completed while approaching the child. This is completed using the Pediatric Assessment Triangle which consists of appearance, work of breathing, and circulation to the skin. The primary assessment consists of assessment of the airway with cervical spine stabilization or maintenance of *spinal immobilization* when trauma is suspected, breathing, circulation, and disability or neurologic status. Interventions to correct any life-threatening conditions are performed before the assessment is continued. The interventions are listed in order of priority.

Airway

ASSESSMENT

Inspect the child's airway. Because partial or total airway obstruction may threaten the patency of the upper airway, assess for the following:

- Vocalization: Can the child talk or cry?
- Tongue obstructing the airway in an unresponsive child.
- Loose teeth or foreign objects, such as gum or small toys, in the oropharynx or hypopharynx.
- Vomitus, bleeding, or other secretions in the mouth.
- Edema of the lips and/or tissues of the mouth.
- Preferred posture. For example, the tripod position is characterized by the child sitting up, leaning forward, with the neck extended and head tilted up in an effort to maximize the airway.
- Drooling.
- Dysphagia.
- Abnormal airway sounds such as stridor, snoring, or gurgling.

INTERVENTIONS

- For any child whose mechanism of injury, symptoms, or physical findings suggest a possible cervical spine injury, manually stabilize the cervical spine or maintain spinal immobilization if completed in the prehospital environment. (Nursing diagnosis: Injury).
- If a child is awake and breathing, he or she may have assumed a position that maximizes the ability to maintain a spontaneous airway. Allow the child to maintain this position or a position of comfort. (Nursing diagnosis: Ineffective airway clearance).
- If the child is unresponsive and/or unable to maintain a spontaneous airway, position the child and manually open the airway. (Nursing diagnoses: Ineffective airway clearance; aspiration; ineffective breathing pattern). Techniques to open or clear an obstructed airway during the primary assessment include:
  - *Jaw thrust.*
  - *Head tilt-chin lift* (difficult to do in the younger child). Do not use this technique if trauma is suspected.
    - Infants and young children have a large occiput; positioning them supine on a bed or backboard may cause their cervical vertebrae to flex anteriorly. Flexion may contribute to compromise of the airway or decrease the effectiveness of the jaw thrust or chin lift maneuvers.
    - To provide neutral alignment of the cervical spine and a neutral position for the child's airway, place padding under the child's shoulders to bring the shoulders into horizontal alignment with the external auditory meatus.[2]

- Suction the oropharynx with a rigid tonsil suction to remove debris. Vomitus or other secretions should be removed immediately (usually prior to manually opening the airway) by suctioning the patient. Suctioning or other interventions must be done in a manner to prevent stimulation of the gag reflex, which may cause subsequent vomiting or aspiration.

- If the child is unable to maintain a patent airway after positioning. (Nursing diagnosis: Ineffective airway clearance):

    - Insert a nasopharyngeal airway if the child is conscious without evidence of facial trauma or skull fracture.

    - Insert an oropharyngeal airway if the child is unconscious or does not have a gag reflex. Proper positioning of the head and jaw must be maintained even in the presence of a patent airway.

- Prepare for endotracheal intubation. (Nursing diagnosis: Aspiration).

Breathing

Once a patent airway has been established, assess for the following:

ASSESSMENT

- Level of consciousness.

- Spontaneous respirations.

- Rate and depth of respirations.

- Symmetric chest rise and fall.

- Presence and quality of bilateral breath sounds.

- Presence of indicators of work of breathing:

    - Nasal flaring.

    - Substernal, subcostal, intercostal, supraclavicular, or suprasternal retractions.

    - Head bobbing.

    - Expiratory grunting.

    - Accessory muscle use.

- Jugular vein distension and tracheal position.

- Paradoxical respirations due to a flail segment.

- Soft tissue and bony chest wall integrity.

INTERVENTIONS

- Position the child to facilitate respiratory effectiveness and comfort. (Nursing diagnosis: Ineffective breathing pattern).

- In the spontaneously breathing child, deliver supplemental oxygen, as indicated by the child's clinical condition. (Nursing diagnoses: Ineffective breathing pattern; impaired gas exchange).

  - Administer oxygen at the highest concentration in a manner the child will tolerate.

  - Consider using a nonrebreather mask at a flow rate sufficient to keep the reservoir bag inflated; usually requires 12 to 15 liters/minute.

- Assist ventilation with 100% oxygen via a bag-valve-mask device, as indicated, for apnea or hypoventilation. Assess effectiveness of assisted ventilation by observing chest rise and fall and auscultating for the presence of breath sounds. (Nursing diagnosis: Ineffective breathing pattern).

- Prepare for endotracheal intubation, as indicated. (Nursing diagnoses: Ineffective breathing pattern; impaired gas exchange).

  - Indications for intubation include:

    - Respiratory arrest.

    - Anticipated need for prolonged airway control.

    - Severe head injury with decreasing level of consciousness or *Pediatric Coma Scale* score or *Glasgow Coma Scale score* (GCS) ≤ 8.

    - Shock (to maximize oxygen delivery to tissues and decrease work of breathing).

    - Respiratory failure.

  - Confirm endotracheal tube placement at the time of insertion and each time the patient is moved.

    - Observe chest rise and fall.

    - Listen for breath sounds in the axilla and epigastric area.

    - Assess for change or improvement of skin and mucous membrane color.

    - Assess end-tidal CO_2 by monitor or device (if available) and oxygen saturation by pulse oximeter.

    - Obtain chest radiograph.

  - Document endotracheal tube size, cuff versus uncuffed tube, and depth by assessing location of tube at the lip, gum, or tooth line.

- Administer medications to facilitate intubation procedure, as ordered. (Nursing diagnoses: Pain; anxiety).

  - If neuromuscular blocking agents are used, a sedative agent must also be administered to provide sedation.

  - Resuscitation equipment must be available at the bedside prior to administration of neuromuscular blocking agents.

- Decompress tension pneumothorax via needle thoracentesis, as indicated. (Nursing diagnosis: Impaired gas exchange). This may be indicated if the patient is in severe respiratory distress or is intubated and not improving with other interventions.

Circulation

Once adequate breathing is established, assess for the following:

ASSESSMENT

- Central and peripheral pulse rate and quality.

- Skin color (e.g., pale, mottled, dusky, cyanotic) and temperature.

- Capillary refill. Normal capillary refill is 2 seconds or less in a warm ambient environment. Capillary refill time is one component used in the evaluation of peripheral perfusion. Factors that may affect capillary refill time, not related to an alteration in general tissue perfusion, include a cool ambient environment and injury with vascular compromise.

- Uncontrolled external bleeding.

INTERVENTIONS

- Control any uncontrolled external bleeding by applying direct pressure over the bleeding sites. (Nursing diagnoses: Fluid volume deficit; cardiac output, decreased; altered tissue perfusion).

- Obtain vascular access by inserting the largest bore catheter that the vessel can accommodate and initiating an intravenous infusion, as indicated by the child's illness or injury. (Nursing diagnoses: Cardiac output, decreased; altered tissue perfusion; fluid volume deficit):

  - In the unconscious child, if peripheral vascular access is unsuccessful after three quick attempts or more than 90 seconds, consider intraosseous access.

  - Administer a 20 ml/kg fluid bolus of a crystalloid solution (0.9% normal saline or lactated Ringer's solution) as indicated by the child's perfusion status.

  - Repeat the bolus if reassessment findings indicate inadequate tissue perfusion. If symptoms of shock persist, the child may need additional crystalloid boluses, blood for hemorrhagic losses, or colloid solutions.

- Initiate cardiac compressions if the pulse rate is less than 60 beats/minute and perfusion is ineffective. (Nursing diagnosis: Cardiac output, decreased).

- Initiate drug therapy, as indicated by the illness or injury and perfusion status. (Nursing diagnosis: Cardiac output, decreased).

- Initiate *defibrillation* or *synchronized cardioversion*, as indicated by dysrhythmia. (Nursing diagnosis: Cardiac output, decreased).

Disability – Brief Neurologic Assessment

After the primary assessment of airway, breathing, and circulation, conduct a brief neurologic assessment to determine the degree of disability, as measured by the child's level of consciousness. The findings must be interpreted based on the child's age and developmental level.

ASSESSMENT

- Determine the child's level of consciousness by assessing the child's response to verbal and/or painful stimuli using the AVPU mnemonic:

  - **A** = Awake and Alert.

  - **V** = Only responsive to **V**erbal stimuli.

  - **P** = Only responsive to **P**ainful stimuli.

  - **U** = Completely **U**nresponsive.

- In children with chronic neurologic impairment, assess responsiveness in relation to their normal or typical status (ask the caregiver the typical level of responsiveness for the child).

- Assess pupil size, shape, equality, and reactivity to light.

INTERVENTIONS

- If the disability assessment indicates a decreased level of consciousness, conduct further investigation during the secondary assessment. (Nursing diagnosis: Altered tissue perfusion).

- Initiate pharmacologic therapy as prescribed. (Nursing diagnosis: Altered tissue perfusion).

- Consider the need for endotracheal intubation to maintain airway and/or ensure adequate ventilation and oxygenation. (Nursing diagnoses: Aspiration; ineffective breathing pattern).

SECONDARY ASSESSMENT

Exposure and Environmental Control

ASSESSMENT

Undress the child to examine and identify any underlying injury or additional signs of illness. Infants and children have a larger body surface area-to-body weight ratio and are at a greater risk to rapidly lose body heat when exposed. Initiate methods to maintain a normothermic state or to warm the patient. Cold stress in critically ill or injured infants can increase metabolic demands, exacerbate the effects of hypoxia and hypoglycemia, and affect responses to resuscitative efforts.

INTERVENTIONS

- Provide measures to maintain normal body temperature or to warm the patient. (Nursing diagnosis: Hypothermia).

  - Warm blankets.

  - Overhead warming lights or other warming device.

  - Warm ambient environment, increasing the room temperature as needed.

  - Warm intravenous fluids via fluid warmer when bolus volumes of intravenous fluids are administered. There are a variety of commercially available fluid warmers specifically intended to warm intravenous fluids. In the febrile child, consider administering the intravenous fluids at normal body temperature.

  - Warm humidified oxygen.

- Provide measures to maintain normal body temperature or to cool the patient. (Nursing diagnoses: Hyperthermia; hypothermia).

  - Remove excessive clothing or blankets.

  - Administer antipyretics per protocol.

Full Set of Vital Signs

ASSESSMENT

Vital signs may be obtained prior to the secondary assessment phase, especially when a team of providers is involved in providing care simultaneously. If a complete set of vital signs has not yet been obtained, it should be done now. Recognizing subtle and significant alterations in vital signs is an important part of analyzing the assessment data. Obtaining serial measurements is needed to identify these trends. The following vital signs should be assessed in all pediatric patients:

- Respirations: Assess the rate and depth of respirations.

- Pulse or heart rate: Auscultate an apical pulse as a baseline rate in infants and younger children and in any critically ill infant, child, or adolescent:

  - Compare central and peripheral pulses bilaterally for strength and equality.

  - Palpate a brachial pulse as the central pulse in the infant.

  - When evaluating central and peripheral perfusion, palpate the peripheral pulse on an uninjured extremity.

- Blood pressure: Measure the blood pressure by auscultation, palpation, ultrasonic flow meter, or noninvasive blood pressure monitor:

  - Blood pressure cuff size can affect the accuracy of readings. An appropriately sized blood pressure cuff bladder covers one half to two thirds of the child's upper arm.

  - Auscultate the initial blood pressure in infants, children, and adolescents with signs of poor perfusion.

- The blood pressure in a child may be within normal limits for the child's age despite significant blood loss.

- A noninvasive, automated blood pressure monitor should be used with caution on critically ill or injured children. Some models are not accurate for extremely high or low blood pressures.[3] Abnormal readings or significant changes in readings should be validated by auscultation or another manual method.

- Typical systolic pressure in children 2 years of age or older is 90 + (2 × age in years). The diastolic pressure is two thirds of the systolic pressure. See Appendix J for blood pressure listings by age.

- Temperature: Obtain temperature via appropriate route (oral, rectal, axillary), considering the child's age and condition. Appendix K is a conversion table of centigrade and fahrenheit temperatures.

- Weight in kilograms: Obtain a measured weight whenever possible. If circumstances do not permit obtaining a measured weight:

  - Ask the caregiver the child's last weight.

  - Use a length-based resuscitation tape, such as the *Broselow™ tape,* to estimate the child's weight if 35 kg or less.

- Normal pediatric vital signs are listed in Table 6. Factors affecting heart rate and respiratory rate are listed in Table 7.

- Consider application of cardiac, cardiorespiratory, or pulse oximeter monitors, as appropriate, for the child's condition.

Table 6

	VITAL SIGNS BY AGE		
Age	Respiratory Rate/Minute	Pulse Beats/Minute	Blood Pressure (Systolic) (mm Hg)
Birth to 1 week	30 to 60	100 to 160	50 to 70
1 to 6 weeks	30 to 60	100 to 160	70 to 95
6 months	25 to 40	90 to 120	80 to 100
1 year	20 to 30	90 to 120	80 to 100
3 years	20 to 30	80 to 120	80 to 110
6 years	18 to 25	70 to 110	80 to 110
10 years	15 to 20	60 to 90	90 to 120

Adapted from Seidel J, Henderson D, eds. *Prehospital Care of Pediatric Emergencies.* Los Angeles, Calif: Los Angeles Pediatric Society; 1987:10. Used with permission.

Table 7

FACTORS AFFECTING HEART RATE AND RESPIRATORY RATE		
Increased Heart Rate and Respiratory Rate	**Decreased Respiratory Rate**	**Decreased Heart Rate**
Fear, anxiety, agitation Crying Fever Hypoxia Hypovolemia Shock Medications	Hypoxia Hypothermia Increased intracranial pressure Respiratory muscle fatigue Medications	Vagal stimulation Hypoxia Hypothermia Cardiac pathology End-stage shock Medications

- Serial blood pressure measurements are useful in identifying subtle changes and a *widening pulse pressure*. Widening pulse pressure can occur secondary to increased intracranial pressure, early septic shock, and early hypovolemic shock.

  - Hypotension is defined by age and can occur secondary to significant fluid or blood losses and certain medications. Hypotension is a late sign of shock in the pediatric patient.

  - The formula used to approximate the lowest acceptable limit of systolic blood pressure, by age, in children older than 2 years of age is 70 + (2 × age in years).

  - Hypertension is defined as blood pressure at or above the 95th percentile for age (see Appendix J).

- Temperature variations that may indicate a serious condition and influence triage decisions include:

  - Rectal temperature >38°C (100.4°F) in infants younger than 2 or 3 months of age.

  - Rectal temperature ≥40°C (104°F) in infants 3 months to 2 years of age with no localized signs of infection.

  - Rectal temperature <36°C (96.8°F).

Family Presence

- Assess the needs of the family taking into consideration cultural variances. (Nursing diagnosis: Anxiety/fear).

- Facilitate and support the family's involvement in the child's care.[4] (Nursing diagnosis: Anxiety/fear).

- Assign a health care professional to provide explanations about procedures and to be with the family in the emergency department. (Nursing diagnosis: Anxiety/fear).

- Assign a staff member to provide family support. (Nursing diagnosis: Anxiety/fear).

Give Comfort Measures

Initiate comfort measures based on chief complaint or obvious injury. (Nursing diagnosis: Pain).

- Evaluate presence and level of pain.
- Stabilize suspected fractures.
- Apply cold to injury sites.
- Dress open wounds.
- Provide a wheelchair or stretcher.
- Consider nonpharmacologic techniques to reduce pain.

Head-to-Toe Assessment

Information from the head-to-toe assessment is collected primarily through inspection, auscultation, and palpation. The order and type of information collected in the secondary assessment may vary based on the child's developmental level, chief complaint, or clinical appearance.

GENERAL APPEARANCE

The general appearance of the child can assist the nurse in discerning problems that need further investigation. The child's physical appearance, general nutritional status, appropriateness of clothing for the season or environment, and reactions to caregivers are important factors in the overall assessment of the child. The Pediatric Assessment Triangle, which looks at general appearance, work of breathing, and circulation, facilitates obtaining this information. Body position and alignment, guarding or self-protective movements, muscle tone, and unusual odors, such as alcohol, gasoline, chemicals, urine, and feces, may be identified during the secondary assessment.

HEAD/FACE/NECK

During the secondary assessment, a more complete neurologic assessment is completed. A Pediatric Coma Scale score or GCS score may be determined at this time. Observe for:

- Eye opening.
- Best motor response.
- Best verbal response.
- Inability to be consoled or comforted; unusual irritability.
- Activity level, as appropriate, for age or developmental level.
- Orientation to person, place, and time in older children, or the ability to recognize caregivers in preverbal and young children.

Inspect

- Lacerations, abrasions, ecchymosis, or edema.
- Petechiae, subconjunctival hemorrhage.
- Loose teeth or material in the mouth.
- Bony deformities or angulation.
- Symmetry of facial expressions.
- Jugular vein distention.

Palpate

- Anterior and posterior fontanelles in infants for fullness, bulging, or depression.
- Tracheal position.
- Bony depressions.

EYES/EARS/NOSE

Inspect

- Eye and eyelid position, ear position:
  - Color of sclera and conjunctiva. Evaluate for subconjunctival hemorrhage.
  - *Hyphema.*
  - Ptosis.
- Drainage or bleeding.
- Lacerations, abrasions, or edema.
- Ecchymosis or bruising:
  - Periorbital ecchymosis or *raccoon's eyes.*
  - Postarticular ecchymosis or *Battle's sign,* which is bleeding behind the ears.
- Eyeglasses or contact lenses.
- Pupils, including size, shape, equality, reactivity to light, and opacity.
- Extraocular eye movements:
  - Observe the child's ability to follow your finger in all six directions.
  - Observe the infant or toddler's tracking of an object in all six directions.

Palpate

- Periorbital tenderness or pain.
- Auricle tenderness or pain.
- Nasal tenderness or pain.

CHEST

Inspect

- Breathing rate, depth, work of breathing, use of accessory muscles, abdominal muscles, paradoxical chest wall movement.
- Symmetry of chest wall movements.
- Lacerations, abrasions, contusions, puncture wounds, impaled objects, ecchymosis, swelling, scars, or presence of central venous access devices.
- Scars from healed chest tube sites, central lines, surgical incisions, or penetrating wounds.

Auscultate

- Equality of breath sounds.
- Adventitious sounds such as wheezes, crackles, and friction rubs.
- Heart sounds for rate, rhythm, and adventitious sounds such as murmurs, gallops, and friction rub.

Palpate

- Chest wall tenderness.
- Crepitus.
- Subcutaneous emphysema.
- Bony deformities.

ABDOMEN

Inspect

- Use of abdominal muscles for breathing.
- Lacerations, abrasions, contusions, impaled objects, or ecchymosis (seat belt sign).
- Distention.
- Feeding tubes.
- Scars from healed surgical incisions or penetrating wounds.

Auscultate

- Bowel sounds in all quadrants.

Palpate

- All four quadrants for rigidity, tenderness, and guarding. In the infant or young child who is crying, evaluation for firmness or rigidity is more difficult. Palpating the abdomen on inspiration allows for palpation when the abdominal muscles are more relaxed.

PELVIS AND GENITALIA

Inspect

- Lacerations, abrasions, or edema.
- Drainage from the meatus or vagina.
- Scrotal bleeding or edema.
- Priapism.

Palpate

- Pelvic stability.
- Anal sphincter tone.
- Femoral pulses.

EXTREMITIES

Inspect

- Signs of congenital anomalies such as a club foot, length discrepancies, or *clubbing* of digits.
- Angulation, deformity, open wounds with evidence of protruding bone fragments, edema, ecchymosis, *purpura,* and *petechiae.*
- Color.
- Abnormal movement.
- Position.
- Scars or venous access devices.

Palpate

- Skin temperature.
- Symmetry and quality of distal pulses. Compare bilateral peripheral pulses for strength and equality. There may be neurovascular compromise in an injured extremity.
- Bony crepitus.
- Muscle strength and range of motion.
- Sensation.

INSPECT POSTERIOR SURFACES

Inspect

- Bleeding, abrasions, wounds, hematomas, or ecchymosis.
- Rashes, petechiae, edema, or purpura.
- Patterned injuries or injuries in various stages of healing.

Palpate

- Tenderness and deformity of the spine.
- *Costovertebral angle tenderness.*

History

The history is obtained from the caregiver of the infant or young child or from both the caregiver and older child or adolescent. The history is another important piece of the puzzle that assists the health care provider in analyzing assessment findings, formulating nursing diagnoses, and making a triage decision. The MIVT mnemonic (i.e., mechanism of injury, injuries sustained, vital signs, and treatment), can be used to elicit a history from prehospital providers. The CIAMPEDS mnemonic describes the components of the basic pediatric assessment:

C	Chief Complaint	Reason for the child's ED visit and duration of complaint (e.g., fever lasting for 2 days).
I	Immunizations	Evaluation of the child's current immunization status: • The completion of all scheduled immunizations for the child's age must be evaluated. The most current immunization recommendations are published by the American Academy of Pediatrics. • In Australia, the immunization guidelines are published yearly in the Australian Immunization Handbook, National Health and Research Council. • If the child has not received immunizations due to religious or cultural beliefs, document this information.
	Isolation	Evaluation of the child's exposure to communicable diseases (chickenpox, shingles, mumps, measles, whooping cough, tuberculosis): • A child with active disease or who is potentially infectious, based on a history of exposure and the disease incubation period, must be placed in respiratory isolation on arrival in the emergency department. • Immunosuppressed or compromised children can develop active disease even when previously immune. These children must also be protected from inadvertent exposure to viral and bacterial illnesses while in the emergency department and placed in *protective* or *reverse isolation.* • Other exposures that may be evaluated include exposures to meningitis (with or without evidence of purpura), pneumonia, scabies.
A	Allergies	Evaluation of the child's previous allergic or hypersensitivity reactions: • Document reactions to medications, foods, products (e.g., latex), and environmental allergens. The type of reaction must also be documented.
M	Medications	Evaluation of the child's current medication regimen including prescription and over-the-counter medications: • Dose administered. • Time of last dose. • Duration of medication use.

P	Past Medical History	A review of the child's health status, including prior illnesses, injuries, hospitalizations, surgeries, and chronic physical and psychiatric illnesses. Use of alcohol, tobacco, drugs or other substances of abuse must be evaluated, as appropriate:
		• The past medical history of the infant must include the prenatal and birth history:
		  ■ Complications during pregnancy or delivery.
		  ■ Number of days infant remained in hospital postbirth.
		  ■ Infant's birth weight.
		• The past medical history of the menarche female includes the date and description of last menstrual period.
		• The past medical history for sexually active patients may include:
		  ■ Type of birth control used.
		  ■ *Barrier protection.*
		  ■ Prior treatment for sexually transmitted diseases.
		  ■ Gravida (pregnancies) and para (births, miscarriages, abortions, living children).

	Parent's/Caregiver's Impression of the Child's Condition	Identification of the child's primary caregiver. Consider cultural differences that may affect the caregiver's impressions. Evaluation of the caregiver's concerns and observations of the child's condition.

E	Events Surrounding the Illness or Injury	Evaluation of the onset of the illness or circumstances and mechanism of injury:
		• Illness:
		   ■ Length of illness, including date and day of onset and sequence of symptoms.
		   ■ Exposure to others with similar symptoms.
		   ■ Treatment provided prior to ED visit.
		   ■ Examination by primary care provider.
		• Injury:
		   ■ Time and date injury occurred.
		   ■ M: Mechanism of injury, including the use of protective devices such as seat belts and helmets.
		   ■ I: Injuries suspected
		   ■ V: Vital signs in prehospital environment
		   ■ T: Treatment by prehospital providers
		   ■ Description of circumstances leading to injury.
		   ■ Witnessed or unwitnessed.

D	Diet	Assessment of the child's recent oral intake and changes in eating patterns related to the illness or injury: • Changes in eating patterns or fluid intake. • Time of last meal and last fluid intake. • Regular diet: Breast milk, type of formula, solid foods, diet for age, and developmental level, and cultural differences. • Special diet or diet restrictions (e.g., American Dietetic Association diet).
D	Diapers	Assessment of the child's urine and stool output: • Frequency of urination over last 24 hours; changes in frequency. • Time of last void. • Changes in odor or color of urine. • Last bowel movement; color and consistency of stool. • Change in frequency of bowel movements.
S	Symptoms Associated with the Illness or Injury	Identification of symptoms and progression of symptoms since the onset of the illness or injury event.

Additional history, including social and family histories, may also be needed.

Diagnostic Procedures

- The necessity of laboratory and radiographic studies is determined by the child's clinical presentation, pattern of injury, history, and specific institution protocols.

- Because of the infant and toddler's risk of hypoglycemia with serious or critical illness or injury, obtain a whole blood glucose (bedside glucose test) or serum glucose.

- The need for continuous physiologic monitoring is determined by the child's condition, risk for deterioration, or need to evaluate physiologic responses to treatment. A combination of cardiac, pulse oximetry, and noninvasive blood pressure monitoring may be indicated. When available, invasive blood pressure and end-tidal CO_2 monitoring are additional valuable adjuncts for the care of the critically ill or injured child.

NURSING DIAGNOSES, INTERVENTIONS, AND EXPECTED OUTCOMES

The initial assessment provides information to evaluate the patient's responses to the illness or injury event. The specific nursing diagnoses are determined by the analysis of these assessment data and observations. Each nursing diagnosis is derived through diagnostic reasoning. Priorities of intervention are then determined. Each diagnosis represents an actual health problem or one that may develop because of the presence of risk factors.[5] The problem may be corrected by the nurse or require a collaborative intervention with other health care professionals. The identification of expected outcomes corresponds to the interventions and goals formulated to correct the health problem described by the nursing diagnosis.[6]

In each chapter, the nursing diagnoses are listed in two ways. After each intervention, the applicable nursing diagnosis will be listed in parentheses. The correlation of the nursing diagnoses, interventions, and expected outcomes is presented in a table format. The nursing diagnoses, interventions, and expected outcomes for common problems that may be identified during the primary or secondary assessments or as related to the caregiver or family are listed in this table.

Nursing Diagnoses, Interventions, and Expected Outcomes

NURSING DIAGNOSIS	INTERVENTIONS	EXPECTED OUTCOMES
Airway clearance, ineffective, related to: • Edema of the airway, vocal cords, epiglottis, and upper airway • Irritation of the respiratory tract • Laryngeal spasm • Altered level of consciousness secondary to hypoxia • Inability to remove oropharyngeal secretions • Fatigue • Pain	• Position supine or maintain position of comfort • Open and clear the airway • Insert airway adjunct	The child will maintain a patent airway, as evidenced by: • Regular rate, depth, and pattern of breathing • Symmetric chest expansion • Effective cough and gag reflex • Absence of signs and symptoms of airway obstruction: Stridor, dyspnea, and hoarse voice • Clear sputum of normal amount without abnormal color or odor • Absence of signs and symptoms of retained secretions: Fever, tachycardia, and tachypnea

Aspiration, risk of, related to:
• Altered level of consciousness
• Impaired cough or gag reflex secondary to hypoxia
• Structural defect to head, face, or neck
• Secretions and debris in airway
	• Position supine
	• Open and clear the airway
	• Consider endotracheal intubation
	• Insert a gastric tube
	• Give nothing by mouth
		The child will not experience aspiration, as evidenced by:
		• Patent airway
		• Clear and equal breath sounds
		• Regular rate, depth, and pattern of breathing
		• ABG values within normal limits:
		  ■ PaO_2 80 to 100 mm Hg (10.0 to 13.3 KPa)
		  ■ SaO_2 >95%
		  ■ $PaCO_2$ 35 to 45 mm Hg (4.7 to 6.0 KPa)
		  ■ pH between 7.35 and 7.45
		• Chest radiograph without abnormality
		• Ability to handle secretions independently

NURSING DIAGNOSIS	INTERVENTIONS	EXPECTED OUTCOMES

Breathing pattern, ineffective, related to:
• Pain
• Musculoskeletal impairment
• Unstable chest wall segment
• Lung collapse
• Respiratory infection
• Neurologic impairment
	• Position supine or maintain a position of comfort
	• Open and clear the airway
	• Administer oxygen
	• Assist ventilation, if needed
	• Consider endotracheal intubation
	• Initiate cardiopulmonary resuscitation, if needed
		The child will have an effective breathing pattern, as evidenced by:
		• Regular rate, depth, and pattern of breathing
		• Clear and equal breath sounds
		• Absence of use of accessory muscles or nasal flaring
		• Symmetric chest expansion
		• ABG values within normal limits:
		  ■ PaO_2 80 to 100 mm Hg (10.0 to 13.3 KPa)
		  ■ SaO_2 >95%
		  ■ $PaCO_2$ 35 to 45 mm Hg (4.7 to 6.0 KPa)
		  ■ pH between 7.35 and 7.45
		• Absence of stridor, dyspnea, and cyanosis
		• Trachea midline
		• Chest radiograph without abnormality

Gas exchange, impaired, related to:
• Ineffective breathing pattern
• Ineffective airway clearance
• Aspiration
• Shock
• Decreased ventilatory drive from head injury
• Chest injury
	• Administer oxygen
	• Assist ventilation, if needed
	• Consider endotracheal intubation
	• Investigate causes of altered consciousness
	• Decompress tension pneumothorax
		The child will maintain adequate gas exchange, as evidenced by:
		• Oxygen saturation >95% by pulse oximetry
		• ABG values within normal limits:
		  ■ PaO_2 80 to 100 mm Hg (10.0 to 13.3 KPa)
		  ■ SaO_2 >95%
		  ■ $PaCO_2$ 35 to 45 mm Hg (4.7 to 6.0 KPa)
		  ■ pH between 7.35 and 7.45
		• Skin normal color, warm, and dry
		• Improved level of consciousness
		• Regular rate, depth, and pattern of breathing
		• Symmetric chest expansion
		• Clear and equal breath sounds

Fluid volume deficit related to: • Hemorrhage • Fluid shifts • Alteration in capillary permeability	• Control bleeding • Obtain vascular access and initiate fluid therapy • Initiate intraosseous access, if needed • Insert indwelling urinary catheter • Monitor intake and output	The child will have an effective circulating volume, as evidenced by: • Stable vital signs appropriate for age • Urine output of 1 to 2 ml/kg/hour • Urine specific gravity within normal limits • Strong, palpable peripheral and central pulses • Improved level of consciousness • Skin normal color, warm, and dry • Hematocrit of 30 ml/dl or hemoglobin of 12 to 14 gm/dl or greater • External hemorrhage is controlled • Moist mucous membranes
Cardiac output, decreased, related to: • Decreased venous return secondary to acute blood loss, massive peripheral vaso-dilation, or myocardial compromise • Dysrhythmia	• Control bleeding • Obtain vascular access and initiate fluid therapy • Administer blood • Initiate cardiopulmonary resuscitation, if needed • Initiate drug therapy • Perform defibrillation or synchronized cardioversion, if needed	The child will maintain adequate circulatory function, as evidenced by: • Strong, palpable peripheral and central pulses • Adequate blood pressure for age • Pulse rate appropriate for age • Absence of dysrythmias • Skin normal color, warm, and dry • Improved level of consciousness • Urine output of 1 to 2 ml/kg/hour

NURSING DIAGNOSIS	INTERVENTIONS	EXPECTED OUTCOMES
Tissue perfusion, altered cerebral, peripheral, renal, and visceral, related to: • Decreased perfusion related to hypovolemia, hypoxia, or hypercarbia • Altered cerebral perfusion related to cerebral edema, swelling, or primary injury	• Control bleeding • Obtain vascular access and initiate fluid therapy • Administer blood • Investigate causes of altered consciousness • Initiate pharmacologic therapy for altered consciousness • Remove jewelry or constricting clothing	The child will maintain adequate tissue perfusion, as evidenced by: • Strong, palpable peripheral and central pulses • Adequate blood pressure for age • Appropriate apical pulse for age • Skin normal color, warm, and dry • Improved level of consciousness • Urine output of 1 to 2 ml/kg/hour
Injury, risk of, related to: • Instability of vertebral column fracture • Altered level of consciousness • Potential for spinal column injury • Inadequate or absent spinal precautions • Seizures • Child maltreatment	• Manually stabilize the cervical spine • Maintain spine stabilization or immobilization • Position the patient • Evaluate for indicators of child maltreatment	The child will be free from injury, as evidenced by: • Absence of iatrogenic extension of injury • Minimization of movement of neck by proper alignment and immobilization of the spinal column • Child's verbalization and demonstration of an understanding of need to avoid movement of neck • Absence of increase in extent of original injury • Management and control of the child's seizure activity
Hypothermia related to: • Rapid infusion of intravenous fluids • Decreased tissue perfusion • Exposure	• Initiate warming measures	The child will maintain a normal core body temperature, as evidenced by: • Core temperature measurement of 36 to 37.5°C (96.8 to 99.5°F) • Absence of shivering, cool skin, pallor • Skin normal color, warm, and dry
Hyperthermia related to: • Infectious process • Dehydration • Ineffective temperature regulation	• Initiate cooling measures to decrease temperature • Initiate fluids • Evaluate child for source of infection	The child will maintain a normal core body temperature, as evidenced by: • Core temperature measurement of 36 to 37.5°C (96.8 to 99.5°F) • Skin normal color, warm, and dry
Pain related to: • Soft tissue injury and edema • Fractures • Pleural irritation • Stimulation of nerve fibers • Invasive procedures	• Administer pain medications • Administer medications to facilitate intubation • Initiate comfort measures • Stabilize impaled objects • Distract child with music, toys	The child will experience relief of pain, as evidenced by: • Diminishing or absent level of pain, indicated by patient's self-report using an objective measurement tool in the verbal child • Absence of physiologic indicators of pain: Tachycardia, tachypnea, pallor, diaphoretic skin, and increasing blood pressure • Absence of nonverbal cues of pain: Crying, grimacing, inability to assume position of comfort, and guarding • Ability to cooperate with care, as appropriate

NURSING DIAGNOSIS	INTERVENTIONS	EXPECTED OUTCOMES
Infection, risk of, related to: • Impaired skin integrity • Contamination of wound from initial injury or instrumentation • Interruption in perfusion • Failure to obtain immunizations	• Stabilize impaled objects • Apply sterile dressings • Administer antibiotics • Obtain immunization status • Administer vaccines • Initiate isolation measures	The child will be free from infection, as evidenced by: • Core temperature measurement of 36 to 37.5°C (96.8 to 99.5°F) • Absence of systemic signs of infection: Fever, tachypnea, tachycardia • Wounds free from redness, swelling, purulent drainage, or odor • Urine output of 1 to 2 ml/kg/hour • Negative blood cultures • White blood cell count and differential within normal limits • Improved level of consciousness
Anxiety and fear (child and caregiver) related to: • Unfamiliar environment • Unpredictable nature of condition • Invasive procedures • Possible disfigurement or scarring • Knowledge deficit	• Facilitate family presence • Assess the needs of the family • Keep family informed • Provide psychosocial support • Administer medications to facilitate intubation	The child and caregiver will experience decreasing anxiety and fear, as evidenced by: • Orientation to surroundings • Ability to describe reasons for equipment and procedures used in treatment • Ability to verbalize concerns and ask questions of health care team • Use of effective coping skills • Vital signs returning to within normal limits

PLANNING AND IMPLEMENTATION

Interventions for life-threatening conditions are performed as soon as the condition is identified. Those interventions are listed with each component of the primary assessment. Additional interventions may be identified during or following the secondary assessment. These interventions may include the following:

- Prepare for admission or transfer to a pediatric tertiary care center, as indicated by the clinical condition.

- Obtain vascular access for administration of maintenance fluids or medication. (Nursing diagnoses: Fluid volume deficit; infection).

- Administer maintenance fluids. (Nursing diagnosis: Fluid volume deficit).

  - The administration of maintenance intravenous fluids, including the type of fluid and rate, is tailored to the specific needs of the child. Once circulating volume is restored, maintenance intravenous fluids are administered to accommodate for insensible losses and ongoing fluid needs. The glucose, sodium, and potassium needs of the patient, as well as ongoing losses, will be used to determine the appropriate fluid. The solution is often 5% dextrose/0.2% or 0.45% normal saline. In Australia, 4% dextrose in 1/4 or 1/5 normal saline is used.

- Based on the patient's weight, fluid requirements per hour can be calculated using the following formula[7,8]:

    4 ml/kg/hour for the first 10 kg of body weight (100 ml/kg/24 hours)

    +2 ml/kg/hour for the second 10 kg of body weight (50 ml/kg/24 hours)

    +1 ml/kg/hour for each additional kg of body weight over 20 kg (20 ml/kg/24 hours).

    Ex: The hourly maintenance fluid need for a 15-kg child would be:

    $$4 \text{ ml} \times 10 \text{ kg} = 40 \text{ ml/hour}$$
    $$\underline{+2 \text{ ml} \times\ 5 \text{ kg} = 10 \text{ ml/hour}}$$
    $$15 \text{ kg} = 50 \text{ ml/hour}$$

    Ex: The hourly maintenance fluid need for a 25-kg child would be:

    $$4 \text{ ml} \times 10 \text{ kg} = 40 \text{ ml/hour}$$
    $$+2 \text{ ml} \times 10 \text{ kg} = 20 \text{ ml/hour}$$
    $$\underline{+1 \text{ ml} \times\ 5 \text{ kg} =\ 5 \text{ ml/hour}}$$
    $$25 \text{ kg} = 65 \text{ ml/hour}$$

- In some circumstances, maintenance fluids may be restricted (i.e., patients with increased intracranial pressure, pulmonary contusion). Restricted rates are calculated by the following method:

    ♦ Maintenance volume/hour × desired degree of restriction.[8]

    ♦ For a 15-kg patient who is being placed on two thirds maintenance, the hourly rate is: 50 ml/hour (maintenance) × 2/3 (restricted) = 33 ml/hour.

- Insert a gastric tube to decompress the stomach as indicated. (Nursing diagnosis: Aspiration). Consult a chart or length-based resuscitation tape to ascertain the correct tube size. See Appendix L for a listing of tube sizes based on age.

- Insert an indwelling urinary catheter, as indicated by condition, unless urethral injury is suspected. Consult a chart or length-based resuscitation tape to ascertain the correct catheter size. (Nursing diagnosis: Fluid volume deficit). See Appendix L for a listing of tube sizes based on age.

    - Normal hourly urine output varies with the size and age of the child. (Nursing diagnosis: Fluid volume deficit):

        ♦ Infant   2 ml/kg/hour.

        ♦ Child   1 to 2 ml/kg/hour.

        ♦ Adolescent   0.5 to 1 ml/kg/hour.

- Determine the need to keep the child without food or drink. (Nursing diagnosis: Aspiration).

- Monitor the child's intake and output, as indicated by condition. (Nursing diagnosis: Fluid volume deficit).

- Administer medications (e.g., antibiotics, vaccines, pain medications) as prescribed. (Nursing diagnoses: Infection; pain).

- Initiate appropriate isolation measures. (Nursing diagnosis: Infection).

- Facilitate family presence in the treatment area, as guided by the assessment of family needs. (Nursing diagnosis: Anxiety/fear):

    - Provide timely and clear explanations of procedures and treatment plan.

    - Assign a health care professional to provide ongoing explanations and support.

- Provide psychosocial support to help the child cope with fear of treatment procedures. (Nursing diagnosis: Anxiety/fear).

- Evaluate for indicators of child maltreatment (see Chapter 9, "Child Maltreatment"). (Nursing diagnosis: Injury).

EVALUATION AND ONGOING ASSESSMENT

The evaluation phase of the nursing process occurs when the nurse evaluates the patient's responses to the interventions and the continued effects of the illness or injury event. The achievement of expected outcomes is evaluated, and the treatment or intervention plan is adjusted as needed to attain unmet outcomes. If the child's condition deteriorates, the primary assessment must be repeated. General evaluation of the patient's progress includes ongoing assessment of the following:

- Airway patency.

- Breathing effectiveness.

- Level of consciousness, activity level.

- Skin temperature and color, color of mucous membranes.

- Pulse rate and quality.

- Intake and output.

- Vital signs.

- Pain.

- Body systems, as appropriate, based on nursing diagnoses and desired outcomes.

PEDIATRIC TRIAGE

Triage, which means to pick, sort, or choose, is a process used to set priorities and determine the urgency of need for emergency care. The objectives of a triage system are to evaluate all incoming patients, to classify patients in terms of severity of illness (the triage decision), and to initiate appropriate interventions at the patient's entry point into the emergency department.[7-10] The triage or acuity decision is based on the initial assessment and history. The four components of pediatric triage include:

- The Pediatric Assessment Triangle which is an "across-the-room assessment" or an "as you approach the child assessment."

- Initial assessment.

- History.

- Triage or acuity decision.

Pediatric Assessment Triangle

The Pediatric Assessment Triangle is a method to rapidly and accurately complete an initial or "across-the-room" assessment. This method facilitates rapid determination of the severity of the child's illness or injury, regardless of diagnosis. It also identifies a general category of the physiologic problem.

The Triangle encompasses the overall appearance of the child, work of breathing, and circulation to the skin (see Figure 6). It is done by direct observation, before touching the child and starting the primary assessment. The child should be observed for the following:

- Appearance.
    - Tone.
    - Interactibility.
    - Consolability.
    - Look or gaze.
    - Speech or cry.
- Breathing.
    - Nasal flaring.
    - Retractions.
    - Abnormal airway sounds.
    - Position of comfort.
    - Altered respiratory rate.
- Circulation to skin.
    - Pallor.
    - *Mottling*.
    - Cyanosis.

The visual or observational assessment continues during the nurse's initial interaction with the patient and caregiver.

Figure 6
PEDIATRIC ASSESSMENT TRIANGLE

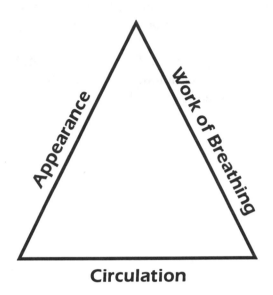

Initial Assessment in Triage

The triage initial assessment starts with a rapid evaluation of the primary assessment, as previously discussed in this chapter. If the child does not have a patent airway, is not breathing adequately, does not have adequate perfusion, or has decreased responsiveness or is unresponsive, the remainder of the triage assessment is interrupted and appropriate interventions are initiated. If the child is not compromised, the initial assessment is continued.

Following the primary assessment, the secondary assessment is completed, as discussed earlier in this chapter. In some circumstances, modification of the secondary assessment may be necessary in the triage area because of limitations in space, privacy, or time. However, adequate assessment data must be obtained to make an accurate triage decision (e.g., vital signs, history, focused head-to-toe assessment). Any components of the secondary assessment not completed during the triage process may be completed when the patient is placed in the treatment area.

Triage History

Obtaining the history is part of the secondary assessment. The triage or acuity history follows the CIAMPEDS format. Information may be obtained from a variety or sources, including prehospital providers, the caregiver, and the child. The history yields important information that assists the nurse in making the triage decision. Table 8 provides sample questions to elicit information delineated by the CIAMPEDS mnemonic.

Page 84   CHAPTER 4

Table 8

TRIAGE HISTORY	
Format	**Questions**
(C) Chief Complaint	Why was the child brought to the emergency department? What is the primary problem or concern and duration of complaint?
(I) Immunizations	Are they up to date? When were they last given?
Isolation	Has the child recently been exposed to any communicable diseases?
(A) Allergies	Does the child have any known allergies? Is the child allergic to any medications? What was the child's reaction to the medication?
(M) Medications	Is the child taking any prescription drugs or over-the-counter drugs (e.g., acetaminophen)? When was the last dose administered and how much was given? Is the child on immunosuppressive medications?
(P) Past Medical History	Does the child have a history of any significant illness, injury, or hospitalization? Does the child have a known chronic illness?
Parents Impression of Child's Condition	What is different about the child's condition that concerns the caregiver?
(E) Events Surrounding the Illness or Injury	How long has the child been ill? Was the onset rapid or slow? Has anyone else in the family been ill? If the emergency visit is for an injury, when did the injury occur, was it witnessed, and what happened?
(D) Diet	How much has the child been eating and drinking? When was the last time the child ate or drank?
Diapers	When was the child's last void? How much was it? When was the child's last bowel movement? What did it look like and how large was the stool?
(S) Symptoms Associated with the Illness or Injury	What other symptoms are present? When did the symptoms begin? Has the condition gotten better or worse?

Triage or Acuity Decision

Once the initial assessment is completed, the triage decision is made. The triage or acuity decision is derived from the analysis of assessment data including history and physical findings. The patient is classified based on the severity of illness. Although there are several types of categorization systems in the United States, the most common system categorizes patients using the following groups and criteria[10,11]:

EMERGENT   Pediatric patients with life- or limb-threatening conditions who require resuscitation or immediate intervention to avoid loss of life or permanent disability. Additionally, patients with potentially life- or limb-threatening illness, injury, or psychologic crisis, who are at risk for deterioration and require immediate intervention, are also classified as emergent (e.g., cardiopulmonary arrest, multisystem injury, moderate-to-severe respiratory distress, compensated or decompensated shock, suicide attempt, extremity injury with neurovascular compromise, altered neurologic status).

URGENT   Pediatric patients with illness, injury, or mental health conditions requiring prompt but not immediate care. For these patients, treatment delays of up to 2 hours will not compromise life or limb. These patients must be periodically reassessed to assure there has not been any deterioration in condition (e.g., mild wheezes with mild-to-no respiratory distress, mild-to-moderate dehydration, suspected fracture of the forearm).

NONURGENT   Pediatric patients with minor, stable illness or injury. These patients may safely wait more than 2 hours without an increased risk of morbidity or mortality (e.g., ear discomfort, minor wounds, isolated soft tissue injury, sore throat).

In Australia and Canada, a 5-category triage system is used. Levels 1 and 2 equate to the emergent category, levels 3 and 4 equate to the urgent category, and level 5 equates to the nonurgent category.

Occasionally, the triage nurse may feel uncomfortable about a patient's clinical appearance or subtle assessment findings. In general, it is preferable to place the potentially ill or injured patient in a higher triage category to prevent the possibility of delays in treatment. If, during any part of the triage assessment, the nurse determines that the child has an emergent condition, the triage process is interrupted and appropriate interventions are initiated. Pediatric patients waiting in the emergency department must be monitored frequently. Serial, timely reassessment is essential to identify the deterioration of the urgent or nonurgent patient.

The triage decision also includes prioritizing among patients based on a variety of factors (i.e., acuity category, severity of alteration in primary assessment findings, and department activity and resources). The goal of triage is to expeditiously evaluate and initiate treatment for all patients. Although the assessment and priority of interventions for the individual patient are based on alterations in airway, breathing, circulation, and disability, prioritizing among patients may be based on the severity of the alteration and number of systems involved. For example, an emergent patient with signs of decompensated shock may be treated before an emergent patient with moderate-to-severe respiratory distress. Your clinical decision is based on the patient who is at greatest risk. Table 9 contains a list of signs, symptoms, pediatric behaviors, or history that may signal a serious illness or injury.

Table 9

TRIAGE RED FLAGS[9,12]		
• Apnea • Choking • Drooling • Stridor • Grunting • Sternal retractions • Irregular respiratory patterns • Absence of breath sounds • Cyanosis	• Diaphoresis • Tachycardia • Hypotension • Bradycardia • Petechia • Purpura • Hypothermia • Fever in an infant younger than 3 months of age >38°C (100.4°F), or temperature >40 to 40.6°C (104 to 105°F) at any age	• Pain • Decreased tearing • Sunken or bulging fontanelles • History of a chronic illness • Child who acts as a surrogate parent • History of a family crisis • Signs and symptoms of maltreatment • Return ED visit within 24 hours

SUMMARY

The initial assessment of ill or injured pediatric patients involves a systematic process that recognizes life-threatening conditions, identifies injuries, and determines priorities of care. Recognition of life-threatening conditions requires knowledge of normal growth and development as well as the anatomic and physiologic characteristics unique to infants, children, and adolescents. The initial assessment, the triage process, and the prioritization of care are fundamental pieces of the pediatric emergency care puzzle.

REFERENCES

1. Emergency Nurses Association. *Emergency Nursing Core Curriculum*. 4th ed. Philadelphia, Pa: WB Saunders; 1994.

2. Nypaver M, Treloar DF. Neutral cervical spine positioning in children. *Ann Emerg Med*. 1994;23:208-211.

3. Derrico D. Comparison of blood pressure measurement methods in critically ill children. *Dimen Crit Care Nurs*. 1993;12:31-39.

4. Emergency Nurses Association. *Presenting the Option for Family Presence*. Park Ridge, Ill: Author; 1995.

5. North American Nursing Diagnosis Association. *Nursing Diagnoses: Definitions and Classifications, 1995-1996*. Philadelphia, Pa: Author; 1996.

6. Emergency Nurses Association. *Emergency Nurses Guide to Nursing Diagnosis*. Park Ridge, Ill: Author; 1992.

7. Weigle CG, Yaster M. Electrolyte, metabolic and endocrine disorders. In: Nichols DG, Yaster M, Lappe DG, Haller JA, eds. *Golden Hour – The Handbook for Advanced Pediatric Life Support*. 2nd ed. St. Louis, Mo: Mosby-Year Book; 1996:197-216.

8. Aoki BY, McCloskey K. Renal metabolic endocrine disorder. In: Aoki BY, McCloskey K, eds. *Evaluation, Stabilization, and Transport of the Critically Ill Child*. St. Louis, Mo: Mosby-Year Book Inc; 1992:133-224.

9. Soud TE, Andry C. Pediatric triage. In: Soud TE, Rogers JS, eds. *Manual of Pediatric Emergency Nursing*. St. Louis, Mo: Mosby-Year Book; 1998:89-106.

10. Murphy KA. Introduction to pediatric triage. In: Murphy KA, ed. *Pediatric Triage Guidelines*. St. Louis, Mo: Mosby-Year Book; 1997:2-7.

11. Emergency Nurses Association. *Triage: Meeting the Challenge*. Park Ridge, Ill: Author; 1992.

12. Fredrickson J. Triage. In: Kelley SJ, ed. *Pediatric Emergency Nursing*. 2nd ed. Norwalk, Conn: Appleton & Lange; 1994:11-16.

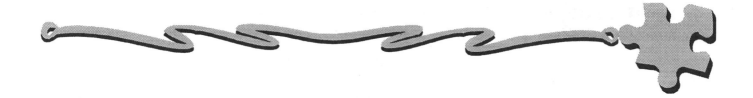

CHAPTER 5

Respiratory Distress and Failure

OBJECTIVES

On completion of this lecture, the learner should be able to:

+ Identify the anatomic and physiologic characteristics of the respiratory system as a basis for the signs and symptoms of respiratory distress or failure.

+ Identify the most frequent causes of respiratory distress and failure in children.

+ Identify the appropriate nursing diagnoses and expected outcomes based on the assessment findings.

+ Delineate the specific interventions needed to manage the child with respiratory distress or failure.

+ Evaluate the effectiveness of nursing interventions related to patient outcomes.

+ Identify health promotion strategies related to respiratory distress and failure.

INTRODUCTION

Respiratory disorders are a major cause of morbidity and mortality in the pediatric population.[1] Children are unique in their responses to respiratory problems because of their anatomic, physiologic, and developmental characteristics. Respiratory compromise in children can be caused by upper and lower respiratory tract infections, sedative medications, central nervous system disorders, musculoskeletal deformities, or congenital anomalies and disorders.

Respiratory distress is part of a continuum that, if left untreated, results in respiratory failure. Respiratory failure is the most common pathway to cardiopulmonary arrest in children. The outcomes for children following cardiopulmonary arrest are poor; thus, early recognition and treatment of the child in respiratory distress are critical.[2]

ANATOMIC, PHYSIOLOGIC, AND DEVELOPMENTAL CHARACTERISTICS AS A BASIS FOR SIGNS AND SYMPTOMS

The respiratory center is located in the brain stem and controls the rate of ventilation by responding to changes in arterial carbon dioxide ($PaCO_2$) and hydrogen ion concentrations (H^+). An excess of either substance causes a direct excitatory effect on the respiratory center, resulting in an increased rate of ventilation.

$$\uparrow PaCO_2 \text{ or } \uparrow H^+ = \uparrow \text{Respiratory Rate}$$

Oxygen (O_2) does not have a significant effect on the respiratory center but instead acts on chemical receptors or chemoreceptors located in the carotid and aortic bodies. Chemoreceptors indirectly control the rate of ventilation by sending signals to the respiratory center through afferent nerves. Although chemoreceptors are sensitive to $PaCO_2$ and H^+ levels, they are most strongly stimulated when arterial PaO_2 falls below 60 mm Hg.[3]

$$\downarrow PaO_2 = \uparrow \text{Respiratory Rate (early sign) and } \downarrow \text{Respiratory Rate (late sign)}$$

In the infant, the central nervous system and peripheral nerves are not well developed, and there are fewer peripheral chemoreceptors. Although healthy infants and children will compensate for hypercarbia, hypoxia, and acidosis by hyperventilating, younger infants are less able to compensate for these stressors. Premature infants, rather than responding with hyperventilation, may initially respond with tachypnea followed by bradypnea and apnea.[4]

The child's ventilatory system is in a constant state of growth and development until approximately 7 to 8 years of age, when it is similar to that of the adult. Table 10 summarizes key anatomic characteristics and their clinical significance to respiratory distress and failure.

DEFINITIONS OF RESPIRATORY DISTRESS AND FAILURE

Respiratory distress is a clinical state characterized by increased work of breathing. *Respiratory failure* is a clinical diagnosis often characterized by inadequate elimination of carbon dioxide or inadequate oxygenation of the blood.[3] Therefore, respiratory distress and failure represent the two ends of a continuum of ventilatory dysfunction. **The clinical manifestations of progression on this continuum can be subtle and are often not recognized early.**

Respiratory failure is frequently described in the physiologic terms of the concentration of partial pressure of oxygen (PaO_2) or carbon dioxide ($PaCO_2$). Unfortunately, blood gas values alone may be easily subject to misinterpretation and are not always available when intervention is required. Respiratory failure occurs when the child can no longer compensate to maintain adequate gas exchange. Fatigue from excess work of breathing is often a precipitating factor. **Work of breathing and an evaluation of ventilatory effectiveness may be more helpful to determining the child's potential for respiratory failure than blood gas results alone. Ventilatory assistance must never be delayed while blood gas results are awaited because rapid deterioration and respiratory arrest may occur.**

Table 10

KEY ANATOMIC CHARACTERISTICS	
CHARACTERISTICS	**CLINICAL SIGNIFICANCE**
Nares have little supporting cartilage.	Nasal flaring is an early sign of distress.
Infants younger than 4 months of age are obligate nasal breathers.	Nasopharyngeal secretions or nasogastric tubes can cause airway obstruction.
Head is large in proportion to body with weak supporting musculature and occipital prominence.	Flexion of airway occurs when child is supine; head bobbing occurs when he or she is distressed.
Tongue is large in proportion to oropharynx.	Tongue can easily occlude airway when supine.
Epiglottis is U-shaped, higher, and more anterior in the airway.	Epiglottis is more prone to infection and trauma.
Larynx is positioned more anteriorly and cephalad.	Position of larynx increases risk for aspiration.
Cricoid cartilage is narrowest part of the airway, and the trachea is funnel shaped.	Provides an anatomic cuff for endotracheal tubes and a frequent site of foreign-body obstruction.
Airway diameter is proportional to child's size.[5] The infant's tracheal diameter approximates the diameter of the little finger.	Airway obstruction can quickly develop in infants and small children. Small amount of edema or secretions can markedly increase airway resistance and result in partial or complete airway obstruction.
Tracheal length is proportional to the child's size. The length for an infant is approximately 7 cm.	Correct depth of endotracheal tube insertion varies with size of child. Right mainstem intubation occurs when endotracheal tube is inserted beyond tracheal length.
Tracheal and bronchial cartilaginous support rings are C shaped rather than O shaped.	Allows airway collapse that can be exacerbated during illness or when the neck is hyperextended or flexed.
Alveoli number approximately 24 million, compared to 300 million in adults.[6] Alveoli have less elastic recoil and less supportive elastic tissue.	Normal respiratory rate is dependent on child's age; a child requires faster respiratory rates for normal function. Respiratory rate increases with distress. Alveoli are more prone to collapse at the end of expiration.
Lung (tidal) volume is approximately 10 ml/kg (e.g., 100 ml in a 10-kg child) compared to that in the adult, which is 500 ml.	Results in low residual capacity and oxygen reserve. Variation in tidal volume must be considered when bag-valve-mask ventilation is performed to avoid overinflation or underinflation.
Metabolic rate is twice that of adults with twice the oxygen consumption.	Hypoxia occurs more rapidly when the child is in respiratory distress. Other factors that increase metabolic rate (e.g., fever) contribute to increased respiratory demands.
Rib orientation is more horizontal than vertical.	Chest diameter is maximally expanded at baseline and cannot be increased with distress (barrel chested).
Ribs are cartilaginous and intercostal muscles are immature.	Allows chest wall collapse rather than expansion during distress causing retractions.
Chest wall is thin; thorax is small with organs in close proximity.	Allows transmitted breath sounds. Breath sounds from one area are heard in other areas of the chest and not easily differentiated.
Diaphragm is the major muscle of breathing.	Ventilation is directly affected when diaphragmatic excursion is impeded by pressure from above, such as with the hyperexpansion seen in asthma, or from below, as with abdominal distension from gastric insufflation. Abdominal breathing is common.
Hemoglobin concentrations are approximately 75% that of the adult, or 10.5 to 12 gm/100 ml.[7]	Cyanosis develops when 5 gm of hemoglobin are desaturated or when as much as 50% of the child's blood is deoxygenated. Therefore, cyanosis is a late sign of distress.

CAUSES OF RESPIRATORY DISTRESS AND FAILURE

In the child, the most common causes of respiratory distress and failure are upper or lower airway obstructive disorders. Other causes of respiratory failure include central nervous system depression, musculoskeletal disorders, and thoracic disorders (see Table 11). It is not always necessary to identify the cause of the distress immediately. It is more important to recognize that respiratory distress exists and to initiate the proper interventions to prevent the deterioration to respiratory failure or arrest.

NURSING CARE OF THE CHILD WITH RESPIRATORY DISTRESS OR FAILURE

The child who is in respiratory distress or failure requires simultaneous assessment and the initiation of critical interventions. Refer to Chapter 4, "Initial Assessment and Triage," for a review of a comprehensive primary and secondary assessment. Additional or specific history data important to the evaluation of respiratory distress are listed below. Assessment findings that may indicate respiratory distress or failure are listed in the signs and symptoms section.

Assessment

ADDITIONAL HISTORY

- Time of onset.

- Characteristic of onset (rapid or gradual).

- Previous episodes of respiratory distress.

SIGNS AND SYMPTOMS

- Altered level of consciousness. Any alteration in the level of consciousness is considered a result of cerebral hypoxia until proven otherwise.

    - Inability to recognize caregivers.

    - Decreased level of response to environment.

    - Restlessness.

    - Anxiety.

    - Confusion.

    - Inability to be consoled.

Table 11

CAUSES OF RESPIRATORY DISTRESS AND FAILURE	
SYSTEMS	**EXAMPLES**
Central nervous system depression: • Immaturity • Infection • Intoxication • Anoxia or increased intracranial pressure	• Apnea of prematurity • Sepsis • Meningitis • Shock • Electrolyte imbalances • Sedatives • Narcotics • Abusive substances • Head trauma • Near-drowning • Reye's syndrome • Encephalopathies
Musculoskeletal disorders: • Neuromuscular • Skeletal	• Muscular dystrophies • Guillain-Barré syndrome • Poliomyelitis • Scoliosis/kyphosis • Severe pectus excavatum • Congenital thoracic dystrophy
Thoracoabdominal disorders	• Dysfunctional diaphragm • Diaphragmatic hernia • Severe constipation • Peritoneal dialysis • Gastric insufflation • Hepatomegaly • Ascites
Respiratory tract disorders: • Upper airway obstruction • Lower airway obstruction	• Croup • Retropharyngeal abscess • Epiglottitis • Foreign body • Bacterial tracheitis • Subglottic stenosis • Tracheomalacia • Smoke inhalation • Trauma • Vascular rings • Asthma • Bronchiolitis • Pneumonia • Pulmonary contusion • Pneumothorax/hemothorax • Pleural effusion • Acute respiratory distress syndrome • Pulmonary edema • Atelectasis • Aspiration • Bronchomalacia • Smoke inhalation • Foreign body • Trauma

- Increased work of breathing.

  - Nasal flaring.

  - Retractions (see Figure 7).

  - Head bobbing.

  - Grunting. Created by premature closure of the glottis in an attempt to increase the physiologic positive end expiratory pressure. It is a compensatory mechanism to relieve collapsing alveoli.

- Tripod position. Leaning forward while sitting up allows the tongue to remain forward and open the airway.

- Paradoxical respirations. Often called "seesaw" breathing and represents increased dependence on diaphragm to breathe.

- Pallor.

- Cyanosis. Late sign; represents significant hypoxia.

- Unusual drooling. Inability to swallow may indicate pharyngeal obstruction.

- Decreased gag reflex. May be from decreased level of consciousness or muscle tone.

- Altered respiratory rate.

  - Tachypnea.

  - Bradypnea or a sudden decrease in respiratory rate. Late sign; represents fatigue and impending arrest.

  - Apnea. Apnea is usually considered pauses in breathing of more than 15 to 20 seconds. Periodic breathing which occurs in neonates, is irregular breathing with pauses of less than 15 seconds.

- Altered heart rate.

  - Tachycardia.

  - Bradycardia. Late sign; represents impending arrest.

- Snoring. Represents partial obstruction of nasopharyngeal space.

- Stridor. Inspiratory sound representing partial obstruction or collapse of the trachea.

- Adventitious breath sounds. Wheezing and crackles are common in reactive airway disease, asthma, bronchiolitis, pneumonia, and pulmonary edema.

- Decreased, absent, or unequal breath sounds. Physical examination findings may vary over time because of secretions, bronchoconstriction, fluid shifts, or airway collapse.

Figure 7
LOCATION OF RETRACTIONS

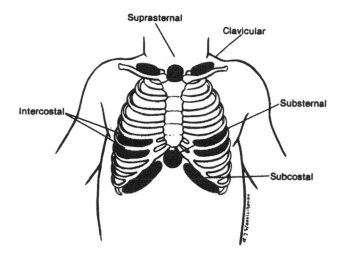

From Wong DL. The child with disturbance of oxygen and carbon dioxide exchange. In: Wong DL, ed. *Whaley & Wong's Nursing Care of Infants and Children.* 5th ed. St. Louis, Mo: Mosby-Year Book; 1995:1340. Reprinted with permission.

DIAGNOSTIC PROCEDURES

A variety of radiographic, imaging, and laboratory studies may be indicated based on the suspected etiology of the child's condition. Definitive diagnostic testing is performed during the resuscitation effort or after the child is stabilized. The following procedures or studies may be indicated for the child with respiratory distress or failure.

Monitors

- Pulse oximeter.
    - Poor perfusion may impede the monitor's ability to obtain an accurate reading.
    - A normal reading does not negate the child's need for supplemental oxygen.
- Cardiac monitor, as indicated.
- Capnography, as indicated.

Radiographic Studies

- Chest radiograph to determine the presence of enlarged heart, foreign body, pulmonary infection, pulmonary edema, hyperexpansion, or pneumothorax or hemothorax.
- Lateral radiograph of the neck or thorax to evaluate the presence of a foreign body or pleural effusions.
- Other radiographic and imaging studies may be indicated based on the etiology of the respiratory compromise.

Laboratory Studies

- Arterial or capillary blood gas may be obtained, depending on the child's condition and clinical concern. Capillary blood gas may be used to evaluate pH and CO_2 levels. A decreasing pH indicates a worsening of the cellular oxygen debt as metabolic acidosis develops because of anaerobic metabolism and lactic acid production. An elevated $PaCO_2$ indicates respiratory acidosis and impaired ventilation of the alveoli. A low PaO_2 indicates hypoxia.

- Increasing carbon dioxide retention represents hypoventilation. This can be measured with blood gases and monitored or trended with the use of capnography.

- Other laboratory studies including cultures may be indicated based on the child's condition and treatment plan.

Nursing Diagnoses, Interventions, and Expected Outcomes

NURSING DIAGNOSIS	INTERVENTIONS	EXPECTED OUTCOMES
Airway clearance, ineffective, related to: • Edema of the airway, vocal cords, epiglottis, and upper airway • Irritation of the respiratory tract • Laryngeal spasm • Altered level of consciousness or muscle weakness or fatigue • Inability to remove oropharyngeal secretions • Anatomic abnormalities • Fatigue • Pain	• Position supine or elevate head of bed • Suction airway • Allow position of comfort • Clear nasal secretions with bulb syringe • Use jaw thrust or chin lift maneuver • Insert nasopharyngeal or oropharyngeal airway • Prepare for endotracheal intubation	The child will maintain a patent airway, as evidenced by: • Regular rate, depth, and pattern of breathing • Symmetric chest expansion • Effective cough and gag reflex • Absence of signs and symptoms of airway obstruction: Stridor, dyspnea, and hoarse voice • Clear sputum of normal amount without abnormal color or odor • Absence of signs and symptoms of retained secretions: Fever, tachycardia, and tachypnea

Breathing pattern, ineffective, related to:
• Exacerbation of underlying chronic disease
• Muscular or skeletal deformities
• Age-related characteristics
• Inactivity or immobility
• Altered level of consciousness or muscle weakness or fatigue
• Poor positioning
• Diaphragmatic impedance
• Infection
• Lung collapse
• Pain
	• Position supine or elevate head of bed
	• Suction airway
	• Allow position of comfort
	• Clear nasal secretions with bulb syringe
	• Use jaw thrust or chin lift maneuver
	• Insert nasopharyngeal or oropharyngeal airway
	• Decompress abdomen
	• Administer oxygen
	• Assist ventilations
	• Prepare for endotracheal intubation
	• Obtain peak expiratory flow measurement
		The child will have an effective breathing pattern, as evidenced by:
		• Regular rate, depth, and pattern of breathing
		• Clear and equal breath sounds
		• Absence of use of accessory muscles or nasal flaring
		• Symmetric chest expansion
		• ABG values within normal limits:
		  ▪ PaO_2 80 to 100 mm Hg (10.0 to 13.3 KPa)
		  ▪ SaO_2 >95%
		  ▪ $PaCO_2$ 35 to 45 mm Hg (4.7 to 6.0 KPa)
		  ▪ pH between 7.35 and 7.45
		• Absence of stridor, dyspnea, and cyanosis
		• Trachea midline
		• Chest radiograph without abnormality
		• Peak expiratory flow >70% of predicted value

NURSING DIAGNOSIS	INTERVENTIONS	EXPECTED OUTCOMES

Gas exchange, impaired, related to:
• Ineffective breathing pattern
• Ineffective airway clearance
	• Position supine or elevate head of bed
	• Suction airway
	• Allow position of comfort
	• Clear nasal secretions with bulb syringe
	• Use jaw thrust or chin lift maneuver
	• Insert nasopharyngeal or oropharyngeal airway
	• Administer oxygen
	• Administer medications
	• Assist ventilations
	• Prepare for endotracheal intubation
	• Relieve conditions that impede diaphragmatic excursion
		The child will maintain adequate gas exchange, as evidenced by:
		• Oxygen saturation >95% by pulse oximetry
		• ABG values within normal limits:
		  ■ PaO_2 80 to 100 mm Hg (10.0 to 13.3 KPa)
		  ■ SaO_2 >95%
		  ■ $PaCO_2$ 35 to 45 mm Hg (4.7 to 6.0 KPa)
		  ■ pH between 7.35 and 7.45
		• Skin normal color, warm, and dry
		• Improved level of consciousness
		• Regular rate, depth, and pattern of breathing
		• Symmetric chest expansion
		• Clear and equal breath sounds

Triage or Acuity Decisions

The following are used as triage guidelines for children with respiratory distress or failure[8]:

EMERGENT   Pediatric patient with signs and symptoms indicating moderate-to-severe respiratory distress or impending respiratory failure such as agitation, lethargy, altered level of consciousness; adventitious, absent, unequal, or decreased breath sounds; decreased air exchange or entry; moderate-to-severe retractions, nasal flaring, head bobbing, expiratory grunting; extreme tachypnea, bradypnea, or apneic episodes; tachycardia or bradycardia; poor muscle tone; unusual drooling, dysphonia, dysphagia; pallor, dusky, gray color, cyanosis; tripod position.

URGENT   Pediatric patient with signs and symptoms indicating mild-to-moderate respiratory distress; mild-to-moderate retractions, nasal flaring; crackles, wheezing, or other adventitious sounds; paroxysmal coughing; history of choking with color change, gagging, or vomiting; history of cyanotic or apneic episode at home; history of chronic pulmonary or cardiac condition with respiratory symptoms.

NONURGENT   Pediatric patient with mild respiratory symptoms without respiratory distress; normal breath sounds, normal color. May have rhinorrhea, nasal congestion, or cough.

Planning and Implementation

Refer to Chapter 4, "Initial Assessment and Triage," for a description of the general nursing interventions for the pediatric patient. After a patent airway, breathing, and circulation are assured, the following interventions are initiated, as appropriate, for the child's condition.

ADDITIONAL INTERVENTIONS

- Position the child to facilitate respiratory effectiveness and comfort. (Nursing diagnoses: Ineffective airway clearance; ineffective breathing pattern; impaired gas exchange).

  - Raise the head of the bed to the most comfortable angle.

  - Try to avoid invasive procedures or actions that may upset the child until the airway is secured (e.g., patients with partial airway obstruction from a foreign body or epiglottis).

- Suction the infant's nares with a bulb syringe when secretions are present. (Nursing diagnosis: Ineffective airway clearance).

- Administer supplemental oxygen by the most appropriate method, delivering the highest concentration of oxygen, as appropriate, for the child's condition. Refer to Pediatric Considerations: Respiratory Interventions and Diagnostic Procedures, Oxygen Delivery at the end of Chapter 5.

- Give nothing by mouth, as appropriate. (Nursing diagnosis: Aspiration).

  - Children with extreme tachypnea, severe respiratory distress, or impending failure must be given nothing by mouth because of the risk of aspiration and potential need for intubation.

  - Feeding may also compound the respiratory problem in infants because it increases metabolic demand and oxygen requirements.

  - For those with mild distress, encourage oral intake because tachypnea can lead to increased insensible fluid losses. If the child is to receive nothing by mouth for a significant period, intravenous fluids are required.

- Relieve any conditions that are impeding diaphragmatic excursion. (Nursing diagnosis: Ineffective breathing pattern; impaired gas exchange).

  - Insert a gastric tube to reduce gastric distention. Air in the stomach from swallowing air or bag-valve-mask ventilation will result in gastric distention, which can impede ventilatory efforts.

  - If a gastrostomy tube is in place for feeding, decompression via the gastrotomy tube may be needed.

- Prepare and administer medications, per protocol, including antipyretic. (Nursing diagnosis: Impaired gas exchange).

- Anticipate the need and prepare for assisted ventilation, intubation, and other advanced support measures, as appropriate. (Nursing diagnoses: Ineffective airway clearance; ineffective breathing pattern; impaired gas exchange). Refer to Pediatric Considerations: Respiratory Interventions and Diagnostic Procedures, Airway Adjuncts and Providing Assisted Ventilation at the end of Chapter 5.

  - Assess endotracheal tube placement:

    - Observe for symmetric chest rise.

    - Auscultate for breath sounds bilaterally at the midaxillary areas and over the epigastrium. Compare pitch, intensity, and location of the sounds.

    - When available, an end-tidal CO_2 detector can be used to confirm tube placement.

- ◆ Confirm endotracheal tube positioning with a chest radiograph.

- ◆ Record position of endotracheal tube at level of the gum, lip, or teeth.

- ■ *Rapid sequence induction* for intubation may be required for the child in impending or actual respiratory failure. Refer to Pediatric Considerations: Respiratory Interventions and Diagnostic Procedures, Rapid Sequence Induction at the end of Chapter 5.

- ■ Prepare for alternative airway and breathing support measures, if indicated:

  - ◆ A needle cricothyrotomy is indicated only in cases of complete upper airway obstruction when all other interventions have failed to produce an adequate airway.

  - ◆ An emergency tracheostomy is rarely indicated in children and must be performed only by experienced physicians.

- ■ Prepare for needle decompression of tension pneumothorax.

Evaluation and Ongoing Assessment

Pediatric patients with respiratory emergencies require meticulous and frequent reassessment of airway patency, breathing effectiveness, perfusion, and mental status. The etiologies of respiratory distress and failure encompass a broad range of disorders. Initial improvements may not be sustained, and additional interventions may be required. The patient's response to interventions and trending of the patient's condition must be closely monitored for achievement of desired outcomes. To evaluate the patient's respiratory progress, monitor the following:

- Airway patency.

- Level of consciousness and activity.

- Work of breathing.

- Breath sounds and quality of air exchange.

- Peak flow measurements.

- Oxygen saturation and end-tidal CO_2, as indicated.

- Vital signs.

SELECTED EMERGENCIES

Upper Airway

Respiratory distress and failure can result when structures of the upper airway are occluded by edema, secretions, foreign bodies, or anatomic defects. Examples of these emergencies include croup, epiglottitis, bacterial tracheitis, foreign-body obstruction, obstructive sleep apnea, and tracheomalacia or vascular rings. Croup, epiglottitis, and foreign-body obstruction are further compared in Table 12.

Table 12

COMPARISON OF UPPER AIRWAY EMERGENCIES		
CROUP[9-11,13]	**EPIGLOTTITIS**[9,12,13]	**FOREIGN-BODY OBSTRUCTION**[14]
Acute viral illness; usually causes partial airway obstruction because of tracheal narrowing.	Acute bacterial illness; if untreated, usually progresses to complete airway obstruction because of cellulitis of the epiglottis, arytenoids, and aryteno-epiglottic structures.	Acute tracheobronchial obstruction; may be partial or complete.
Caused by parainfluenza virus type I or III, adenovirus, or respiratory syncytial virus.	Most commonly caused by *Haemophilus influenzae* type b, however, eradication in some communities due to immunization has occurred. May also be caused by *Streptococcus pneumoniae*, *Staphylococcus aureus*, and group A and group C beta-hemolytic streptococci.	Most often caused by food items, especially peanuts, but may also be caused by toys, coins, latex balloons, and small disc batteries. Frequently follows history of gagging.
Occurs most commonly in children 6 months to 3 years of age.	Occurs in children younger than 2 years of age 25% of the time, but may occur in any age group.	Occurs most commonly in children 9 months to 5 years of age but may occur in any age group.
Peak incidence in late fall and early winter.	No seasonal preference.	No seasonal preference.

• Presents with gradual onset of stridor, a "barking cough" that is worse at night, hoarse voice, tachypnea, nasal flaring, and retractions following an upper airway infection.
• Low-grade fever is common, and wheezing is occasionally reported.
• Neck radiograph may reveal tracheal narrowing, referred to as the "steeple sign."
	• Presents with several hours of high fever, sore throat, muffled voice, and drooling, which lead quickly to respiratory distress.
	• May keep mouth open and use tripod positioning to maintain airway patency.
	• May have toxic appearance because of concurrent bacteremia.
	• Lateral neck radiograph may reveal epiglottic and aryteno-epiglottic swelling, referred to as the "thumb sign" and the "posterior triangle."
	• Most blood cultures are positive for the causative agent.
		• Presentation of respiratory distress varies depending on:
		  ■ When the aspiration occurred.
		  ■ Whether the item is inert, caustic, or organic.
		  ■ Whether the item is in the esophagus and pressing on the airway or is in the airway itself.
		• Signs and symptoms may include drooling, stridor, asymmetric wheezing or breath sounds, or chest pain.
		• Anterior-posterior, lateral, and decubitus view chest radiographs may reveal radiopaque or obstructing items.
		• Partially obstructing, nonradiopaque items can be very difficult to evaluate by radiograph.
		• Direct visualization by deep laryngoscopy or bronchoscopy may be required for definitive diagnosis.

COMPARISON OF UPPER AIRWAY EMERGENCIES		
CROUP[9-11,13]	**EPIGLOTTITIS**[9,12,13]	**FOREIGN-BODY OBSTRUCTION**[14]

• Provide cool mist.
• Encourage fluids.
• Administer oral or parenteral dexamethasone sodium phosphate to reduce airway edema, as ordered.
• Administer nebulized racemic epinephrine, as ordered. Children must be monitored for 4 to 6 hours because effect of medication may not be sustained causing a rebound effect.
	• Place in position of comfort and do not separate from caregiver.
	• Do not perform procedures until airway is stabilized. These include:
	  ■ Throat examination as it can precipitate gagging and complete obstruction.
	  ■ Rectal temperature.
	  ■ Blood work or intravenous access.
	• Provide blow-by oxygen, as tolerated.
	• Anticipate endotracheal intubation in surgery.
	• Complete intravenous access, radiographs, laboratory work, and antibiotics once the airway is stabilized.
		• Initiate pediatric basic life-support techniques to relieve choking, as appropriate.
		• Place in position of comfort and do not separate from caregiver.
		• Do not perform invasive procedures until airway is stabilized. These include:
		  ■ Throat examination.
		  ■ Rectal temperature.
		  ■ Blood work or intravenous access.
		• Provide blow-by oxygen, as needed.
		• Complete intravenous access and radiographs once airway is stabilized.

Lower Airway

Respiratory distress and failure can also result when structures of the lower airway are occluded by edema, bronchoconstriction, secretions, foreign bodies, weak muscle walls, or anatomic defects. Examples of these emergencies include asthma, bronchiolitis, pneumonia, foreign-body obstruction, bronchomalacia, muscular dystrophy, and scoliosis or kyphosis.

REACTIVE AIRWAY DISEASE (ASTHMA)

Asthma is the most common chronic illness in children, and the worldwide incidence is rising.[15,16] It is a chronic, obstructive, inflammatory disorder of the lower airways in which a variety of pulmonary cells and their mediators play a role. The disease is characterized by hyperreactiveness of the airway, widespread inflammatory changes, and mucous plugging. Recurrent episodes, which may include wheezing, breathlessness, chest tightness, or coughing, are common. Exacerbations of asthma are often precipitated by seasonal and environmental allergies, exercise, infections, medications, irritants, weather changes, smoking, exposure to secondhand smoke, and emotions.

Confirmation of the diagnosis of asthma is usually delayed until the child has had repeated episodes of wheezing and is older than 1 year of age. Diagnosing asthma in infants is often difficult, and under-recognition and undertreatment are common problems in this age group. Treatment is best directed toward long-term control rather than episodic emergency care.[17]

In Australia, over 30% of children will have symptoms of asthma before 8 years of age. By 12 years of age, over 45% of children will have been affected by asthma.[18] This translates to lost school days by the child and lost work days by the caregiver.

Additional History

- Frequent coughing, especially at night.

- Recurrent wheezing.

- Recurrent breathlessness.

- Recurrent chest tightness.

- Known triggers or exposure to any of the following prior to this illness:

  - Exercise.

  - Viral infection.

  - Animals with fur or feathers.

  - Housedust mites.

  - Molds or pollen.

  - Smoke from tobacco or wood.

  - Weather changes.

  - Strong emotional expression such as laughing or crying hard.

  - Airborne chemicals or dust.

  - Medications such as salicylates or nonsteroidal anti-inflammatory drugs.

- Atopic dermatitis or eczema.

- Previous history of reactive airway disease, asthma, previous wheezing episodes:

  - Frequency of symptoms.

  - Number of school days missed.

  - Present medications including dose, route, and frequency.

  - Morning baseline peak flow volumes.

  - Number of ED visits per year.

  - Number of hospitalizations; date of last hospitalization.

  - Number of critical care admissions; date of last admission to critical care unit.

  - Number of endotracheal intubations; date of last intubation.

- Management by a primary care provider, pulmonologist, or an allergy specialist.

Signs and Symptoms

- Wheezing.

- Prolonged expiratory phase.

- Decreased or unequal breath sounds.

- Tachypnea.

- Retractions.

- Coughing, especially at night and early morning.

Diagnostic Procedures

Laboratory Studies

- Theophylline levels: Only required for children receiving theophylline preparations. Serum levels must be between 10 and 20 mg/L. Higher levels are associated with headache, nausea or vomiting, and dysrhythmia formation.[17]

- Arterial blood gas for severe exacerbations. A $PaCO_2$ >42 mm Hg or PaO_2 <90 mm Hg with signs of muscle fatigue or a declining level of consciousness, despite maximal therapy, may indicate impending respiratory failure and the need for endotracheal intubation.[17]

Additional Interventions

- Deliver supplemental oxygen per protocol. Monitor oxygen saturation until a clear response to bronchodilator therapy has occurred.[17]

- Obtain peak expiratory flow or forced expiratory volume measurement. See Pediatric Considerations Supplement, peak expiratory flow measurement. Record the percentage of predicted best (see Figure 8 for normal values).

Figure 8

PEAK FLOW CURVE VALUES

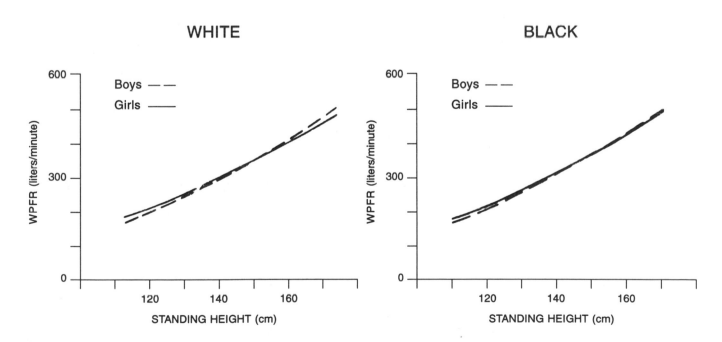

From Johnson K, ed. *The Harriet Lane Handbook: A Manual for Pediatric House Officers.* St. Louis, Mo: Mosby-Year Book; 1993:336. Reprinted with permission.

- Administer medications, as ordered (see Figure 9 for medications and recommended doses):

    - Short-acting beta$_2$-agonists. May be delivered as nebulized aerosol or metered dose inhaler. See Pediatric Considerations, nebulizer therapy.

    - Nebulizers are usually administered every 20 minutes to a total of three treatments or may be administered continuously depending on patient condition.

    - Anticholinergics may potentiate bronchodilatory effect of beta$_2$-agonists.

    - Systemic corticosteroids. Oral administration of prednisone has been shown to have effects equivalent to those of intravenous methylprednisolone sodium succinate.[17]

- Reassess patient after dose of inhaled bronchodilator and at least every 60 minutes thereafter. More frequent assessment may be required for severe exacerbations.

- Classify the severity of the asthma exacerbation (see Figure 10).

- Prepare for admission or transfer if the child's condition does not improve.[17]

- Prepare for discharge if the child's condition has improved and desired outcomes are achieved (peak expiratory flow $\geq$70% of normal, response sustained 60 minutes after last treatment, no distress, and normal physical examination).[17]

    - Review home management of asthma with caregiver:

        - Medications.

        - Dose, frequency, and purpose.

        - Have the caregiver demonstrate the proper use of the nebulizer or metered dose inhaler and spacer.

    - Review measurement of peak expiratory flow.

        - Have the caregiver demonstrate use of the peak flow meter to assure proper technique and review indications that require a change in the child's treatment.

        - At home, peak expiratory flow is usually obtained in the morning prior to bronchodilator therapy and is used to guide the home therapy plan.[17] Refer to Pediatric Considerations: Respiratory Interventions and Diagnostic Procedures, Peak Expiratory Flow Measurements at the end of Chapter 5.

    - Discuss trigger avoidance with caregiver.

    - Emphasize the need for regular care in an outpatient setting. Refer the patient to a primary care provider.

    - Recommend follow-up appointment with primary care provider or asthma specialist.

Figure 9

DOSAGES OF DRUGS FOR ASTHMA EXACERBATIONS
IN EMERGENCY MEDICAL CARE OR HOSPITAL

DOSAGES			
Medications	**Adults**	**Children**	**Comments**
Inhaled short-acting beta$_2$-agonists			
Albuterol Nebulizer solution (5 mg/mL)	2.5-5 mg every 20 min for 3 doses, then 2.5-10 mg every 1-4 hours as needed, or 10-15 mg/hour continuously.	0.15 mg/kg (minimum dose 2.5 mg) every 20 min for 3 doses, then 0.15-0.3 mg/kg up to 10 mg every 1-4 hours as needed, or 0.5 mg/kg/ hour by continuous nebulization.	Only selective beta$_2$-agonists are recommended. For optimal delivery, dilute aerosols to minimum of 4 mL at gas flow of 6-8 L/min.
MDI (90 mcg/puff)	4-8 puffs every 20 min up to 4 hours, then every 1-4 hours as needed.	4-8 puffs every 20 min for 3 doses, then every 1-4 hours as needed.	As effective as nebulized therapy if patient is able to coordinate inhalation maneuver. Use spacer/ holding chamber.
Bitolterol Nebulizer solution (2 mg/mL)	See albuterol dose.	See albuterol dose, thought to be one-half as potent as albuterol on a mg basis.	Has not been studied in severe asthma exacerbations. Do not mix with other drugs.
MDI (370 mcg/puff)	See albuterol dose.	See albuterol dose.	Has not been studied in severe asthma exacerbations.
Pirbuterol MDI (200 mcg/puff)	See albuterol dose.	See albuterol dose, thought to be one half as potent as albuterol on a mg basis.	Has not been studied in severe asthma exacerbations.
Systemic (injected) beta$_2$-agonists			
Epinephrine 1:1000 (1 mg/mL)	0.3-0.5 mg every 20 min for 3 doses sq.	0.01 mg/kg up to 0.3-0.5 mg every 20 min for 3 doses sq.	No proven advantage of systemic therapy over aerosol.
Terbutaline (1 mg/mL)	0.25 mg every 20 min for 3 doses sq.	0.01 mg/kg every 20 min for 3 doses then every 2-6 hours as needed sq.	No proven advantage of systemic therapy over aerosol.
Anticholinergics			
Ipratropium bromide Nebulizer solution (0.25 mg/mL)	0.5 mg every 30 min for 3 doses then every 2-4 hours as needed.	0.25 mg every 20 min for 3 doses then every 2-4 hours as needed.	May mix in same nebulizer with albuterol. Should not be used as first-line therapy; should be added to beta$_2$-agonist therapy.
MDI (18 mcg/puff)	4-8 puffs as needed.	4-8 puffs as needed.	Dose delivered from MDI is low and has not been studied in asthma exacerbations.
Corticosteroids Prednisone Methylprednisolone Prednisolone	120-180 mg/day in 3 or 4 divided doses for 48 hours then 60-80 mg/ day until PEF reaches 70% of predicted or personal best.	1 mg/kg every 6 hours for 48 hours then 1-2 mg/kg/day (maximum = 60 mg/day) in 2 divided doses until PEF 70% of predicted or personal best.	For outpatient "burst" use 40-60 mg in single or 2 divided doses for adults (children–1-2 mg/kg/day, maximum 60 mg/day) for 3-10 days.

Note: No advantage has been found for higher dose corticosteroids in severe asthma exacerbations, nor is there any advantage for intravenous administration over oral therapy provided gastrointestinal transit time or absorption is not impaired. The usual regimen is to continue the frequent multiple daily dosing until the patient achieves an FEV, or PEF of 50 percent of predicted or personal best and then lower the dose to twice daily. This usually occurs within 48 hours. Therapy following a hospitalization or emergency department visit may last from 3 to 10 days. If patients are then started on inhaled corticosteroids, studies indicate there is no need to taper the systemic corticosteroid dose. If the follow-up systemic corticosteroid therapy is to be given once daily, one study indicates it may be more clinically effective to give the dose in the afternoon at around 3:00 p.m.

Adapted from *Guidelines for the Diagnosis and Management of Asthma. National Asthma Education Program, Expert Panel Report 2.* Washington, DC: US Department of Health and Human Services; July 1997. National Institutes of Health publication 99-4051. Used with permission.

Figure 10

SEVERITY CLASSIFICATION OF ASTHMA EXACERBATIONS

	Mild	*Moderate*	*Severe*	*Respiratory Arrest Imminent*
Symptoms:				
Breathless	While walking	While talking (infant - softer, shorter cry; difficulty feeding)	While at rest (infant - stops feeding)	
	Can lie down	Prefers sitting	Sits upright	
Talks in	Sentences	Phrases	Words	
Alertness	May be agitated	Usually agitated	Usually agitated	Drowsy or confused
Signs:				
Respiratory rate	Increased	Increased	Often > 30/min	
	Guide to rates of breathing in awake children: *Age* < 2 months 2-12 months 1-5 years 6-8 years	*Normal rate* < 60/min < 50/min < 40/min < 30/min		
Use of accessory muscles; suprasternal retractions	Usually not	Commonly	Usually	Paradoxical thoraco-abdominal movement
Wheeze	Moderate, often only end expiratory	Loud; throughout exhalation	Usually loud; throughout inhalation and exhalation	Absence of wheeze
Pulse/min	< 100	100-120	> 120	Bradycardia
	Guide to normal pulse rates in children: *Age* 2-12 months 1-2 years 2-8 years	*Normal rate* < 160/min < 120/min < 110/min		
Pulsus paradoxus	Absent < 10 mm Hg	May be present 10-25 mm Hg	Often present > 25 mm Hg (adult); 20-40 mm Hg (child)	Absence suggests respiratory muscle fatigue
Functional assessment:				
PEF % predicted or % personal best	80%	Approx. 50-80%	< 50% predicted or personal best or response lasts < 2 hrs	
PaO_2 (on air) and/or	Normal (test not usually necessary)	> 60 mm Hg (test not usually necessary)	< 60 mm Hg: possible cyanosis	
PCO_2	< 42 mm Hg (test not usually necessary)	< 42 mm Hg (test not usually necessary)	≥ 42 mm Hg: possible respiratory failure	
SaO_2% (on air) at sea level	> 95% (test not usually necessary)	91-95%	< 91%	
	Hypercapnia (hypoventilation) develops more readily in young children than in adults and adolescents.			

*Notes:
■ The presence of several parameters, but not necessarily all, indicates the general classification of the exacerbation.
■ Many of these parameters have not been systematically studied, so they serve only as general guides.

Adapted from *Guidelines for the Diagnosis and Management of Asthma. National Asthma Education Program, Expert Panel Report 2.* Washington, DC: US Department of Health and Human Services; July 1997. National Institutes of Health publication 99-4051. Used with permission.

BRONCHIOLITIS

Bronchiolitis is a lower respiratory tract infection in infants younger than 1 year of age and is most commonly caused by the respiratory syncytial virus.[18,19] The airway obstruction is usually gradual and is caused by edema and secretions of the lower respiratory tract. Extensive mucous plugging may progress to atelectasis and pneumonia. It is more often seen in the winter and early spring. Children with cardiac and pulmonary diseases are at greater risk for severe life-threatening manifestations of the virus.[20]

Additional History

- Symptoms of upper respiratory tract infection.

- History of vomiting and poor fluid or food intake.

- Pre-existing conditions such as chronic pulmonary insufficiency, congenital heart disease, or pulmonary hypertension.

Signs and Symptoms

- Cough.

- Tachypnea.

- Grunting.

- Wheezing.

- Prolonged expiratory phase.

- Decreased air entry or exchange.

- Retractions.

- Apnea spells.

- Low-grade fever common in early infection.

Additional Interventions

- Place in contact isolation.

- Consider nasal washing for respiratory syncytial virus antigen test. Nasal lavage has a positive predictive value of 95.6% and a negative predictive value of 92.5%.[21]

- Administer medications, as ordered. Although still somewhat controversial, recent studies indicate that the use of beta$_2$-agonists and systemic corticosteroids do not shorten the course of illness, alter its severity, or decrease the length of hospital stays.[22,23] When admitted to the hospital, certain infants may be candidates for ribavirin which is an antiviral aerosol medication: Those with complicated congenital heart disease, cystic fibrosis, infants younger than 6 weeks of age, born at less than 37 weeks gestational age, taking immunosuppressive medication, or requiring mechanical ventilation.[24]

PNEUMONIA

Pneumonia is a lower respiratory tract infection caused by a viral, bacterial, parasitic, or fungal organism.[25] Most pneumonias in children are viral in origin. Pneumonia can occur in any age group and can vary in etiology and severity, depending on the child's age and immune status. It may be a primary condition or result secondary to other respiratory problems such as asthma or bronchiolitis. It presents as an acute inflammatory reaction in the lung tissue. As fluid and cellular debris accumulate in the areas of infection, compliance and vital capacity decrease and work of breathing increases.

Additional History

- Worsening of symptoms of upper respiratory tract infection.

- Abrupt onset of fever and chills with bacterial pneumonia.

- History of vomiting and poor fluid or food intake.

- Pre-existing conditions such as chronic pulmonary insufficiency, congenital heart disease, or pulmonary hypertension.

Signs and Symptoms

- Cough.

- Tachypnea.

- Grunting.

- Unequal breath sounds.

- Crackles.

- Wheezes.

- Retractions.

- Chest pain.

- Apnea spells.

- Fever.

- Abdominal pain which is more common in children with lower lobe pneumonia and may include abdominal distension and tenderness.

Additional Interventions

- Administer antimicrobial medications.

HEALTH PROMOTION

- Instruct caregivers to protect young children from foods or objects that commonly cause airway obstruction.

- Provide anticipatory guidance on childproofing the environment to avoid aspiration of small objects.

- Encourage caregiver to obtain training in pediatric basic life-support techniques.

- Provide caregivers with information on childhood immunizations, especially pertussis and *Haemophilus influenzae* vaccine, and the importance of keeping the child up-to-date. Provide referral and resources for immunizations, as appropriate.

- For children with asthma, provide information regarding precipitating triggers to avoid, such as tobacco smoke, aspirin, dust, pollen, molds, and animal fur or feathers.

- Instruct caregivers to administer medication to their children, as ordered by the physician.

- Provide referral or information on obtaining a primary care provider if one is not already established.

SUMMARY

This chapter has outlined the child's unique responses to respiratory problems because of specific anatomic, physiologic, and developmental characteristics. Respiratory compromise in children can occur during upper and lower respiratory tract infections, when they receive sedation for procedures, from muscular skeletal deformities, or even from congenital anomalies. Selective respiratory emergencies, including croup, epiglottitis, foreign-body obstruction, asthma, bronchiolitis, and pneumonia have been reviewed.

Respiratory distress is part of a continuum that results in respiratory failure if left untreated, and respiratory failure is the most common pathway to cardiopulmonary arrest in children. Further interventions for the child with respiratory compromise have been delineated in this section. In addition, suggestions for health promotion strategies directed at altering the adverse outcomes of respiratory distress and failure have been offered. A collaborative, systematic approach to care reduces fragmentation and enhances the opportunity to improve outcome.

REFERENCES

1. Few B. Respiratory problems. In: Curley MAQ, Bloedel-Smith J, Maloney-Harmon P, eds. *Critical Care Nursing of Infants and Children*. Philadelphia, Pa: WB Saunders; 1996:619-655.

2. Curley MAQ, Ead N. Resuscitation of infants and children. In: Curley MAQ, Bloedel-Smith J, Maloney-Harmon P, eds. *Critical Care Nursing of Infants and Children*. Philadelphia, Pa: WB Saunders; 1996:963-988.

3. Chameides L, Hazinski MF, eds. *Pediatric Advanced Life Support*. Dallas, Tex: American Heart Association; 1997.

4. American Academy of Pediatrics. *Workbook for Advanced Pediatric Life Support: Recognition and Initial Stabilization – The First Thirty Minutes*. Chicago, Ill: Author; 1993.

5. Sigda M, Wright-Lott J. Concepts of altered health in children. In: Mattson-Porth C, ed. *Pathophysiology: Concepts of Altered Health*. Philadelphia, Pa: JB Lippincott; 1994:103-123.

6. Hunsberger M, Feegan L. Altered respiratory function. In: Betz CL, Hunsberger M, Wright S, eds. *Family Centered Nursing Care of Children*. Philadelphia, Pa: WB Saunders; 1994:1167-1275.

7. Shafer FE, Seibel NL, Reaman GH. Hematologic disorders. In: Holbrook PR, ed. *Textbook of Pediatric Critical Care*. Philadelphia, Pa: WB Saunders; 1993:743-772.

8. Thomas DO. Pediatric triage and assessment. In: Sheehy SB, ed. *Emergency Nursing: Principles and Practice*. 3rd ed. St. Louis, Mo: Mosby-Year Book; 1992:657-669.

9. Cressman WR, Myer CM. Diagnosis and management of croup and epiglottitis. *Pediatr Clin North Am*. 1994;41:265-276.

10. Kunkel NC, Baker MD. Use of racemic epinephrine, dexamethasone, and mist in the outpatient management of croup. *Pediatr Emerg Care*. 1996;12:156-159.

11. Milner AD. The role of corticosteroids and croup. *Thorax*. 1997;52:595-597.

12. Repasky TM. Emergency: epiglottitis. *Am J Nursing*. 1995;95:52.

13. Schroeder LL, Knapp JF. Recognition and emergency management of infectious causes of upper airway obstruction in children. *Semin Respir Infect*. 1995;10:21-30.

14. Wolach B, Raz A, Weinberg J, Mikulski Y, Ben Ari J, Sadan N. Aspirated foreign bodies in the respiratory tract of children: eleven years experience with 127 patients. *Int J Pediatr Otorhinolaryngol*. 1994;30:1-10.

15. Gay JC, Muldoon JH, Neff JM, Wing LJ. Profiling the health service needs of populations: description and uses of the NACHRI classification of congenital and chronic health conditions. *Pediatr Ann*. 1997;26:655-663.

16. *Global Initiative for Asthma*. Bethesda, Md: National Heart, Lung, and Blood Institute and World Health Organization; 1995. National Institutes of Health publication 95-3659.

17. *Guidelines for the Diagnosis and Management of Asthma. National Asthma Education Program, Expert Panel Report 2*. Washington, DC: US Department of Health and Human Services; 1997. National Institutes of Health publication 99-4051.

18. Robertson CF, Heycock E, Bishop J, Nolan T, Olinsky A, Phelan PD. Prevalence of asthma in Melbourne school children: Changes over 26 years. *BMJ*. 1991;302:116.

19. McFarlane K. RSV and bronchiolitis. *Paediatr Nurs*. 1995;7:32-37.

20. Moler FW, Khan AS, Meliones JN, Custer JR, Palmisano J, Shope TC. Respiratory syncytial virus morbidity and mortality estimates in congenital heart disease patients: a recent experience. *Crit Care Med*. 1992;20:1406-1413.

21. Balfour-Lynn I, Girdhar D, Aitken C. Diagnosing respiratory syncytial virus by nasal lavage. *Arch Dis Child*. 1995;72:58-59.

22. Roosevelt G, Sheehan K, Grupp-Phelan J, Tanz R, Listernick R. Dexamethasone is ineffective in the treatment of bronchiolitis. *Pediatr Emerg Care.* 1995;11:327-328.

23. Dobson JV, Stephens-Groff SM, McMahon SR, Stemmler MM, Brallier SL, Bay C. The use of albuterol in hospitalized infants with bronchiolitis. *Pediatrics.* 1998;101:361-368.

24. American Academy of Pediatrics. Reassessment of the indications for ribavirin therapy in respiratory syncytial virus infections. *Pediatrics.* 1996;97:137-140.

25. Coakley-Maller C, Shea M. Respiratory infections in children: preparing for the fall and winter. *Adv Nurse Pract.* 1997;5:20-27.

Pediatric Considerations:
Respiratory Interventions and Diagnostic Procedures

AIRWAY AND BREATHING INTERVENTIONS IN THE PRIMARY ASSESSMENT

Opening the Airway

- Techniques to manually open the airway include the head tilt–chin lift and jaw thrust maneuvers. Maintaining the airway in a neutral position during these maneuvers is important. Flexion or hyperextension of the neck may compromise the child's airway or decrease the effectiveness of the head tilt–chin lift or jaw thrust maneuvers. The oropharynx should be suctioned immediately if secretions, vomitus, blood, or other debris are present.

- Head tilt–chin lift[1,2] (used only in children without head or neck trauma) (see Figure 11):

  - Place one hand on the forehead and tilt the head into a neutral position in an infant and slightly farther back in the child.

  - Place fingers of the other hand under the bony part of the lower jaw at the chin. Lift the chin upward.

  - Take care not to push the mouth closed or compress the tissues under the chin.

- Jaw thrust (see Figure 12)[1,2]

  - Place two or three fingers on each side of the child's lower jaw.

  - Gently lift the jaw without tilting the head.

  - Place the thumbs at the chin and displace the chin downward to open the mouth.

- Oropharyngeal suctioning:

  - Use a rigid tonsil tip suction to remove thick secretions and particulate matter.

  - Avoid stimulating the child's gag reflex, which could result in vomiting.

  - Avoid prolonged suctioning. In infant's, vagal stimulation may occur during suctioning, resulting in a decrease in heart rate.

Figure 11
HEAD TILT–CHIN LIFT MANEUVER

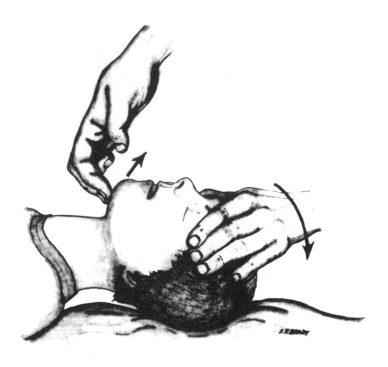

Figure 12
JAW THRUST MANEUVER

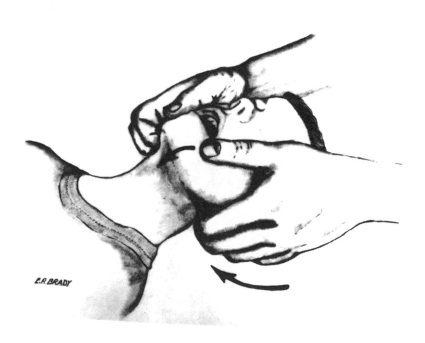

Airway Adjuncts

Airway adjuncts may be required to maintain a patent airway in the child with a decreased level of consciousness, copious secretions, or edema of the upper airway.

- Oropharyngeal airway[1-3]:

  - Indicated for the unconscious, spontaneously breathing child with an impaired gag reflex to relieve obstruction from the tongue. May be used to maintain an open airway during bag-valve-mask ventilation.

  - Determine size by placing the airway next to the child's face with the flange at the level of the teeth. The tip of the airway should end at the angle of the jaw (see Figure 13):

    - An airway that is too small may push the tongue into the oropharynx.

    - An airway that is too large may obstruct the trachea.

  - Insert the oropharyngeal airway using a tongue blade to depress and displace the tongue forward. Insert the airway, curve down, over the tongue (see Figure 13):

    - Do not insert the airway in the inverted position and rotate as is done in the adult.

    - Rotating the airway during insertion may traumatize the soft tissue structures of the oropharynx or cause injury to the teeth.

- Nasopharyngeal airway[1-3]:

  - Indicated for conscious children because it does not stimulate the gag reflex. Useful in children with nasopharyngeal edema or copious nasal secretions.

  - Available in infant through adult sizes.

  - Select a nasopharyngeal airway that has a diameter slightly smaller than the diameter of the child's nares. The length should be equal to the distance from the nares to the tragus of the ear.

  - Lubricate the tip of the airway prior to insertion.

  - Angle the bevel of the nasopharyngeal airway toward the septum.

  - Insert the airway by gently pushing in a posterior direction, perpendicular to the facial plane (see Figure 14).

Oxygen Administration

Initially and during resuscitation, the spontaneously breathing pediatric patient with respiratory distress and/or signs of shock requires oxygen to be delivered in the highest possible concentration. A nonrebreather mask with oxygen at 12 to 15 liters/minute is the preferred method unless the child requires ventilatory assistance. Other methods of oxygen delivery are discussed later in this section.

Bag-Valve-Mask Ventilation

If the patient is not breathing adequately once a patent airway is established, manual ventilation with a bag-valve-mask device and 100% oxygen must be initiated. The bag-valve-mask device most frequently used in the emergency department includes a self-inflating resuscitation bag with a reservoir and a face mask. Table 13 describes two types of resuscitation bags commonly available.

Figure 13

SIZING AND INSERTION OF AN ORAL AIRWAY

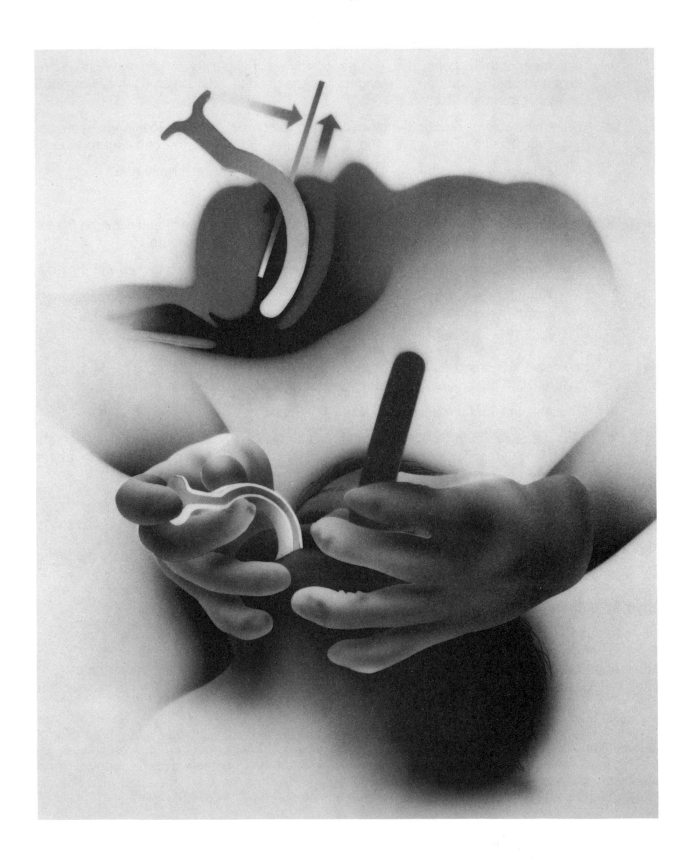

Figure 14
INSERTION OF A NASOPHARYNGEAL AIRWAY

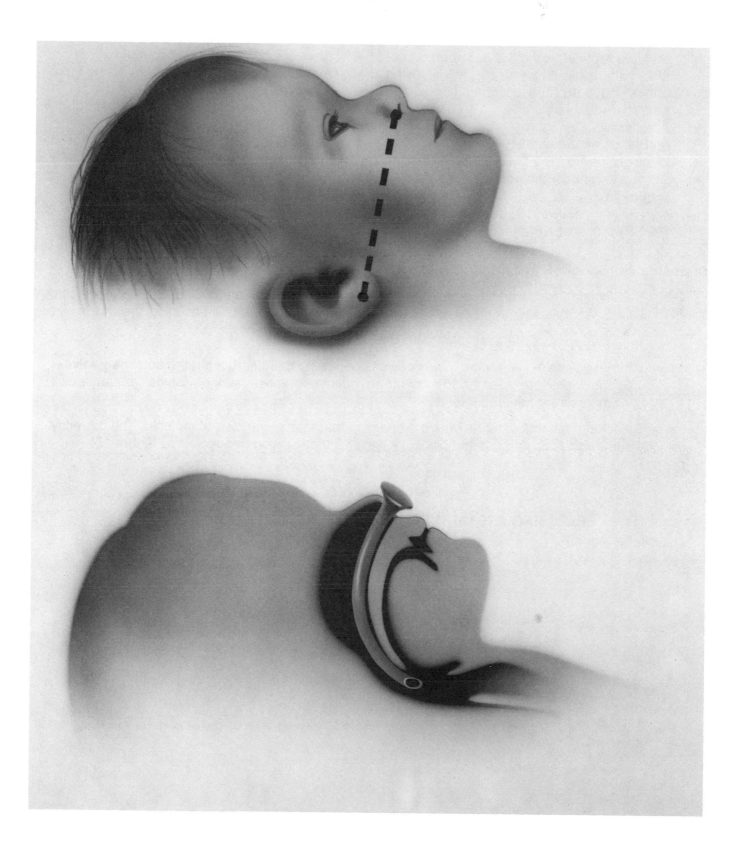

Table 13

MANUAL RESUSCITATION BAGS	
Self-Inflating Bags	**Flow-Inflating Bags**
• Delivers room air without a gas source. • Ideally there should be no pop-off valve; if a pop-off valve is present, it should be able to be bypassed easily. • Administers 100% oxygen if a gas source and reservoir are used. • Does not deliver free-flow oxygen. • Difficult to monitor the pressure or volume of inspired air. • Can deliver positive end expiratory pressure (PEEP) with a PEEP attachment.	• Requires continuous gas source. • A manometer should be used. • Administers 100% oxygen. • Oxygen flow continues between manual inflation. • Bag is compliant, making it easy to measure lung compliance. • Can deliver PEEP.

Choosing the Correct-Sized Bag-Valve-Mask Device

- Self-inflating resuscitation bags are used most frequently and are available in several sizes. Use a bag that is large enough to deliver an adequate tidal volume based on the child's size.

  - The appropriate tidal volume is 10 to 15 ml/kg.

  - The pediatric bag-valve-mask device delivers up to 500 ml of air; the adult bag-valve-mask delivers up to 1,500 ml of air. An infant bag-valve-mask device delivers at least 450 ml of air for full-term infants.

- Select a mask that extends from the bridge of the nose to the cleft of the chin. The correctly sized mask fits tightly without placing excessive pressure on the eyes (see Figure 15).

Figure 15

SELECTING THE CORRECT MASK FOR ASSISTED VENTILATION

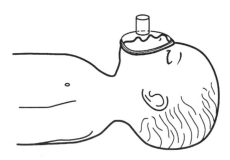

From French JP. Oxygenation and ventilation. In: French JP, ed. *Pediatric Emergency Skills*. St. Louis, Mo: Mosby-Year Book; 1995:86. Reprinted with permission.

Providing Assisted Ventilation

- While maintaining an open airway, deliver manual ventilations (see Figure 16):

    - One-handed procedure: Press the mask against the bridge of the nose and chin with the thumb and index finger, respectively, to maintain a seal. Rest the middle finger on the mandible, lifting it up. Use the other hand to squeeze the bag.[1,3]

    - Two-handed/two-person procedure: One person holds the mask to the face using the technique described above. Two hands may be used to obtain a good seal. The second person provides the ventilation by squeezing the bag.[1,3]

Figure 16

BAG-VALVE-MASK VENTILATION

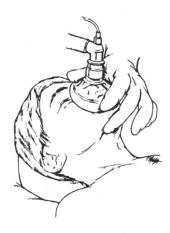

From Yaster M, Maxwell LG. Airway management. In: Nichols DG, Yaster M, Lappe DG, Haller JA, eds. *Golden Hour: The Handbook of Advanced Pediatric Life Support*. St. Louis, Mo: Mosby-Year Book; 1996:25. Reprinted with permission.

- Assess for adequate ventilation by observing for rise and fall of the chest, bilateral breath sounds during ventilation, and improvement in skin or mucous membrane color.

- The application of cricoid pressure (Sellick maneuver) may minimize gastric inflation during bag-valve-mask ventilation (see Figure 17):

    - To perform cricoid pressure, apply pressure to the cricoid cartilage, pushing it posteriorly. This compresses the esophagus between the cricoid cartilage and the cervical spine.[1,3]

    - In infants, use one fingertip to apply cricoid pressure.

    - In older children, use the thumb and index finger to apply cricoid pressure.

- Insertion of a gastric tube to alleviate gastric distension is recommended when the patient requires bag-valve-mask ventilation[1]:

    - Gastric distention predisposes the child to regurgitation and increases the risk of aspiration.

    - Gastric distention may impede adequate ventilation by limiting the downward movement of the diaphragm.

Figure 17
CRICOID PRESSURE

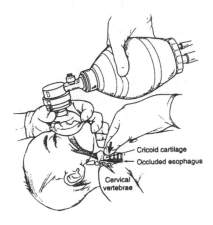

From Chameides L, Hazinski MF, eds. *Pediatric Advanced Life Support*. Dallas, Tex: American Heart Association; 1997:4-11. Reprinted with permission.

Endotracheal Intubation

- Assemble the equipment for intubation:

  - Obtain the correct size laryngoscope handle and blades (see Appendix L).

  - Choose the correct size and type of endotracheal tube:

    - Use uncuffed endotracheal tubes in children younger than 8 years of age. In these children, the cricoid ring is the narrowest portion of the airway and acts as a natural cuff.

    - Use a length-based resuscitation tape that lists tube and equipment sizes (e.g., Broselow™ tape).[4]

    - Use the formula 16 + patient's age in years ÷ 4 to estimate the appropriate tube size.[1]

    - Have available an endotracheal tube that is 0.5 mm smaller and 0.5 mm larger than the estimated tube size.

  - Determine the depth of endotracheal tube insertion.[5] The formula for estimating oral endotracheal tube depth (length of tube at the lip) is:

    - Newborn (>2 kg to 5 kg)   9 to 10 cm

    - 6 months   11 cm

    - 1 year   12 cm

    - Older than 1 year of age   12 +1/2 age in years = cm length at the tip

    - The length-based resuscitation tape includes information on estimated depth of endotracheal tube insertion (length of tube at lip) for each weight grouping.

- If a stylet is used, it must not extend past the distal tip of the endotracheal tube:
    - Lubricate the stylet before insertion into the tube to assist with removal.[3]
    - Never use the stylet to force the endotracheal tube into the trachea.[3]
    - Cooling the tube prior to use may eliminate the need for a stylet.
- Have suctioning equipment available and ready. A tonsil tip suction and appropriate-sized suction kits that are compatible with the endotracheal tube size should be available.
- Prepare medications, as indicated.

- Assist with the intubation procedure:
    - Place the child on a cardiac monitor, pulse oximeter, and noninvasive blood pressure monitor.
    - Ensure that the child is well oxygenated prior to the intubation attempt.
        - Apply cricoid pressure, as indicated.
        - Ventilate using a bag-valve-mask device with reservoir and 100% oxygen prior to the intubation attempt.
    - Administer medications if rapid sequence induction is being used.
    - Monitor the child's heart rate, oxygen saturation, and color continuously during the intubation.
        - Avoid prolonged intubation attempts. Intubation attempts lasting longer than 30 seconds can result in profound hypoxia.[1]
        - If the heart rate or pulse oximeter begins to decrease, or pallor or cyanosis is observed, interrupt the intubation attempt and ventilate the child with a bag-valve-mask device and 100% oxygen. Young infants are particularly sensitive to decreases in oxygen saturation and vagal stimulation, resulting in a precipitous drop in heart rate.

- Confirm endotracheal tube placement:
    - Observe for bilateral symmetric chest rise and fall.
    - Auscultate for breath sounds bilaterally at the midaxillary areas and epigastrium. Compare the pitch, intensity, and location of sounds:
        - Listen for low-pitched gurgling and observe for distention of the epigastrium with ventilation, which indicates esophageal intubation.
        - Observe for clinical signs of improvement (e.g., color, perfusion, oxygen saturation).
        - When available, use an end-tidal CO_2 detector to confirm tube placement. In arrest situations, CO_2 may not be detected even when the tube is placed correctly in the trachea because of a lack of pulmonary circulation.
        - Obtain a chest radiograph to confirm endotracheal tube position.
        - Record the position of the endotracheal tube at the level of the gum, lip, or teeth.

- Secure the endotracheal tube. A suggested method to tape the tube (see Figure 18) is as follows[6]:

  - Cut two pieces of 1-inch-wide tape (approximately 6 inches in length). Cut or tear the pieces in half lengthwise for approximately 4 inches (leave an intact 2-inch length that remains the full width).

  - Lightly paint the upper lip, cheeks, and endotracheal tube with tincture of benzoin. Avoid contact with mucous membranes.

  - Apply the intact piece of adhesive tape to the cheek and adhere one length of the torn portion across the upper lip.

  - Wrap the second length of the torn portion around the tube at least two or three times.

  - Apply the second strip in a similar fashion from the opposite direction and the other cheek.

  - Document the location of the endotracheal tube at the lip or gum line.

- Maintain endotracheal tube placement by:

  - Restraining the child's arms with soft restraints.

  - Administering medications, as indicated.

  - Applying towel rolls laterally to the head to maintain the head in the midline.

- Suction the endotracheal tube as needed to maintain patency:

  - Use sterile technique to reduce the likelihood of airway contamination.[1]

  - The suction device should provide a vacuum of more than −300 mm Hg when the tube is clamped. However, −80 to −120 mm Hg is usually the maximum vacuum needed when an infant or child is suctioned.[7]

Figure 18
SECURING AN ENDOTRACHEAL TUBE

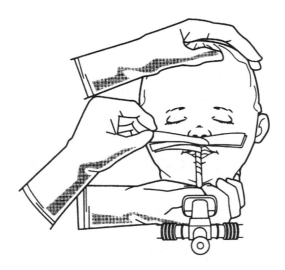

From French JP. Oxygenation and ventilation. In: French JP, ed. *Pediatric Emergency Skills*. St. Louis, Mo: Mosby-Year Book; 1995:118. Reprinted with permission.

- Tracheal suction catheters should have a Y-piece, T-piece, or lateral opening between the suction tube and the suction power control.[1]

- Insert the suction catheter, without suction applied, to a length just beyond the end of the endotracheal tube. Apply suction for no longer than 5 seconds as the catheter is withdrawn using a rotating, twisting motion.[1]

- Ventilate the child with 100% oxygen before and after suctioning to avoid hypoxemia.

- Monitor the child for the development of bradycardia, decreased oxygen saturation, and changes in skin color during the procedure.

Rapid Sequence Induction

Rapid sequence induction is endotracheal intubation performed following the administration of selected sedative/hypnotics, analgesics, and neuromuscular blocking agents. The induction of sedation or general anesthesia and paralysis is used in both emergent and elective intubation in children. Table 14 describes the procedure and medications commonly used. The following are considerations for rapid sequence induction:

- Rapid sequence induction can and should be done on children even if they are unresponsive.

- The medications and sequence will be influenced by the patient's hemodynamic status and condition (e.g., head trauma versus respiratory distress).

- Specific medications and sequence may vary among institution, physician, and protocols.

- Ensure that all supplies, equipment, and personnel are prepared prior to the administration of the medications.

- Monitor the patient for effects of the medications. The procedure sequence and physiologic monitoring are as described for endotracheal intubation.

- Someone skilled in pediatric intubation should perform the intubation procedure.

RESPIRATORY INTERVENTIONS

Oxygen Delivery

Supplemental oxygen should be administered to any child who has a patent airway and is in respiratory distress. Because children have fewer and smaller alveoli than adults, oxygen reserves can be rapidly depleted. The oxygen delivery method chosen should deliver the concentration most appropriate for the patient's condition and oxygen need. Table 15 provides an overview of oxygen delivery methods utilized in the emergency care setting.

Table 14

TECHNIQUE FOR RAPID SEQUENCE INDUCTION

1. Obtain all necessary equipment: Bag-valve-mask device, laryngoscope, suction equipment, endotracheal tubes and stylet, oxygen equipment, and resuscitation medications. Place the child on a cardiac monitor and pulse oximeter.[8]

2. In the spontaneously breathing child, preoxygenate with high-flow oxygen for 4 to 5 minutes using a nonrebreather mask.[8]

3. If the child is hypoventilating or apneic, hyperventilate with a bag-valve-mask with 100% oxygen. Perform cricoid pressure to decrease the possibility of aspiration.[9]

4. The following drugs may be used (the exact drugs and the order in which they are administered will vary by institution):
   a. Pancuronium bromide (Pavulon): Neuromuscular blocking agent, administered to decrease fasciculation if succinylcholine chloride will be used. This step is not necessary in children younger than 5 years of age.[3,10]
   b. Atropine sulfate: Indicated in children younger than 7 years of age to decrease the development of bradycardia.[10] Atropine sulfate will reduce secretions if ketamine is used.[9]
   c. Lidocaine hydrochloride: Indicated in children with increased intracranial pressure because it blunts the systemic and intracranial hypertension associated with endotracheal intubation and suctioning.[3,11]
   d. Thiopental (Pentothal): Short-acting sedative/amnestic agent that produces general anesthesia; contraindicated in the presence of hypotension (may cause hypotension) and status asthmaticus.[11] Thiopental is indicated in cases of isolated head injury (without hypotension) because the drug lowers intracranial pressure.[11] Has no analgesic properties.[3]
   e. Midazolam hydrochloride (Versed): Short-acting sedative/amnestic agent. Used as an alternative to thiopental if hypovolemia exists. Has no analgesic properties.[3]
   f. Ketamine (Ketalar): Sedative/amnestic agent; contraindicated in children with increased intracranial pressure or ocular injury.[3,9] Indicated in children with hypotension and/or hypovolemia (without head injury) and asthma.[8] Atropine sulfate may help to diminish the increased secretions that occur with ketamine.[9]
   g. Succinylcholine chloride (Anectine): Neuromuscular blocking agent/depolarizing muscle relaxant.[11] Administer 1 to 3 minutes after pancuronium bromide.[8] Contraindicated in the presence of neuromuscular disease, significant ocular injury, burns, spinal cord injury, increased intracranial pressure, hyperkalemia, or more than 24 hours after major injury.[3,9] Side effects include hyperkalemia and significant cardiac dysrhythmias. Premedication with atropine sulfate may decrease the risk of bradycardia.[9] No longer used in routine intubation in children.[3]
   h. Vecuronium bromide (Norcuron): Neuromuscular blocking agent/nondepolarizing muscle relaxant.[3] Action differs from other nondepolarizing agents. Vecuronium bromide does not release histamine, which may dilate the cerebral vasculature, elevate intracranial pressure, and decrease systemic blood pressure and cerebral perfusion pressure.[12]
   i. Additional medications include diazepam (sedative/amnestic agent) and fentanyl citrate (Sublimaze).[9] Both medications will help control discomfort and the development of increased intracranial pressure in response to endotracheal intubation.[11]

5. Orally intubate the child, verify the position, and release cricoid pressure. Consider the insertion of a nasogastric or orogastric tube following the intubation procedure.

6. Provide continued sedation as needed.[8]

Table 15

| | | | OVERVIEW OF OXYGEN DELIVERY METHODS | | |

Device	Flow Rate	Concentration Delivered	Considerations
Nonrebreather mask	12 to 15 liters/ minute	60 to 90%	• Used in spontaneously breathing patients who require highest concentration of oxygen available such as those in respiratory distress and shock. • Need to assure adequate flow rate to keep reservoir bag inflated. • With a snug fit, delivers highest oxygen concentration available by mask. • Pediatric- and adult-sized masks available. • Partial rebreathers are used in neonates. • Requires humidification.
Nasal cannula	1 to 6 liters/minute	Up to 50%	• Least restrictive. • Does not require humidification. • Used in infants and children on home oxygen therapy. • To avoid frightening the child, slowly start the flow of oxygen after the cannula is secured.
Simple face mask	6 to 10 liters/ minute	35 to 60%	• Infant-, pediatric-, and adult-sized masks available. • Adequate minimum flow rate should be used to flush the mask. • Requires humidification.
Blow-by oxygen	6 to 10 liters/ minute	Dependent on flow rate and proximity to face	• Indicated for infant or young child requiring oxygen who will not tolerate an oxygen mask on the face. • Start the oxygen flow through a simple mask, corrugated tubing, or O_2 tubing threaded through the bottom of a cup. Hold the delivery device as close to the child's nose and mouth as tolerated.
Oxygen hood	10 to 15 liters/ minute	Up to 90%	• Minimum rate of 10 liters/minute. Rate $\geq$10 liters/minute required to assure carbon dioxide flushed from inside hood. • Oxygen concentration can be continuously monitored via meter. • Can achieve high concentrations of oxygen (80% to 90% with high flow rates).[13] Used in neonates and young infants <10 kg who will not tolerate a mask on the face. • Requires humidification.
Bag-valve-mask device with a reservoir	15 liters/minute	100%	• Choose correct-sized mask and bag-valve device. • Mask should fit snugly and have a small under-mask volume to decrease dead space.

Gaining Cooperation

Children may be frightened and/or resist the application of an oxygen mask directly on the face. It is important to gain the child's cooperation through explanation and a nonthreatening approach:

- Allow the child to hold the mask before placing it on the face and allow him or her to feel the oxygen flow.

- Gain cooperation by describing the mask as a "space mask" or a Santa Claus beard (nonrebreather).[13]

- Use stickers or other age-appropriate distraction techniques.

- If a child struggles against having a mask directly on the face, do not force the child to wear the mask. Use blow-by technique with a higher flow rate if the child will not tolerate the mask being placed directly on the face.

Sizing and Securing the Oxygen Delivery Device

Correct sizing of the oxygen delivery device is important for the patient's comfort and accurate delivery of the desired oxygen concentration:

- Select a mask that extends from the bridge of the nose to the cleft of the chin. The correctly sized mask fits tightly without placing excessive pressure on the eyes.[2]

- Place the mask over the child's face, starting from the nose downward, and adjust the nose clip and head strap.[2]

- Secure a nasal cannula to the child's face by using a transparent occlusive dressing on each cheek.

Administering Inhaled Agents to Children

- Nebulized pharmacologic agents:

  - Indicated for children with respiratory distress from a lower airway disease (e.g., asthma or reactive airway disease).

  - Obtain an apical heart rate and respiratory rate prior to administering the treatment. If the child's heart rate exceeds the normal limits for age, notify the physician.

  - Assess the child's respiratory status, including level of consciousness, work of breathing, and breath sounds, before and after the aerosol treatment.

  - Dilute medication with normal saline to a total volume of 3 ml.

  - Deliver with at least a 6 liters/minute continuous flow of oxygen.

  - Encourage the caregiver to hold the infant or younger child to facilitate administration of the treatment.

  - Have the child breathe through his or her mouth using the mouthpiece or mask.

  - Monitor the child during and following the treatment for any changes in the child's condition.

- Metered-dose inhaler:

  - Typically used in children older than 2 years of age but can be used in infants with a face mask.

  - Always use with an aerosol chamber or "spacer."

  - Allow several breaths between medication delivery puffs.

  - The technique is extremely important in assuring delivery of the medication. Therefore, two adults may be required to secure the mask and deliver the medication.

  - Obtain an apical heart rate and respiratory rate prior to administering the medication.

  - Assess the child's respiratory status, including level of consciousness, work of breathing, and breath sounds, before and after the delivery of the medication.

DIAGNOSTIC TESTS AND MONITORING

Peak Expiratory Flow (PEF) Measurements

Results can be categorized using traffic light metaphors for a home plan of care[14]:

- Green zone – Greater than 80% predicted best result = no additional therapy is required.

- Yellow zone – 50 to 80% of predicted best result = additional, immediate therapy is required.

- Red zone – Less than 50% predicted best result = serious exacerbation and emergency care is required.[14]

Pulse Oximetry

Pulse oximetry is a diagnostic tool used to measure the percent of hemoglobin saturated with oxygen. Pulse oximetry is used to monitor oxygenation status during procedures, monitor clinical condition, and evaluate response to therapy.[15] There are several important points to remember about pulse oximetry:

- Readings must be interpreted in relation to the patient's clinical status.

- Poor perfusion and/or vasoconstriction will also effect the reliability of the reading.[15]

- Evaluate the correlation of the pulse signal reading on the oximeter to the patient's apical heart rate:

  - Poor correlation may indicate an inaccurate saturation reading.

  - Ensure that the sensor probe is functioning properly; replace probe as needed.

End-Tidal CO_2 Monitoring

End-tidal CO_2 monitoring is most commonly used in the emergency care setting to monitor intubated patients via a mainstream end-tidal CO_2 analyzer or a disposable CO_2 detection device.[16] End-tidal CO_2 readings are used to:

- Detect inadvertent displacement of the endotracheal tube or placement of the endotracheal tube in the esophagus.

- Monitor effectiveness of cardiopulmonary resuscitation.

- Monitor selected patients when ventilation is being controlled (e.g., head trauma).

Endotracheal tube placement must always be confirmed clinically. The end-tidal CO_2 device is used as an adjunct to confirm placement and monitor the patient's ventilations.[16] Side-stream sampling methods may be used in nonintubated patients to monitor end-tidal CO_2 during conscious or deep sedation.

Points to Remember:

- Administer oxygen and aerosol treatments by any method the anxious child will tolerate.

- Allow the child to assume a position of comfort to facilitate breathing and decrease agitation.

- Always have appropriate-sized airway equipment available if the child is exhibiting signs of respiratory distress. The equipment should accompany the child during transport within the hospital.

- Treat primary respiratory arrest with ventilation and oxygen first.

- When breathing is ineffective or a respiratory arrest occurs, always perform bag-valve-mask ventilation prior to intubation.

- Administer 100% oxygen prior to intubation procedures.

REFERENCES

1. Chameides L, Hazinski MF. *Textbook of Pediatric Advanced Life Support.* Dallas, Tex: American Heart Association; 1997.

2. Manley LK. Procedures involving the respiratory system. In: Bernardo LM, Bove MA, eds. *Pediatric Emergency Nursing Procedures.* Boston, Mass: Jones & Bartlett; 1993:63-81.

3. Yaster M, Maxwell LG. Airway management. In Nichols DG, Yaster M, Lappe DG, Haller JA, eds. *Golden Hour: The Handbook of Advanced Pediatric Life Support.* 2nd ed. St. Louis, Mo: Mosby-Year Book; 1996:9-57.

4. Lubitz D, Seidel J, Chameides L, Luten R, Zaritsky A, Campbell F. A rapid method for estimating weight and resuscitation drug dosages from length in the pediatric age group. *Ann Emerg Med.* 1988;17:576-581.

5. Hauersperger KR. *Pediatric Emergency and Critical Care Handbook.* Columbus, Ohio: Children's Hospital; 1998.

6. Zander J, Hazinski MF. Pulmonary disorders. In: Hazinski MF, ed. *Nursing Care of the Critically Ill Child.* 2nd ed. St. Louis, Mo: Mosby-Year Book; 1992:423.

7. Emergency Cardiac Care Committee and Subcommittees, American Heart Association. Guidelines for cardiopulmonary resuscitation and emergency cardiac care. *JAMA.* 1992;268:2276-2281.

8. Yamamoto LG, Yim GK, Britten AG. Rapid sequence anesthesia induction for emergency intubation. *Pediatr Emerg Care.* 1990;6:200-213.

9. Aoki BY, McCloskey K. *Evaluation, Stabilization, and Transport of the Critically Ill Child.* St. Louis, Mo: Mosby-Year Book; 1992:412-413.

10. Fitzmaurice L. Approach to multiple trauma. In: Barkin RM, ed. *Pediatric Emergency Medicine.* St. Louis, Mo: Mosby-Year Book; 1992:183.

11. Nakayama DK, Waggoner T, Venkataraman ST, Gardner M, Lynch JM, Orr RA. The use of drugs in emergency airway management in pediatric trauma. *Ann Surg.* 1992;216:205-211.

12. Lennon RL, Olson RA, Gronert GA. Atracurium or vecuronium for rapid sequence endotracheal intubation. *Anesthesiology.* 1986;64:510-513.

13. Thomas D. Tips for oxygen administration in the child. In: Thomas D, ed. *Quick Reference to Pediatric Emergency Nursing.* Rockville, Md: Aspen Publishers; 1991:98.

14. US Department of Health and Human Services. *Guidelines for the Diagnosis and Management of Asthma. National Asthma Education Program. Expert Panel Report 2.* Washington, DC: National Institutes of Health; 1997.

15. Fuerst RS. Use of pulse oximetry. In: Henreitig FM, King C, eds. *Textbook of Pediatric Emergency Procedures.* Baltimore, Md: Williams & Wilkins; 1997:823-828.

16. Gonzalez del Ray JA. End-tidal CO_2 monitoring. In: Henreitig FM, King C, eds. *Textbook of Pediatric Emergency Procedures.* Baltimore, Md: Williams & Wilkins; 1997:829-837.

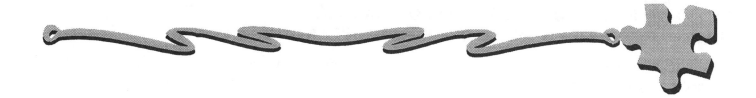

CHAPTER 6

Pediatric Trauma

OBJECTIVES

On completion of this lecture, the learner should be able to:

✦ Identify the anatomic and physiologic characteristics of the pediatric trauma patient as a basis for the signs and symptoms associated with trauma.

✦ Identify the causes, types, mechanisms, and patterns of injury associated with pediatric trauma.

✦ Identify the appropriate nursing diagnoses and expected outcomes based on the assessment findings.

✦ Delineate the specific interventions needed to care for the pediatric trauma patient.

✦ Evaluate the effectiveness of nursing interventions related to patient outcome.

✦ Identify health promotion strategies related to pediatric trauma.

INTRODUCTION

Trauma has a greater impact on morbidity and mortality than any other disease. Each year nearly one child in four receives treatment for an injury.[1] Approximately 21,000 people, 0 to 24 years of age, are killed each year by preventable injuries.[2] Almost 22 million children are injured each year, and 600,000 of these children require hospitalization.[3] Common mechanisms of injury are motor vehicle crashes, bicycle crashes, auto-pedestrian incidents, drowning, firearms, burns, and falls. In Australia, injury and poisoning are the leading causes of death in people 1 to 44 years of age. These deaths are attributed to motor vehicle crashes, suicide, falls, drowning, poisoning, burns, suffocation, and choking.[4]

ANATOMIC, PHYSIOLOGIC, AND DEVELOPMENTAL CHARACTERISTICS AS A BASIS FOR SIGNS AND SYMPTOMS

The trauma nursing process associated with the care of the pediatric trauma patient is based on knowledge of pediatric anatomy and physiology and the child's response to injury. Inherent to this process is the recognition of the distinct anatomic and physiologic characteristics of the pediatric patient.[5]

Cardiovascular Characteristics

- Children have a healthy cardiovascular system and the physiologic ability to initially compensate for hypovolemia.

- It is critical to remember that hypotension related to hypovolemia in the pediatric trauma patient is a late sign and may indicate a loss of at least 25% of the circulating blood volume.

Temperature Regulation

- Children have a less mature thermoregulatory mechanism.

- Children are susceptible to heat loss because of their high ratio of body surface area to body mass, large head in proportion to the rest of their body, and small amount of subcutaneous tissue.

- Hypothermia can impede the child's response to resuscitative measures.

- Factors that can lead to hypothermia in the pediatric trauma patient include:

  - Prehospital environmental exposure.

  - Leaving the child uncovered for even a short period of time.

  - Cool ambient temperature of emergency vehicle and trauma room.

  - Wet or moist dressings.

  - Fluid-saturated clothing from blood, secretions, vomitus, perspiration, or other causes.

  - Poor perfusion status.

Other Anatomic and Physiologic Characteristics

- The infant and child's center of gravity is higher. The center of gravity in the infant is at vertebral level T-11 to T-12, while in the adult it is at L-4 to L-5. Because of their higher center of gravity and underdeveloped muscles, it is more difficult for toddlers to keep their balance.[6]

- The head is large and heavy, and the neck muscles are weak, predisposing the child to head and neck trauma.

- The protruberant abdomen, immature abdominal muscles, and small pelvis of the child offer little protection to the underlying solid and hollow organs. Therefore, abdominal organs are prone to injury.[6]

- The cranium is thin and more pliable in young children.

Developmental Characteristics

Children are prone to injury because of psychosocial and cognitive aspects of development:

- Children are easily distracted, impulsive, have little concept of danger, and lack experience with similar situations.

- Children have difficulty determining the speed or the distance of an oncoming vehicle.

- Children have difficulty localizing sound and their visual field tends to focus on a single object similar to their own height.[6]

- They often believe that, because they see the car, the driver must see them.

CAUSES, TYPES, MECHANISMS, AND PATTERNS OF INJURY IN CHILDREN

Blunt Injuries

Isolated and multisystem injury may occur with blunt trauma. Injury occurs first to the outer skin and soft tissue and then to the underlying structures. Initially, injury to one or more solid organs may be obscured in the pediatric patient.[1] Therefore, cautious evaluation with a high index of suspicion for injury is required for all children with blunt trauma.

MOTOR VEHICLE CRASHES

The largest number of trauma deaths in children are the result of motor vehicle crashes. During a motor vehicle crash, four separate collisions occur.[6] The first collision occurs when the vehicle strikes another object. Even though the vehicle has decelerated or stopped, the body continues to travel at the original speed. The second is the collision of the body with something in the car. The third collision involves the organs striking other organs, muscle, bone, or other supporting structures. The fourth collision will occur if there are loose objects in the vehicle that become projectile forces.

Head trauma is a common injury for unrestrained children involved in a motor vehicle crash.[7] Until 9 or 10 years of age, the head is significantly larger in proportion to the remainder of the child's body. When an unrestrained child is involved in a motor vehicle crash, the large head acts like a missile, leading the torso throughout the vehicle cabin. Children who are front-seat passengers are at risk for hitting the dashboard with significant force. In a front-end crash at approximately 30 mph, an unrestrained child will hit the dashboard with the same force as the impact of falling three stories to a solid surface. Although mechanisms of pediatric injury vary, the part of the child's body that most commonly comes in contact with an unyielding object is the head.

Most states within the United States have mandated the use of car seats for young children. Regardless of geographic region, compliance and proper use of pediatric safety restraint devices continue to be problematic. Participation in safety restraint education programs is important for all health care workers who care for children.

Improper use of restraint systems can also lead to injury. These patterns of injury vary by the child's size, location in the vehicle, and the type and method of restraint used. The infant has a higher center of gravity. During a motor vehicle crash, infants have a greater risk of cervical fracture at the level of C-1 to C-3 when in a safety restraint seat that is positioned facing forward in the vehicle. Placement of the infant in a rear-facing restraint seat, secured in the rear seat of the vehicle, can potentially prevent this type of injury by minimizing the fulcrum effect of the infant's head whipping forward.

The use of lap belts in children has been associated with severe flexion-distraction injuries of the lumbar spine and hollow viscous injury. However, the use of lap belts has been proven to decrease the fatal injuries that could be sustained. The use of a shoulder belt and lap belt is even more effective in decreasing the incidence of injury.[8]

AIR BAG INJURIES

Air bags are standard equipment in almost all new cars and are designed to supplement the protection provided by safety belts in frontal crashes. Federal safety standards require that all new passenger cars and light trucks be equipped with both driver- and passenger-side air bags by 1999. Although air bags have a good overall safety record and have saved an estimated 1,200 lives as of the end of 1995, they pose several risks for children. Children who are unbelted, improperly belted, or are too close to the dashboard when an air bag inflates are at risk for injury. Because of an increasing number of child deaths related to air bag deployment, individualized deactivation measures are being explored.

The inflating air bag can violently impact the child with such force that it may injure or even kill the child. Injuries associated with air bag deployment include facial trauma, upper extremity fracture, intra-abdominal injury, abrasions and chemical irritation of the skin or eyes, cervical spine injury, and partial to complete decapitation.

To ensure that children ride safely, NHTSA recommends the following:

- Never place a rear-facing infant safety seat in the front seat of the vehicle with a front passenger-side air bag.

- Infants younger than 1 year of age and weighing less than 9 kg (20 lbs) must always ride in a rear-facing infant safety seat.[9]

- The rear seat is the safest place for children of any age to ride.

PEDESTRIAN INJURIES

In the United States, a pedestrian struck by a car is more likely to sustain left-sided injuries because cars are driven on the right side of the road. Head and musculoskeletal injuries are most prevalent. The abdominal structures most commonly injured, listed in the order of frequency, are the spleen, genitourinary system, gastrointestinal tract, liver, pancreas, pelvis, and major vessels.[10] Preschool children may be injured when they play around parked cars. Older children may be injured while running across the street.[11] Pedestrians who are struck by automobiles often have one or more injuries.[12,13] The biomechanics of the child pedestrian who is struck by a vehicle include the following:

- Classically, the injuries occur as the child impacts the vehicle and is thrown away from the vehicle. The child's body becomes a projectile, led by the head, which hits the ground and results in a head injury.

- Toddlers and preschoolers may be knocked down and dragged under the vehicle. The vehicle's front bumper may cause chest, abdomen, pelvic, or femur injuries.

- Older preschool-aged and school-aged children may sustain femur fractures from the bumper and chest injuries from the hood.

- If the child is thrown onto the hood of the vehicle and strikes the windshield, head and facial injuries may occur. When the car decelerates or stops, the child slides or rolls to the street, usually striking his or her head on the pavement.

Children struck by motor vehicles are at high risk for multisystem injury. The pattern of injury sustained is dependent on the relationship among variables, such as the speed of the vehicle, point of initial impact, additional points of impact, the child's height and weight, and landing surfaces. A thorough trauma assessment is essential to identify all injuries.

FALLS

Falls account for more than one third of childhood injuries requiring medical evaluation. The factors that contribute to the injuries sustained from a fall include the velocity of the fall, the child's body orientation at the time of impact, the type of impact surface, and the time that the force is applied to the body on impact.[14] In early childhood, children are prone to falls because of their higher center of gravity, increased mobility, and a limited perception of danger.

- Infants more commonly sustain falls from low objects, such as high chairs, baby walkers, shopping carts, countertops, changing tables, beds, and tables.

- Toddlers and preschoolers sustain falls from low objects. However, they are at increased risk for falls from heights such as windows, balconies, and stairs.

- The school-aged child is often involved in a fall related to a sports or recreational activity such as tree climbing, bicycling, playground equipment, skating, and organized sports activities.

RECREATIONAL INJURIES

Injuries related to sports are responsible for a significant number of ED visits. Those sports responsible for the highest number of emergency visits are basketball, bicycle riding, football, baseball, and softball. Roller skating and soccer injuries are also common.[2] The injuries that occur from these sports include extremity injuries, head trauma, abdominal injury particularly in football and soccer, and spinal cord or vertebral column injury.

Bicycle-related injuries have risen in recent years. Approximately 653,675 people were treated in 1996 for bicycle-related injuries.[2] The most common injury related to bicycle incidents is head trauma.[15] One fourth of injured bicyclists treated in the emergency department have sustained head trauma.[16] This includes skull fractures, concussions, and subdural hematomas. The use of bicycle helmets has reduced the mortality related to bicycle incidents; however, compliance with wearing a helmet is reported at only 5%.[16] Compliance with wearing a helmet is enhanced by state legislation and municipal enforcement. Blunt abdominal trauma, including pancreatic injury, small bowel injury, and solid-organ injury, has been reported with bicycle incidents.

The resurgence of skateboarding has been linked to an increase in extremity and head injuries. It was estimated that approximately 35,750 people were treated in the emergency department in 1996 for skateboarding injuries.[2] Of these injuries, 74% were injuries to an extremity and 21% were injuries to the head or neck. The 5- to 14-year-old age group is most frequently injured.[17] The pattern of injury differs, depending on the age and size of the child. Younger children more commonly sustain head trauma because of their higher center of gravity and limited ability to break the fall. Older children usually sustain extremity trauma as they try to break their fall. Death from skateboarding injuries most commonly occurs when the child collides with a motor vehicle.[18]

Snowboarding is popular in many areas of the world. One study reported the age range of snowboarders to be 10 to 48 years of age with a mean age of 19.8 years.[19] The injuries associated with snowboarding include upper extremity injuries, particularly fractures and shoulder dislocations; concussion; spinal strain; abdominal injury; and lower extremity injuries. Injuries to the upper extremity are the most common.[19] In contrast, skiers have a higher incidence of lower extremity injury. Skiing injuries often are related to the collision of two skiers or with a stationary object. These collisions can result in severe injuries to the head, chest, or abdomen.

The use of personal watercrafts has increased in recent years. A personal watercraft is less than 4 meters (13 feet) in length and allows the person operating the craft to sit, stand, or kneel on the craft rather than being confined within a hull. Approximately 7.4% of children between 0 and 14 years of age sustain personal watercraft-related injuries each year. In the 1- to 24-year-old age group, approximately 38% sustained injuries. The injuries sustained, listed in order of frequency, occur to the leg, head, and lower trunk. Lacerations and contusions are the most common injuries. Additional injuries include fractures, internal injuries, and dental and joint injuries.[20]

Asphyxiation and Submersion Injuries

ASPHYXIATION

Asphyxiation and suffocation are among the leading causes of death in children; they may result from inhalation injuries sustained during a fire, mechanical suffocation, foreign-body obstruction or inhalation, or hanging. In addition to the hypoxia sustained during a hanging injury, the child may also sustain a spinal cord injury, cerebral injury, laryngeal edema, and pulmonary edema. Vertebral injury is uncommon in hanging incidents.

SUBMERSION

Drowning is a common cause of death in the pediatric patient.[21] About 40 to 50% of deaths related to drowning occur in children 1 to 4 years of age.[21] In Australia, 26% of drowning deaths occurred in children 0 to 4 years of age. Overall, drowning accounted for 36% of injury deaths of Australian children 0 to 4 years of age.[4] Drowning is not isolated to pools and ponds but may occur in bathtubs, buckets, or water that is greater than 1 or 2 inches in depth. Males drown three times more often than females.[22]

Near-drowning is defined as survival or temporary survival following asphyxia caused by submersion episode.[21] Immersion in water with ice is associated with a better outcome than prolonged immersion in warm or cold water without ice. The length of time the child is submerged and the water quality will affect the length of resuscitation and the outcome.

Although the pathophysiology differs, symptoms of near-drowning by salt or fresh water are similar. Large amounts of fluid are rarely aspirated. The signs and symptoms may be delayed in onset and are associated with cerebral hypoxia and pulmonary injury. These may vary in severity from minimal or no symptoms to cardiopulmonary arrest.

Penetrating Injury

The incidence of penetrating trauma in the pediatric population is rising. Penetrating trauma includes stabbing, firearm, and blast injuries. In 1996, there were approximately 10,600 deaths from firearms in the 1- to 24-year-old age group.[2] Firearms are the fourth leading cause of death in the 5- to 24-year-old age group.[2] The death rate is higher among males than females. The firearm death rate for teenagers 15 to 19 years of age rose 77% between 1985 and 1990. In the 10- to 14-year-old age group, the death rate increased 18%.[23]

The injuries sustained from a penetrating force will depend on the location of the impact and the type of penetrating object. With firearms, the amount of tissue damage is related to the projectile, mass, shape, fragmentation, type of tissue struck, and the striking velocity. The injury sustained from a stab wound is dependent on the length of the instrument, the velocity at which the force was applied, and the angle of entry.

NURSING CARE OF THE PEDIATRIC TRAUMA PATIENT

Primary Assessment

The primary assessment consists of assessment of the airway and simultaneous stabilization of the cervical spine, breathing, circulation, and neurologic status. Interventions to correct any life-threatening conditions are performed before the assessment is continued. Refer to Chapter 4, "Initial Assessment and Triage," for a review of a comprehensive primary assessment. Assessment and intervention components unique to the primary assessment of the pediatric trauma patient are delineated in the following section.

AIRWAY

- Open the airway while manually stabilizing the spine if the child is unconscious. The jaw thrust must be done to manually open the airway and avoid manipulation of the neck. Adequate assessment of the airway of an unconscious patient cannot be accomplished unless the airway is opened first using a jaw thrust maneuver. (Nursing diagnoses: Ineffective airway clearance; aspiration).

- Assess the child's airway while maintaining cervical spine stabilization or immobilization. (Nursing diagnosis: Injury, risk).

    - If the child is not immobilized on arrival, initiate manual cervical spine stabilization by holding the head in a neutral position.

- Cervical spine immobilization includes holding the head in a neutral position, placing bilateral support devices, and using tape to secure the head and the devices. Do not hyperextend, flex, or rotate the neck during these maneuvers. If immediately available, apply a rigid collar before applying the head supports and tape. The child's body movement must be controlled before the head is secured. The tape must extend to the backboard, if present, or to the stretcher, if not.

- Because infants and young children have a large occiput, positioning them supine on a backboard causes their cervical vertebrae to flex and move anteriorly. Flexion may contribute to airway compromise or decreased effectiveness of the jaw thrust or chin lift maneuvers. To provide neutral alignment of the cervical spine, padding is placed under the child's shoulders to bring the shoulders into horizontal alignment with the external auditory meatus.[24]

- If the child is already in a rigid cervical collar and strapped to a backboard, do *not* remove any devices. Check that the devices are placed appropriately.

- Complete spinal immobilization includes cervical immobilization, as defined above, with the application of a backboard and straps or tape across the body.

- Complete spinal immobilization with a backboard and straps must be done at the completion of the secondary assessment, depending on the degree of resuscitation required and the availability of team members. Refer to Pediatric Considerations: Cervical and Spinal Immobilization, Spinal Immobilization at the end of Chapter 6.

- Any child whose mechanisms of injury, symptoms, or physical findings suggest a possible spinal injury must be stabilized or immobilized.

- Position the patient in a supine position. (Nursing diagnoses: Ineffective airway clearance; aspiration; ineffective breathing pattern).

  - If the patient is not already supine, logroll the patient onto his or her back while maintaining cervical spine stabilization.

  - If the patient is awake and breathing, he or she may have assumed a position that maximizes the ability to breathe. Before proceeding with cervical spine stabilization be sure that interventions do *not* compromise the child's breathing status.

  - Remove helmet while maintaining cervical spine stabilization.

- Clear and maintain the airway. (Nursing diagnosis: Ineffective airway clearance).

  - Suction the airway if blood, vomitus, or secretions are present.

  - A nasopharyngeal airway may be inserted if the child is conscious and without evidence of facial trauma or basilar skull fracture.

  - An oropharyngeal airway may be inserted if the child is unconscious.

- Consider endotracheal intubation for definitive airway control for patients who require manual positioning to maintain a patent airway or meet other intubation criteria. (Nursing diagnosis: Aspiration).

  - Because of the differences in pediatric anatomy, maintaining the airway of the child who is immobilized on a backboard is more difficult. Intubation must be performed without manipulation of the cervical spine.

- Preoxygenate the child prior to endotracheal intubation. If the child demonstrates ineffective or absent breathing, ventilate the child with a bag-valve-mask and 100% oxygen prior to endotracheal intubation.

- Rapid sequence induction technique may be needed.

BREATHING

- Administer oxygen via a nonrebreather mask to all multiple trauma patients. A flow rate of 12 to 15 liters/minute is required to keep the reservoir bag of the nonrebreather mask inflated. All multiple trauma patients must receive supplemental oxygen until a complete assessment of the oxygenation and perfusion status is completed. (Nursing diagnoses: Ineffective breathing pattern; impaired gas exchange).

- Prepare for and assist with needle thoracentesis if a tension pneumothorax is present or evident. (Nursing diagnosis: Ineffective breathing pattern).

- Apply an occlusive dressing taped on three sides if an open pneumothorax is present. (Nursing diagnosis: Ineffective breathing pattern).

CIRCULATION

- Control any uncontrolled external bleeding. (Nursing diagnoses: Fluid volume deficit; cardiac output, decreased; inadequate tissue perfusion).

  - Apply direct pressure over the bleeding site.

  - Elevate the extremity.

  - Apply pressure over arterial pressure points.

- Obtain peripheral vascular access and initiate infusions of lactated Ringer's solution or 0.9% normal saline, as indicated. Insert the largest bore catheter that the vessel can accommodate. (Nursing diagnoses: Fluid volume deficit; cardiac output, decreased; inadequate tissue perfusion).

- Establish two peripheral intravenous access sites in critically injured children:

  - If peripheral vascular access is unsuccessful after three quick attempts in less than 90 seconds, consider intraosseous infusion in critically injured children.[25,26]

  - If evidence of inadequate tissue perfusion is present, administer a 20 ml/kg fluid bolus of a crystalloid solution. Repeat the bolus if reassessment findings indicate inadequate tissue perfusion. If symptoms of shock persist, 10 ml/kg of warmed, packed type-specific or O-negative red blood cells may be administered.

- Fluids are administered as rapidly as possible, usually over 5 to 10 minutes, by use of a syringe and stopcock or by opening the flow rate mechanisms on the intravenous blood tubing and elevating the intravenous solution. (Nursing diagnoses: Fluid volume deficit; cardiac output, decreased; inadequate tissue perfusion). A pressure bag may be placed on the intravenous fluid bag to facilitate rapid administration:
  - If available, use a rapid infuser device, as indicated.
    - ◆ The child must weigh more 20 kg, therefore requiring a fluid bolus of approximately 500 ml.
    - ◆ A 20-gauge or larger intravenous catheter must be in place.
  - Use Y-tubing and normal saline when blood administration is anticipated.
- Prepare for and assist with emergency thoracotomy in the emergency department or resuscitation area. Emergency thoracotomies are rarely done for children and are associated with a dismal outcome. Indications for emergency thoracotomy are determined by patient history, patient presentation, and trauma protocol. (Nursing diagnoses: Fluid volume deficit; cardiac output, decreased).
- Obtain blood sample for typing.

DISABILITY

- If the disability assessment indicated a decreased level of consciousness, conduct further investigation during the secondary assessment. (Nursing diagnoses: Impaired gas exchange; altered tissue perfusion).
- Initiate pharmacologic therapy, as ordered. (Nursing diagnosis: Altered tissue perfusion).

Secondary Assessment

Refer to Chapter 4, "Initial Assessment and Triage," for a review of a comprehensive secondary assessment. The identification of multisystem injuries is a critical component of the secondary assessment of the pediatric trauma patient. Assessment and intervention components unique to the secondary trauma assessment are delineated in the following section.

EXPOSURE AND ENVIRONMENTAL CONTROL

- Any clothing that remains on the child must be cut away to allow a complete assessment of all body areas.
  - All clothing must be saved for forensic evidence, to identify the mechanism of injury or suspected injuries, or for the family.
  - Warming methods must be initiated to maintain a normothermic state. This includes a radiant warmer, warmed blankets, overbed warmer, warmed oxygen, and warmed intravenous fluids. (Nursing diagnosis: Hypothermia).

FULL SET OF VITAL SIGNS

- Palpate pulses and auscultate an apical pulse as a baseline rate. Compare bilateral peripheral pulses for strength and equality. There may be neurovascular compromise in an injured extremity; therefore, it is important to palpate pulses on an uninjured extremity when evaluating central perfusion.

- Auscultate an initial blood pressure. Blood pressure in a child may be normal despite significant blood loss. A noninvasive, automated blood pressure monitor must be used with caution on critically injured children. Some models are not accurate with extremely high or low blood pressures.[27]

- Obtain a temperature to monitor for hypothermia. The rectal route must be used in critically injured children unless otherwise contraindicated. This may be deferred until the posterior assessment when the child is logrolled.

FAMILY PRESENCE

- Involve the family as soon as possible in the resuscitation process.

- Facilitate family presence to support the child.

GIVE COMFORT MEASURES

- Initiate pain control measures as soon as possible, including:

  - Age-appropriate nonpharmacologic methods to facilitate coping.

  - Analgesics and other appropriate medications to control procedural pain and pain from injuries.

HEAD-TO-TOE ASSESSMENT

- Refer to Chapter 4, "Initial Assessment and Triage," for a description of the head-to-toe assessment.

HISTORY

- Obtain information from prehospital personnel, as indicated by the injury event. The MIVT mnemonic, which stands for Mechanism of injury, Injuries sustained, Vital signs, and Treatment, can be used.

  - Mechanism and pattern of injury:

    - If the mechanism of injury involved a motor vehicle crash, obtain information regarding the use of restraints, position in the vehicle, site of impact on the vehicle, vehicle speed, ejection, vehicle rollover, air bag deployment, and any fatalities in the vehicle.

    - If the mechanism of injury was penetrating trauma, the type of object should be identified.

- ♦ If the mechanism of injury was a fall, the height from which the child fell is important. Falls of more than three times the child's height are significant.

- ♦ The history for a child who is injured while riding a bicycle should include what the bicycle collided with, whether the child was run over, whether the child was thrown from the bicycle, use of a helmet, and any damage to the vehicle.

- ♦ For the child struck by a motor vehicle, obtain information regarding the speed the vehicle was traveling, whether the child was run over or caught under the vehicle, the type of surface it occurred on, and where on the body the child was struck.

- ■ Injuries suspected. Ask prehospital personnel to describe the patient's general condition, level of consciousness, and apparent injuries.

- ■ Vital signs in the prehospital environment.

- ■ Treatment initiated and patient responses.

INSPECT POSTERIOR SURFACES

- • Refer to Chapter 4, "Initial Assessment and Triage" for a description of posterior surfaces.

DIAGNOSTIC PROCEDURES

- • Indications for laboratory and radiographic studies are determined by the child's clinical presentation, pattern of injury, history, and specific institution protocols.

- • Initiate ongoing cardiac monitoring, pulse oximetry, and capnography monitoring as soon as possible, based on the child's condition.

Nursing Diagnoses, Interventions, and Expected Outcomes

NURSING DIAGNOSIS	INTERVENTIONS	EXPECTED OUTCOMES
Airway clearance, ineffective, related to: • Edema of the airway, vocal cords, epiglottis, and upper airway • Irritation of the respiratory tract • Laryngeal spasm • Altered level of consciousness secondary to hypoxia • Inability to remove oropharyngeal secretions • Fatigue • Pain	• Position supine • Open and clear the airway • Insert airway adjunct	The child will maintain a patent airway, as evidenced by: • Regular rate, depth, and pattern of breathing • Symmetric chest expansion • Effective cough and gag reflex • Absence of signs and symptoms of airway obstruction: Stridor, dyspnea, and hoarse voice • Clear sputum of normal amount without abnormal color or odor • Absence of signs and symptoms of retained secretions: Fever, tachycardia, and tachypnea

Aspiration, risk of, related to:
• Altered level of consciousness
• Impaired cough or gag reflex secondary to hypoxia
• Structural defect to head, face, or neck
• Secretions and debris in airway
	• Position supine
	• Open and clear the airway
	• Consider endotracheal intubation
	• Insert a gastric tube
	• Give nothing by mouth
		The child will not experience aspiration, as evidenced by:
		• Patent airway
		• Clear and equal breath sounds
		• Regular rate, depth, and pattern of breathing
		• ABG values within normal limits:
		  ■ PaO_2 80 to 100 mm Hg (10.0 to 13.3 KPa)
		  ■ SaO_2 >95%
		  ■ $PaCO_2$ 35 to 45 mm Hg (4.7 to 6.0 KPa)
		  ■ pH between 7.35 and 7.45
		• Chest radiograph without abnormality
		• Ability to handle secretions independently

Breathing pattern, ineffective, related to:
• Pain
• Musculoskeletal impairment
• Unstable chest wall segment
• Lung collapse
• Neurologic impairment
	• Position supine
	• Administer oxygen
	• Assist ventilations, if needed
	• Consider endotracheal intubation
	• Initiate cardiopulmonary resuscitation, if needed
	• Perform needle thoracentesis
	• Apply occlusive dressing taped on three sides
		The child will have an effective breathing pattern, as evidenced by:
		• Regular rate, depth, and pattern of breathing
		• Clear and equal breath sounds
		• Symmetric chest expansion
		• ABG values within normal limits:
		  ■ PaO_2 80 to 100 mm Hg (10.0 to 13.3 KPa)
		  ■ SaO_2 >95%
		  ■ $PaCO_2$ 35 to 45 mm Hg (4.7 to 6.0 KPa)
		  ■ pH between 7.35 and 7.45
		• Absence of stridor, dyspnea, or cyanosis
		• Trachea midline
		• Chest radiograph without abnormality
		• Absence of use of accessory muscles or nasal flaring

NURSING DIAGNOSIS	INTERVENTIONS	EXPECTED OUTCOMES

Gas exchange, impaired, related to:
• Ineffective breathing pattern
• Ineffective airway clearance
• Aspiration
• Shock
• Decreased ventilatory drive resulting from head injury
	• Administer oxygen
	• Assist ventilations, if needed
	• Consider endotracheal intubation
	• Investigate causes of altered consciousness
		The child will maintain adequate gas exchange, as evidenced by:
		• Oxygen saturation >95% by pulse oximetry
		• ABG values within normal limits:
		  ■ PaO_2 80 to 100 mm Hg (10.0 to 13.3 KPa)
		  ■ SaO_2 >95%
		  ■ $PaCO_2$ 35 to 45 mm Hg (4.7 to 6.0 KPa)
		  ■ pH between 7.35 and 7.45
		• Skin normal color, warm, and dry
		• Improved level of consciousness
		• Regular rate, depth, and pattern of breathing
		• Symmetric chest expansion
		• Clear and equal breath sounds

Fluid volume deficit related to: • Hemorrhage • Fluid shifts • Alteration in capillary permeability	• Control bleeding • Obtain vascular access and initiate fluid therapy • Administer fluid bolus • Initiate intraosseous access, if needed • Consider emergency thoracotomy • Insert indwelling urinary catheter • Consider pneumatic antishock garment	The child will have an effective circulating volume, as evidenced by: • Stable vital signs appropriate for age • Urine output of 1 to 2 ml/kg/hour • Urine specific gravity within normal limits • Strong, palpable peripheral and central pulses • Improved level of consciousness • Skin normal color, warm, and dry • Hematocrit of 30 ml/dl or hemoglobin of 12 to 14 gm/dl or greater • External hemorrhage is controlled • Moist mucous membranes
Cardiac output, decreased, related to: • Decreased venous return secondary to acute blood loss, massive peripheral vasodilation, or myocardial compromise	• Control bleeding • Obtain vascular access and initiate fluid therapy • Administer fluid bolus • Administer blood • Initiate cardiopulmonary resuscitation, if needed • Consider emergency thoracotomy • Consider pneumatic antishock garment	The child will maintain adequate circulatory function, as evidenced by: • Strong, palpable peripheral and central pulses • Adequate blood pressure for age • Pulse rate appropriate for age • Absence of dysrythmias • Skin normal color, warm, and dry • Improved level of consciousness • Urine output of 1 to 2 ml/kg/hour
Tissue perfusion, altered cerebral, peripheral, renal, and visceral, related to: • Decreased perfusion related to hypovolemia, hypoxia, or hypercarbia • Altered cerebral perfusion related to cerebral edema, swelling, or primary injury	• Control bleeding • Obtain vascular access and initiate fluid therapy • Administer appropriate blood products • Investigate causes of altered consciousness • Initiate pharmacologic therapy for altered consciousness • Remove jewelry or constricting clothing • Consider pneumatic antishock garment	The child will maintain adequate tissue perfusion, as evidenced by: • Strong, palpable peripheral and central pulses • Adequate blood pressure for age • Appropriate apical pulse for age • Skin normal color, warm, and dry • Improved level of consciousness • Urine output of 1 to 2 ml/kg/hour

NURSING DIAGNOSIS	INTERVENTIONS	EXPECTED OUTCOMES
Injury, risk of, related to: • Instability of vertebral column fracture • Altered level of consciousness • Potential for spinal column injury • Inadequate or absent spinal precautions • Pelvic fracture with hemorrhagic shock	• Manually stabilize the cervical spine • Maintain spine stabilization or immobilization • Position the patient	The child will be free from injury, as evidenced by: • Absence of iatrogenic extension of the injury • Minimization of neck by proper alignment and immobilization of the spinal column • Child's verbalization and demonstration of an understanding of need to avoid movement of neck • Absence of increase in extent of original injury
Hypothermia related to: • Rapid infusion of intravenous fluids • Decreased tissue perfusion • Exposure	• Initiate warming measures	The child will maintain a normal core body temperature, as evidenced by: • Core temperature measurement of 36 to 37.5° C (96.8 to 99.5° F) • Absence of shivering, cool skin, pallor • Skin normal color, warm, and dry
Pain related to: • Soft tissue injury and edema • Fractures • Pleural irritation • Stimulation of nerve fibers • Invasive procedures	• Administer pain medications • Stabilize impaled objects • Elevate, splint, apply ice to all fractures	The child will experience relief of pain, as evidenced by: • Diminishing or absent level of pain, indicated by patient's self-report using an objective measurement in the verbal child. • Absence of physiologic indicators of pain: Tachycardia, tachypnea, pallor, diaphoretic skin, and increasing blood pressure • Absence of nonverbal cues of pain: Crying, grimacing, inability to assume position of comfort, and guarding. • Ability to cooperate with care, as appropriate
Infection, risk of, related to: • Impaired skin integrity • Contamination of wound from initial injury or instrumentation • Interruption in perfusion	• Stabilize impaled objects • Apply sterile dressings • Administer antibiotics • Obtain immunization status • Administer vaccines	The child will be free from infection, as evidenced by: • Core temperature measurement of 36 to 37.5° C (96.8 to 99.5° F) • Absence of systemic signs of infection: Fever, tachypnea, tachycardia • Wounds free from redness, swelling, purulent drainage, or odor • Urine output of 1 to 2 ml/kg/hour • Negative blood cultures • White blood count and differential within normal limits • Improved level of consciousness
Anxiety and fear (child and caregiver) related to: • Unfamiliar environment • Unpredictable nature of condition • Invasive procedures • Possible disfigurement or scarring • Knowledge deficit	• Keep family and child informed • Facilitate family presence • Provide psychosocial support	The child and caregiver will experience decreasing anxiety and fear, as evidenced by: • Orientation to surroundings • Ability to describe reasons for equipment and procedures used in treatment • Ability to verbalize concerns and ask questions of health care team • Use of effective coping skills • Vital signs returning to within normal limits

NURSING DIAGNOSIS	INTERVENTIONS	EXPECTED OUTCOMES
Knowledge deficit related to: • Treatment plans or discharge instructions	• Keep family informed • Allow family in room • Provide psychosocial support	The child/caregiver will experience reduced knowledge deficit, as evidenced by: • Ability to identify signs and symptoms requiring medical attention as they relate to the diagnosis • Ability to identify medications: Action and effect, dose, administration time, and side effects • Ability to verbalize understanding of nursing and medical management • Ability to verbalize the need to maintain currency on immunizations and prophylactic care
Powerlessness related to: • Loss of function; uncontrolled pain • Lack of privacy • Lack of knowledge	• Keep family informed • Allow family in room	The child/caregiver will experience an increasing feeling of control over the situational crisis, as evidenced by: • Participation in decision-making activities • Verbalization of questions regarding treatment and course of care • Acceptance of appropriate referrals and resources for support • Use of medical/nursing/allied staff for support and assistance

Triage or Acuity Decisions

EMERGENT   Pediatric patient with actual or potential life- or limb-threatening injury. Any compromise of airway, breathing, or circulation or suspected cervical spine injury (e.g., penetrating injury to head, neck, chest or abdomen; evidence of respiratory distress, shock, or altered level of consciousness; neurovascular compromise of limb).

URGENT   Pediatric patient with no primary assessment deficits but who has injuries requiring treatment within 2 hours (e.g., head trauma without loss of consciousness, suspected extremity fracture without neurovascular compromise).

NONURGENT   Pediatric patient who is awake and alert with no injuries requiring treatment within 2 hours (e.g., minor soft tissue trauma).

Planning and Implementation

Refer to the Chapter 4, "Initial Assessment and Triage," for a list of general interventions. Additional interventions specific to the pediatric trauma patient include:

- Immobilize the spine if not yet completed. (Nursing diagnosis: Risk of injury).

- Consider insertion of a gastric tube if abdominal injury is suspected or gastric distention is present. (Nursing diagnosis: Ineffective breathing pattern).

- Consider insertion of a urinary catheter to monitor fluid status and the effectiveness of fluid resuscitation. (Nursing diagnoses: Fluid volume deficit; inadequate tissue perfusion).

- Facilitate laboratory studies. Blood typing is the highest priority in the critically injured patient.

- Consider the use of pneumatic antishock garment for suspected unstable pelvic fractures with shock. Inflation of the abdominal compartment may decrease respiratory excursion and result in ineffective ventilation because of increased abdominal pressure and elevation of the diaphragm.[25] (Nursing diagnoses: Fluid volume deficit; cardiac output, decreased; altered tissue perfusion).

- Administer antibiotics, as indicated. (Nursing diagnosis: Infection).

- Administer analagesics for pain. (Nursing diagnosis: Pain).

- Administer tetanus vaccine, as indicated. (Nursing diagnosis: Infection).

- Provide psychosocial support to help the child cope with the change in body image and fear of treatment procedures. (Nursing diagnoses: Knowledge deficit; anxiety and fear).

- Evaluate for indicators of child maltreatment (see Chapter 9, "Child Maltreatment").

- Calculate a Pediatric Coma Scale score (see Appendix M) and a Pediatric Trauma Score on admission to and discharge from the emergency department (see Appendix N).

Evaluation and Ongoing Assessment

Children involved in trauma require meticulous and frequent reassessment of airway patency, breathing effectiveness, perfusion, and mental status. Initial improvements may not be sustained, and additional interventions may be needed. The child's response to interventions and trends in the child's condition must be closely monitored for achievement of desired outcomes. The following parameters must be monitored in the pediatric trauma patient:

- Airway patency.

- Endotracheal tube placement, as appropriate.

- Breathing effectiveness and signs of respiratory distress or failure.

- Perfusion.

- Vital signs, including temperature.

- Cardiac rhythm, oxygen saturation, and end-tidal CO_2, as appropriate.

- Pediatric Coma Scale score or Glasgow Coma Scale score, as appropriate for age.

- Volume of intravenous fluids and blood infused.

- Output: Urine, gastric tube, chest tube.

- Ongoing blood loss.

SELECTED INJURIES

Refer to Chapter 4, "Initial Assessment and Triage," for a review of the comprehensive initial assessment and general interventions. Assessment data and interventions specific to the pediatric patient with the particular injury being discussed are delineated in the following sections. Refer to Chapter 7, "Cardiovascular Emergencies," for specific shock management information.

Craniofacial Trauma

Head trauma (e.g., fracture of the vault, traumatic brain injury) is the most common type of pediatric trauma, occurring as a result of mechanisms associated with motor vehicle crashes, falls, assaults, and sports and recreation. Approximately 4,000 children die each year as a result of head injuries. Nearly 50% of these children die within 4 hours after injury.[28]

Anatomic and physiologic differences in children increase the susceptibility to brain injury:

- The head is proportionally larger in regard to both body surface area and weight. This places the pediatric patient at risk for head injury.

- In young children, the cranium is undergoing changes in thickness and elasticity. The child's brain may receive a greater insult because of the thinner and more pliable cranium.

- In young children, small changes in cerebral blood volume and/or cerebral tissue volume can result in significant insult to the brain and rapid decompensation.

- The brain is less myelinated in the infant and young child.

- Young children can accumulate a significant percentage of their blood volume in their cranial vault. Evidence of shock may be present with isolated head trauma in infants.

Specific brain injuries in children differ by age. Infants younger than 1 year of age with head trauma often sustain tears in the subcortical white matter of the temporal and frontal lobes. The white matter is not well myelinated and more susceptible to shearing injury and tears. In children younger than 2 years of age, there is a higher incidence of diffuse brain swelling and a lower incidence of subdural and epidural hematoma formation following head trauma. Other manifestations of head injury in children include impact seizures and diastatic fractures. Approximately 5 to 15% of children seen for head injuries also have associated neck injuries.[28]

ADDITIONAL HISTORY

- Loss of consciousness.

- Temporary amnesia.

- Decreased activity level.

- Inability to recognize caregivers.

- Nausea or emesis since the injury.

- Abnormal behavior for age.

- Seizure following injury.

- Headache.

ASSESSMENT

- Neurologic assessment in the secondary assessment should focus on sensorimotor deficits. Calculate a Pediatric Coma Scale score or Glasgow Coma Scale score, as appropriate for age.

- Test grip strength and equality in older children. In younger children and infants, test strength of extremity movement and withdrawal to touch.

- If the child is comatose, additional assessment of reflexes associated with selected cranial nerves may indicate the integrity of brain stem function (see Appendix O).

- Assess for evidence of neurologic deficit and signs of increased intracranial pressure:

  - Decreased or altered level of consciousness.

  - Pupil dilation with sluggish or absent reaction to light.

  - Vomiting.

  - Slurred speech.

  - Inability to track objects.

  - Ataxia while sitting, crawling, standing, or walking.

  - Bulging anterior fontanelle in infants with an open fontanelle.

  - Sensorimotor deficits.

  - Posturing.

  - Seizures.

  - Bradycardia.

  - Widened pulse pressure.

  - Hypotension, tachycardia, irregular respirations.

ADDITIONAL INTERVENTIONS

Neurologic Deficit Present

- Keep the head in a midline position to promote venous drainage. Maintain spinal immobilization until all radiographs are obtained and cleared.

- Trend neurologic status and vital signs for signs of increased intracranial pressure.

- Assure adequate oxygenation and maintain blood pressure to enhance optimal outcome.

- Prepare for intubation and ventilation with 100% oxygen if Glasgow Coma Scale score is 8 or less.

  - Patients who are unconscious or have signs of increased intracranial pressure must be intubated. Both hypoxia and hypercarbia have potent vasodilatory effects on the cerebral vasculature, resulting in an increased cerebral blood flow and, therefore, an increased intracranial pressure.

  - Ventilate the child to keep the $PaCO_2$ at approximately 30 mm Hg.[24] Rapid sequence induction must be considered if the child is awake or responsive to stimuli or may gag during the intubation procedure. The medications used for rapid sequence induction are selected with considerations for potential effects on intracranial pressure.

- Administer osmotic or loop diuretics, as indicated, to deplete water from the intracellular and interstitial compartments, ultimately resulting in a decrease in cerebral fluid volume and a decreased intracranial pressure.

- Calculate ongoing maintenance fluid needs based on weight and desired degree of fluid restriction as appropriate (see Chapter 4, "Initial Assessment and Triage," planning and implementation).

Neurologic Deficit Absent

- Observe for any change in level of consciousness.

- Provide "head injury" discharge instructions to the caregiver.

SKULL FRACTURES

Signs and symptoms of increased intracranial pressure may be present with a skull fracture due to underlying injury to the brain tissue (cerebral edema and/or intracranial bleeding). The child must be observed for changes in neurologic status and the development of neurologic deficits.

Linear and Depressed Skull Fractures

A linear skull fracture can be described as a nondepressed fracture in any of the bones of the skull. This type of fracture usually heals spontaneously within 2 to 3 months and requires few interventions. Linear fractures associated with serious sequelae include[29]:

- Fractures across the branches of the middle meningeal artery which is located in the temporal area of the cranial vault.

- Occipital bone fractures that extend into the foramen magnum.

- Basilar skull fractures.

A depressed skull fracture is often associated with a direct blow from a solid, heavy object. Depressed skull fracture fragments may require surgical elevation if the depression depth is significant or if fragments pose a threat to underlying cerebral tissue and vasculature.

Signs and Symptoms

- Fracture may or may not be palpable; a depression may be palpable with a depressed skull fracture.

- Pain and tenderness over the fracture site when palpated.

- Cephalohematoma over the fracture site.

- Scalp laceration.

Basilar Skull Fracture

A basilar skull fracture is a linear fracture of any bone that is part of the "base" of the skull: Frontal, ethmoid, sphenoid, temporal, or occipital bones. Fracture of these bones creates a potential for infection and cerebrospinal fluid leak.

Signs and Symptoms

- Otorrhea. If present, suspect a cerebrospinal fluid leak. Test the clear fluid by using a chemical reagent strip. If glucose is present, the drainage is cerebrospinal fluid. This test cannot be used if the cerebrospinal fluid is mixed with blood because blood contains glucose. Another indication of the presence of cerebrospinal fluid in bloody drainage is the halo sign, in which cerebrospinal fluid drainage on linen or gauze forms a dark inner ring and a light outer ring.

- Rhinorrhea.

- Hemotympanum.

- Unilateral hearing loss.

- Postauricular ecchymosis or Battle's sign which may occur hours after injury.

- Periorbital ecchymosis or raccoon's eyes which may occur hours after injury.

Additional Interventions

- If cerebrospinal fluid drainage occurs, do not pack the ears or nose. Apply a nonocclusive sterile dry dressing to absorb the drainage.

CEREBRAL TISSUE INJURY

Concussion

A concussion is a closed-head injury, usually associated with a blow to the head or rapid deceleration, that results in transient neurologic changes. Although symptoms are usually minor, permanent neurologic sequelae, often related to cognitive ability, may occur.

Signs and Symptoms

- Nausea or vomiting.

- Headache.

- Dizziness.

- Brief loss of consciousness.

- Behavior changes.

Diffuse Axonal Injury

Damage to the nerve axon can result from acceleration or deceleration forces that shear or stress the axon. This results in diffuse, microscopic, hemorrhagic lesions. Prolonged coma may result from involvement of the brain stem and *reticular activating system*. The diagnosis of diffuse axonal injury may be delayed for several days. A magnetic resonance imaging scan is used to confirm the diagnosis. The outcome varies, ranging from minimal sequelae to permanent, lifelong disability to death.

Signs and Symptoms

- Immediate unconsciousness that may last as long as several weeks to months.

- Elevated blood pressure.

- Excessive sweating caused by autonomic dysfunction.

- Abnormal posturing.

Contusion

A contusion is a "bruising" of the brain tissue characterized by areas of hemorrhage and edema, commonly caused by a direct blow to the head. Areas of hemorrhage at the site of impact are referred to as a *coup injury;* contusions at sites opposite or distant from the site of impact are referred to as *contrecoup injuries.*

Signs and Symptoms

In addition to those listed for concussion, the child may exhibit:

- Transient or permanent neurologic deficits.

- Transient *retrograde* and/or *antegrade amnesia.*

Intracranial Hemorrhage

Intracranial hemorrhages are uncommon in infants and young children but may occur as a result of a fall, a direct blow to the head, or violent shaking. The types of intracranial hemorrhages are compared in Table 16.

Table 16

COMPARISON OF TYPES OF INTRACRANIAL HEMORRHAGE		
	Epidural Hematoma	**Subdural Hematoma**	**Subarachnoid Hemorrhage**
Definition	• Disruption of middle meningeal artery • Blood collects between skull and dura mater	• Venous bleeding • Blood collects between dura mater and arachnoid mater	• Arterial disruption • Blood collects between arachnoid mater and pia mater
Causes	• Blunt trauma	• May be caused by violent shaking • Consider child maltreatment or *shaken impact syndrome*	• Frequently a result of child maltreatment
Signs and Symptoms	• Initial loss of consciousness, followed by transient consciousness, leading to unconsciousness • Ipsilateral pupil dilation • Contralateral paresis or paralysis • Signs of increased intracranial pressure	• Rapid deterioration in level of consciousness • Signs of increased intracranial pressure	• Stiff neck • Headache • Seizures • Irritability • Signs of increased intracranial pressure

Dental Trauma

FRACTURE OR AVULSION OF A TOOTH

Children may present with fractured or missing teeth resulting from a fall, sports, bicycle crash, or motor vehicle crash. The tooth may be in place but broken, or it may be avulsed from the socket. In certain situations, a permanent tooth may be reimplanted. Primary teeth are generally not reimplanted because of the risk of damage to the *permanent tooth bud*. To ensure optimal results, treatment of the avulsed tooth should begin within 30 minutes of the avulsion.

Signs and Symptoms

- Jagged or broken tooth; loose or missing tooth.
- Sensitivity to cold or fluids.
- Bleeding.
- Soft tissue lacerations, especially of the lower lip and tongue.

Diagnostic Procedures

- Panoramic radiograph including the upper and lower jaw.

Additional Interventions

- Assess airway patency because the tooth or tooth fragment may cause airway compromise or be aspirated.

- A fractured permanent tooth with pulp exposed or deeper dentin involvement is a dental emergency. Refer for immediate dental care.

- Avulsed tooth:

    - Find the permanent tooth.

    - Gently rinse the tooth with water or saline; do not scrub the crown or root.

    - Insert the tooth into the socket or place the tooth in milk until reimplantation.

    - Immediately refer to or contact a dentist or oral surgeon. If the consultant is coming to the emergency department, obtain the necessary supplies to reimplant the tooth.

Vertebral or Spinal Cord Trauma

Approximately 1,000 children sustain injury to the spinal cord each year, and many more sustain injury to the vertebral column.[30] The cervical spine of a child is less protected than that of the adult for a variety of reasons:

- Children have relatively weak muscles of the neck.

- Neck ligaments are more lax.

- Facets of the upper cervical spine are flatter.

- Vertebral bodies are wedged anteriorly and they have a tendency to slide forward with flexion.

The level at which cervical spine injury occurs varies with age. In children who are younger than 8 years of age, injuries are more common to the upper cervical region (C-1 to C-3), whereas older children and adults more commonly have injuries of the lower cervical region.

A phenomenon known as *spinal cord injury without radiographic abnormality* (SCIWORA) occurs almost exclusively among children. Traumatic forces of hyperextension, flexion, and traction may cause SCIWORA. Although the overall prognosis for children with this injury directly relates to the severity of the spinal cord injury, long-term morbidity is common, and the prognosis for functional recovery is considered to be poor.[31] It is important to remember that children may sustain spinal cord injury without an associated vertebral fracture. The use of magnetic resonance imaging has enhanced the diagnosis of spinal cord injury not detected on radiographs or other imaging studies.

The administration of methylprednisolone is indicated in the acutely injured child with a spinal cord injury. The dosing schedule is the same as for an adult.[32]

INJURIES OF THE LUMBAR SPINE ASSOCIATED WITH SAFETY RESTRAINTS

Front-impact motor vehicle crashes accompanied by rapid deceleration forces can cause midlumbar vertebral fractures in children who wear lap safety restraints. Children tend to wear the safety restraint around the abdomen rather than the pelvis. Injuries usually occur between the second and fourth lumbar vertebrae. External abrasions across the lower abdomen are important clues to the injury.

Cardiothoracic Trauma

Significant cardiothoracic trauma rarely occurs alone and is often a component of major multisystem injury. Cardiothoracic trauma in children can be caused by either blunt or penetrating mechanisms. Blunt trauma is more common and can often result in occult injuries to underlying structures. The presence of rib fractures in young children may indicate significant underlying injury. The ribs remain cartilaginous and pliable in children until they are approximately 8 years of age. A significant force may cause injury to underlying structures without concomitant rib fractures. Penetrating injuries are not as common in children, but they may occur as a result of knives, firearms, and high-velocity mechanisms.

ADDITIONAL HISTORY

- Cardiothoracic trauma must be suspected in the child who has sustained the following mechanisms of injury:

  - Rapid deceleration incidents such as motor vehicle crashes.

  - High-velocity impact such as auto-pedestrian crashes.

  - Incidents involving firearms or any penetrating wound to the chest, neck, or abdomen.

  - Significant fall or blow to the chest.

- Chest pain.

ASSESSMENT

- Presence of respiratory distress.

- Physical signs of trauma, such as tire marks, bruising, or open wounds.

- *Paradoxical chest wall movement* with breathing.

- Distended neck veins which is associated with tension pneumothorax or pericardial tamponade. Because of their short neck, this is often difficult to evaluate in infants and small children.

- Deviation of the trachea. In young children, tension pneumothorax may be present without tracheal deviation. Assess for tracheal deviation by palpating the trachea just above the suprasternal notch. It may be difficult to appreciate in infants and small children.

- Percuss for hyperresonance or dullness to percussion; hyperresonance indicates air in the pleural space or pneumothorax; dullness indicates blood in the pleural space or hemothorax.

SIMPLE AND TENSION PNEUMOTHORAX

Pneumothorax is one of the most common forms of pediatric chest trauma and may result from a blunt or penetrating injury. A pneumothorax occurs when air accumulates in the pleural space. The severity of the signs and symptoms is dependent on the percentage of lung collapsed. Children with a small pneumothorax may be asymptomatic.

An open pneumothorax occurs when there is a loss in chest wall integrity and air enters the pleural space through both the wound and the trachea. This is most often associated with penetrating trauma.

A tension pneumothorax develops when air enters the pleural space on inspiration but cannot escape on expiration. The intrathoracic pressure rises, causing collapse of the lung on the side of the injury and a mediastinal shift of the heart, great vessels, and trachea. When enough air accumulates, the unaffected lung collapses. Venous return is impeded, cardiac output falls, and hypotension results.

Signs and Symptoms

- Respiratory distress.
- Diminished or absent breath sounds on the injured side. However, because the chest wall of an infant or young child is so thin, breath sounds are easily referred from other areas of the lung. As a result, decreased breath sounds may not necessarily be heard over involved areas of the lung; instead, a difference in the quality or pitch of the breath sounds over an area of pneumothorax may be noted.[33]
- Tachypnea.
- Tachycardia.
- Pale or cyanotic skin.
- Hyperresonance to percussion.
- Unequal chest expansion.
- In the event of a tension pneumothorax, the child may develop:
  - Severe respiratory distress.
  - Faint peripheral pulses.
  - Hypotension.
  - Distended neck veins and tracheal deviation.
  - Bradycardia.
  - Altered level of consciousness.

Additional Interventions

- If a tension pneumothorax is suspected, immediately prepare for or perform a needle thoracentesis.

- Prepare for chest tube insertion to evacuate the pleural space. A pediatric chest drainage system provides a more accurate measurement of smaller fluid volumes.

- If an open pneumothorax is present, apply a nonporous dressing taped on three sides. Monitor for the development of a tension pneumothorax.

HEMOTHORAX

A hemothorax occurs when blood accumulates in the pleural space. The accumulation of small amounts of blood may be significant enough to produce signs of hypovolemic shock and respiratory distress.

Signs and Symptoms

- Signs of shock.

- Dyspnea.

- Tachypnea.

- Diminished or absent breath sounds on the injured side.

- Dullness to percussion on the injured side.

Additional Interventions

- Prepare for a chest tube insertion.

- Assure fluid resuscitation is initiated prior to chest tube insertion.

- Administer blood, as indicated.

PULMONARY CONTUSION

A pulmonary contusion is a "bruise" of the lung tissue, resulting in alveolar capillary damage. Interstitial and alveolar edema and hemorrhage decrease lung compliance and impair transport of oxygen and carbon dioxide. A pulmonary contusion is identified on a chest radiograph by consolidation and pulmonary infiltrates.

Signs and Symptoms

- Respiratory distress.

- Tachypnea.

- Localized rales or wheezes.

- Hemoptysis.

- Hypoxemia.

Additional Interventions

- Prepare for intubation and assisted ventilation if the contusion is severe; obtain the necessary intubation equipment and supplies.

- If the child is not in shock, restrict intravenous fluids because overhydration during fluid resuscitation can extend the area of contusion.[34]

- If there is no cervical spine injury, elevate the head of the bed.

PERICARDIAL TAMPONADE

Pericardial tamponade is a collection of blood in the pericardial sac. This life-threatening cardiac injury most frequently occurs with penetrating injury but can occur with blunt trauma as well. As blood accumulates in the noncompliant sac, it exerts pressure on the heart and inhibits ventricular filling. Impairment of cardiac function is related to the rate and amount of fluid accumulation in the pericardial sac.

Signs and Symptoms

- Dyspnea.

- Cyanosis.

- Penetrating chest wound, left-sided rib fractures, ecchymosis of the chest wall.

- Signs of shock with hypotension, distended neck veins, muffled heart tones.

- Dysrhythmias: Bradycardia, pulseless electrical activity, asystole.

Additional Interventions

- Prepare for *pericardiocentesis*, as indicated.

- Prepare for possible ED thoracotomy.

- Prepare for operative intervention.

Abdominal Trauma

Abdominal trauma in children is related to a variety of causes, including sports, recreational activities, motor vehicle crashes, and bicycle crashes. There are many physiologic characteristics that increase the child's risk for developing injuries related to abdominal trauma:

- The abdominal muscles are thinner, weaker, and less developed than those of the adult.

- The chest wall is more pliable and does not provide as much protection to abdominal organs.

- The duodenum has an increased vascular blood supply, resulting in larger amounts of blood loss when traumatized.

- The liver and spleen are less protected and are more easily injured.

ADDITIONAL HISTORY

- Abdominal pain or tenderness.

- Nausea or vomiting.

- Last intake of food or liquid.

- Mechanism of injury (e.g., bicycle handlebars, motor vehicle crash with lap safety restraint).

ASSESSMENT

- Location, quality, and radiation of abdominal pain. Pain and apprehension may cause children to tighten their abdominal muscles, making an adequate physical assessment difficult.

- Respiratory pattern and depth:

  - Children are abdominal breathers. Therefore, abdominal pain, such as that caused by peritoneal irritation, may alter the breathing pattern.

  - Children with intra-abdominal bleeding often exhibit an expiratory grunt.

- Palpate for rigidity, guarding, and abdominal distention.

- Evidence of external soft tissue injury (e.g., safety restraint marks).

INTERVENTIONS

- If open abdominal wounds are present, cover with a sterile dressing moistened with sterile saline. Do not attempt to push abdominal contents back into the abdominal cavity.

- Prepare the child for surgery. Children with solid-organ injury resulting in hemodynamic instability and who are unresponsive to fluid resuscitation may require operative intervention.

SPLENIC INJURIES

Trauma of the spleen is often caused by a blunt impact sustained from a sports activity or a fall from a bicycle. Splenic injuries are associated with trauma to the left upper quadrant of the abdomen or left lower chest. Surgical management of splenic trauma is conservative; nonoperative management is the more common approach.

Signs and Symptoms

- Pain in the left upper quadrant of the abdomen that may radiate to the left shoulder.

- Abrasions, contusions to the left upper quadrant.

- Hypoactive or absent bowel sounds.

- Dullness to percussion.

- Signs of shock.

LIVER INJURIES

Liver injury is a major cause of morbidity and mortality in children with abdominal trauma.[35] Management varies and may include surgical intervention or a nonoperative approach.

Signs and Symptoms

- Abrasions or contusions to the right upper quadrant of the abdomen or right lower chest.

- Abdominal distention which is a late sign of extensive intra-abdominal bleeding.

- Right-sided rib fractures.

- Guarding, tenderness, or rigidity to palpation.

- Signs of shock.

SAFETY RESTRAINT-RELATED INJURIES

The possibility of thoracolumbar spine and abdominal injuries has been associated with the use of safety restraints in motor vehicle crashes with a significant impact. Although the number of reported injuries related to appropriate safety restraint use is low, concomitant spinal and abdominal injuries have been reported in young children who were restrained using a lap safety restraint with or without a shoulder harness.

Signs and Symptoms

- Positive "safety belt sign" noted by an area of ecchymosis correlating with the position of the safety restraint across the abdomen.

- Back pain correlating to a lumbar fracture.

- Possible sensorimotor deficits.

- Peritoneal signs such as rigidity, guarding, tenderness, and pain.

- Fever may be present with a hollow organ injury if the presentation is delayed.

Musculoskeletal Trauma

Children often sustain musculoskeletal injuries. These injuries are frequently related to sports and recreational activities, and they occur more often as a child's environment expands to include bicycles, skateboards, trampolines, and automobiles.

Children may sustain a fracture, sprain, subluxation, or dislocation of a joint. Subluxations occur in children as a result of a sudden, forceful, longitudinal pull on an extremity. The most common subluxation is known as "nursemaid's elbow," or subluxation of the radial head. The history is consistent with a sudden longitudinal pulling force on the extremity, such as in a small child who is pulled up by an extended arm.

ADDITIONAL HISTORY

- Mechanism of injury.

- Treatment or splinting done prior to arrival.

- History of previous orthopedic problems.

ASSESSMENT

- Deformity, shortness, or rotation of the affected extremity.

- Edema.

- Tenderness on palpation.

- Reluctance or refusal to move or use an extremity.

- Neurovascular status: Assess for presence of the "5 Ps":

    - Pallor: Are the nailbeds and skin pink? Does blanching occur with pressure? Is the capillary refill less than 2 seconds?

    - Pain: Many children hesitate to complain of pain because they might have been injured while disobeying their caregivers.

    - Pulselessness: Are the peripheral pulses distal to the injury present, strong, and equal?

    - Paresthesia: What is the sensory status of the affected area and the area distal to the injury?

    - Paralysis: Can the child spontaneously move the injured extremity?

ADDITIONAL INTERVENTIONS

- Implement measures to provide optimal tissue perfusion.

    - Always compare the peripheral circulation of the affected extremity to that of the unaffected extremity. What may appear to be impaired circulation in one extremity may actually be present in both extremities and throughout the body, indicating systemic circulatory problems, such as hypovolemia.

    - Evaluate peripheral circulation. If impaired, check the alignment of the extremity, assess the patient's hemodynamic status, and notify the physician. Proper alignment may be needed to restore adequate circulation to the affected extremity.

- Immobilize the injured extremity to include the joints above and below the site of injury. This can be accomplished using:

    - Rigid intravenous boards.

    - Metal or plastic splints.

    - Plaster or fiberglass splints.

- Assess and document the neurovascular status of the affected extremity before and after immobilization.

FRACTURES

Fractures are common in children, but the prognosis for healing is usually excellent. One of the more common types of fractures in children is the greenstick fracture, which is an incomplete fracture through the bone, in which a portion of the cortex and periosteum remains intact. This type of fracture is common in very young children because their bones can sustain a larger amount of buckling and bending. Fractures are not always readily seen in the younger population, making it more difficult to diagnosis the fracture. Problems with healing and future bone growth can occur if the fracture extends through or involves the epiphyseal "growth" plate.

Signs and Symptoms

- Obvious angulation of the extremity may be present.
- Point tenderness.
- Decreased range of motion.
- Edema.
- If the fracture extends completely across the bone, shortening of the extremity may occur.
- Fractured femurs may also exhibit external rotation in addition to shortening.

Additional Interventions

- Administer analgesics.
- Prepare for conscious sedation procedure.
- Prepare for possible closed reduction.
- Discharge teaching:
  - If crutches are given, give the child instructions on walking techniques and assess the return demonstration for correct use.
  - If splints are applied, instruct the caregiver on the signs and symptoms of neurovascular compromise. If appropriate, teach the caregiver how to loosen and reapply the bandages or splints.
  - Instruct the caregiver and child to avoid putting sharp objects inside the cast or splint to relieve itching.
  - Inform the caregiver that if pain continues or increases beyond 48 hours past the injury, the child must be re-examined.

AMPUTATIONS

Fingertip amputations, often caused by a closing door, are one of the most common amputations in children. Many amputated extremities can be successfully reimplanted if the elapsed time from injury to surgery is minimal. Most successful reattachments are guillotine-type amputations which are clean and complete severing of the tissue. Amputations caused by a crushing force are more difficult to reimplant.

Signs and Symptoms

- Partial to complete loss of a limb, hand, foot, finger, or toe.

- Profuse hemorrhage from the limb if vessels are not completely transected.

- Exposed tissue or bone. The bones may be fractured.

Additional Interventions

- If profuse, active bleeding is present, elevate the extremity and apply a pressure dressing.

- When bleeding is contained, apply a sterile nonadhering dressing to the stump and wrap with sterile gauze.

- Care of the amputated part[36]:

    - Gently rinse while avoiding scrubbing the part with sterile saline to remove gross dirt.

    - Wrap the part in gauze slightly moistened with sterile saline, and place the part in a sealable plastic bag.

    - After the bag is sealed, place the bag on ice for transport to surgery or the closest reimplantation center. Remember to label the container.

    - If radiographs are taken, include the parts and the stump.

HEALTH PROMOTION

Prevention measures have an impact on trauma-related morbidity and mortality. Current recommendations include:

- Laws that prohibit children from riding in the cargo areas of pickup trucks.[37]

- No extra seat and no extra rider on farm equipment (e.g., Farm Safety for Kids).

- Community-based education and legislated approaches for the use of bicycle helmets by all children and adults.[38]

- Promote the use of personal flotation devices, parental supervision of children operating a personal watercraft, and safe practices related to personal watercraft.

- Programs that support decreased availability of alcohol and drugs to young people.

- Increased enforcement of existing alcohol and drug use laws.

- Upgrading safety restraint and child passenger safety laws.

- Educating caregivers on firearm safety.

- Educating caregivers and children on the importance of wearing bicycle helmets. Encouraging state and local governments to pass legislation requiring helmet use by all bicyclists and mandating bicycle rental agencies to include helmets as part of the rental contract.

- Encouraging state governments to ban the manufacture and sale of mobile infant walkers or supporting efforts to redesign them. Educating caregivers on the hazards of mobile infant baby walkers. Developing liaisons with other organizations (e.g., National Safe Kids, American Academy of Pediatrics) to discourage the manufacture and sale of baby walkers.

- Identifying appropriate prevention strategies for children with special needs.

Injury prevention must include education, enforcement, and environmental interventions. Other suggested areas for injury prevention are listed in Table 17.[39]

Table 17

INJURY PREVENTION STRATEGIES			
Injury Mechanism	Education/Behavior Change	Enforcement/Legislation	Environment/Technology
Motor Vehicle	Implement media campaign about correct use and positioning of child safety seats; provide consumer training for correct child safety seat use.	Establish/enforce primary restraint laws; improve child safety seat laws; establish child safety seat checkpoints, speed limit and enforcement of driving-under-the-influence programs; create toll-free safety seat hotline to report nonuse of restraints.	Distribute free child safety seats to low-income families; improve signals at problem intersections; reduce speed limits in neighborhoods with children and around schools.
Pedestrian	Motivate medical professionals to counsel parents about traffic dangers; provide pedestrian safety programs at elementary schools.	Enact and enforce pedestrian right-of-way laws.	Improve lighting and crosswalks at problem intersections; distribute reflector tape products.
Bicycle	Conduct bicycle safety rodeos at schools and community fairs; increase bicycle safety information in health curriculums.	Promote bicycle helmet legislation; enforce current bicycle helmet laws.	Distribute free bicycle helmets to low-income families; provide free bicycle repair workshops; increase the number of bicycle lanes and trails.
Fires/Burns	Educate homeowners and rental property owners about scald burn risks and smoke detectors; encourage firefighters to provide school assemblies on fire safety.	Enforce building codes for smoke detector use; encourage building code officials to require hot water heater settings under 48.9°C (120°F).	Promote the use of antiscald device products.
Home (Falls, Poisons)	Educate parents about gates and stairs, sharp-edged furniture, furniture near windows, proper crib construction, miniblind cords, and locking up poisons, medicines, and alcohol.	Prohibit the sale of baby walkers; inspect child care facilities and schools for all hazards.	Distribute no-choke tubes to determine safe objects for small children; encourage use of window guards; distribute cabinet lock products.

INJURY PREVENTION STRATEGIES			
Injury Mechanism	**Education/Behavior Change**	**Enforcement/Legislation**	**Environment/Technology**
Firearms/Violence	Develop media campaign promoting trigger locks and lock boxes; provide conflict resolution, anger management; and other violence prevention programs in schools.	Encourage restrictive licensing for handguns and enforcement of existing firearms laws.	Work with local police on community policing initiative; promote development of product modifications for handguns.
Child Abuse	Provide parent education programs to young and at-risk parents; develop self-help groups.	Work with local officials to maximize effectiveness of child protective services.	Support home visitor programs for new parents; provide affordable day care.
Playgrounds	Provide seminars on playground safety for school officials, park and recreation administrators, and child care providers.	Promote or mandate the use of US Consumer Product Safety Commission standards for playground equipment and surfaces.	Support community development projects that improve playground equipment and surfaces.
Sports	Provide parents, students, and coaches with educational materials on proper sports equipment and physical conditioning.	Promote and mandate the use of proper safety equipment by school and community sports programs.	Promote the use of breakaway bases, mouth guards, and eye protection equipment.
Drowning	Provide information to pool owners about drowning risks and appropriate pool barriers.	Enforce pool barrier codes for community and public pools.	Promote use of pool barriers, including four-sided isolation fencing.

Adapted from Allen K. *Preventing Childhood Emergencies. A Guide to Developing Effective Injury Prevention Initiatives*. Washington, DC: Emergency Medical Services for Children National Resource Center; 1997. Used with permission.

SUMMARY

Care of the pediatric trauma patient requires a coordinated effort from the trauma team and the family. Collaboration by the multidisciplinary team facilitates optimal patient care and integrates the resources that are needed to care for the pediatric trauma patient. Knowledge of normal growth and development, anatomy, mechanisms of injury, and physiologic and psychosocial responses to injury is the foundation of providing trauma nursing care to the pediatric patient. A systematic approach to assessment and intervention contributes to positive patient outcomes through early identification of injuries and recognition of life-threatening conditions. Incorporating the family throughout the care process is important in meeting the psychosocial and emotional needs of the patient and his or her family.

REFERENCES

1. Templeton JM. Mechanism of injury: biomechanics. In: Eichelberger M, ed. *Pediatric Trauma*. St. Louis, Mo: Mosby-Year Book; 1993:20-36.

2. National Safety Council. *Accident Facts, 1998 ed.* Itasca, Ill: Author; 1998.

3. Gallagher S. *Injuries in the School Environment: A Resource Packet, Children's Safety Network.* Washington, DC: National Injury and Violence Prevention Resource Center; 1996.

4. Bordeaux S, Harrison J. Injury mortality Australia, 1995. *Australian Injury Prevention Bulletin.* 1998; 17.

5. Emergency Nurses Association. Pediatric trauma. In: *Trauma Nursing Core Course (Instructor) Manual.* 4th ed. Park Ridge, Ill; Author; 1995:305-324.

6. Pautler MA, Henning J, Buntain WL. Mechanisms and biomechanics of traffic injuries. In: Buntain WL, ed. *Management of Pediatric Trauma*. Philadelphia, Pa: WB Saunders; 1995:10-27.

7. National and Pediatric Trauma Registry. *Pediatric Trauma Registry Report Phase 2*. April, 1993.

8. Dandrinos-Smith S. The epidemiology of pediatric trauma. *Crit Care Nurs Clin North Am.* 1991;3:387-390.

9. National Highway Traffic Safety Administration, National Center for Statistics and Analysis, Traffic Safety Facts. *A Compilation of Motor Vehicle Crash Data from the Fatal Accident Reporting System and General Estimates System.* Washington, DC: US Department of Transportation; 1994.

10. Ziegler MM, Templeton JM. Major trauma. In: Fleisher GR, Ludwig S, eds. *Textbook of Pediatric Emergency Medicine*. 3rd ed. Baltimore, Md: Williams & Wilkins; 1993:1089-1101.

11. Haley K. Multiple trauma. In: Bernardo LM, Thomas DO, eds. *Emergency Nursing Pediatric Core Curriculum*. Park Ridge, Ill: Roadrunner Press; 1998.

12. Waddell JP, Drucker WR. Occult injuries in pedestrian accidents. *J Trauma*. 1971;11:844-852.

13. Haley K, Hammond S, Osborn R, Falcone RE. Pediatric pedestrian versus motor vehicle patterns of injury: debunking the "myth." *Air Med J.* 1997:16:A9.

14. Kottmeier PK. Falls from heights. In: Buntain WL, ed. *Management of Pediatric Trauma*. Philadelphia, Pa: WB Saunders; 1995:450-458.

15. Bergman AB, Rivara FP, Richards DD, Rogers LW. The Seattle children's bicycle helmet campaign. *Am J Dis Child.* 1990;144:727-731.

16. Boyle WE, Bull MJ, Katcher ML, Palmer SD, Rodgers GC, Smith BL, Tully SB. Bicycle helmets. *Pediatrics.* 1995;95:609-610.

17. Rescky J, Jaffe D, Christoffel K. Skateboarding injuries in children, a second wave. *Am J Dis Child.* 1991;145:188-192.

18. Boyle WE, Bull MJ, Katcher ML, Palmer SD, Rodgers GC, Smith BL, Tully SB. Skateboard injuries. *Pediatrics.* 1995;95:611-612.

19. Chow TK, Corbett SW, Farstad DJ. Spectrum of injuries from snowboarding. *J Trauma.* 1996;41:321-325.

20. Branche CM, Conn JM, Annest JL. Personal watercraft-related injuries: A growing public health concern. *JAMA.* 1997;278:663-665.

21. Phelan A. Respiratory emergencies. In: Kelly SJ, ed. *Pediatric Emergency Nursing*. 2nd ed. Norwalk, Conn: Appleton & Lange; 1994:247-279.

22. Thompson A. Environmental emergencies. In: Fleisher GR, Ludwig S, Silverman BK, eds. *Synopsis of Pediatric Emergency Medicine*. Baltimore, Md: Williams & Wilkins; 1996:447-462.

23. Emergency Nurses Association. Epidemiology of trauma: appendix two. In: *Trauma Nursing Core Course (Instructor) Manual*. 4th ed. Park Ridge, Ill: Author; 1995:491.

24. Nypaver M, Treloar DF. Neutral cervical spine positioning in children. *Ann Emerg Med*. 1994;23:208-211.

25. Manley L, Haley K, Dick M. Intraosseous infusion: rapid vascular assess for critically ill or injured infants and children. *J Emerg Nurs*. 1988;14:63-69.

26. Guy J, Haley K, Zuspan SJ. Use of intraosseous infusion in the pediatric trauma patient. *J Pediatr Surg*. 1993:28:158-161.

27. Derrico D. Comparison of blood pressure measurement methods in critically ill children. *Dimens in Crit Care Nurs*. 1993;12:31-39.

28. Tasker RL, Deshpande JK, Carson BS. Head trauma. In: Nichols DG, Yaster M, Lappe DG, Haller JA, eds. *Golden Hour – The Handbook for Advanced Pediatric Life Support*. 2nd ed. St. Louis, Mo: Mosby-Year Book; 1996:217-238.

29. Vernon-Levett P. Head injuries in children. *Crit Care Nurs Clin North Am*. 1991;3:411-422.

30. Dickman CA, Hadley MN, Browner C, Sonntag VK. Neurosurgical management of acute atlas-axis combination fractures: a review of 25 cases. *J Neurosurg*. 1989;70:45-49.

31. Athey A. A three-year-old with spinal cord injury without radiographic abnormality. *J Emerg Nurs*. 1991;17:380-385.

32. Sponseller PD. Orthopedic injuries. In: Nichols DG, Yaster M, Lappe DG, Haller JA, eds. *Golden Hour – The Handbook of Advanced Pediatric Life Support*. 2nd ed. St. Louis, Mo: Mosby-Year Book: 1996;381-397.

33. Soud T, Pieper P, Hazinski MF. Pediatric trauma. In: Hazinski MF, ed. *Nursing Care of the Critically Ill Child*. 2nd ed. St. Louis, Mo: Mosby-Year Book; 1992:829-874.

34. Dickenson CM. Thoracic trauma in children. *Crit Care Nurs Clin North Am*. 1991;3:423-432.

35. Lebet RM. Abdominal and genitourinary trauma in children. *Crit Care Nurs Clin North Am*. 1991;3:433-444.

36. Fultz J. Extremity trauma. In: Kidd PS, Sturt P, eds. *Mosby's Emergency Nursing Reference*. St. Louis, Mo: Mosby-Year Book; 1996:279-312.

37. Woodward GA, Bolte RG. Children riding in the back of pickup trucks: a neglected safety issue. *Pediatrics*. 1990;86:683-691.

38. Sacks JJ, Holmgreen P, Smith S, Sosin DM. Bicycle-associated head injuries and deaths in the United States from 1984 through 1988: how many are preventable? *JAMA*. 1991;266:3016-3018.

39. Allen K. *Preventing Childhood Emergencies: A Guide to Developing Effective Injury Prevention Initiatives*. Washington, DC: Emergency Medical Services for Children National Resource Center; 1997.

Pediatric Considerations:
Cervical and Spinal Immobilization

Spinal Immobilization

Spinal immobilization is performed in children whose mechanism of injury is suspicious for spinal injury. Spinal immobilization should be completed[1]:

- Following acceleration or deceleration injuries (e.g., motor vehicle crashes, pedestrian-related incidents, or crashes in which the child was unrestrained).

- Following injury from vigorous shaking.

- For any unconscious trauma victim.

- Following major trauma with head injury.

The procedure for spinal immobilization is:

- Manually stabilize the cervical spine:

  - For the supine child, place your hands on each side of the child's head. Place the thumbs along the mandible and the fingers behind the head on the occipital ridge.

  - Avoid flexing the neck when the child is placed supine; pressure on the prominent occiput may cause flexion of the neck.

- Apply a rigid cervical collar (see Figure 19):

  - Have a second person assess for and remove any earrings or necklace.

  - Select the appropriate-sized cervical collar using the following technique. (Note: This technique is applicable to the Stifneck™ collar. Other brands have different sizing techniques):

    ♦ Determine the appropriate size by measuring from the patient's chin to the shoulder. Place your fingers on top of the shoulder where the collar will rest and measure the distance to the point of the chin (not the angle of the jaw).

    ♦ Compare this distance on the collar by placing the same number of fingers below the black fastener.

    ♦ The correct-sized collar is based on the measurement between the black fastener and the edge of the rigid plastic at the bottom of the collar (not the foam portion of the collar).

    ♦ Assemble the collar by moving the chin piece up and snapping the black fastener into the hole on the side of the collar.

    ♦ Preform the collar.

- Apply the collar as follows:
  - Slide the back portion of the collar behind and around the child's neck.
  - Slide the chin piece up the chest so that the child's chin is supported by the chin piece.
  - Secure the Velcro® strap.
- The cervical collar fits properly if the chin rests securely in the chin piece, the collar is beneath the ears, and it extends to suprasternal notch, resting on the clavicles.[2]
- Several brands of cervical collars are now available with adjustable chin supports. However, some do not adjust small enough to fit the small child. The WizLoc™, manufactured by Kohlbrat & Bunz Corporation, is adjustable to pediatric sizes. This brand has both an adjustable mandible section and occipital support.
- The smallest rigid cervical collar may be too large for some toddlers and infants. Instead, a towel roll may be used. Continued manual control of the cervical spine may be required if adequate immobilization cannot be achieved.
- Logroll the child onto the backboard or approved immobilization device. The person applying the manual stabilization to the cervical spine is the leader and should inform the assistants of their roles for logrolling the child onto the backboard or immobilization device:
  - One assistant should be at the shoulders and hips; a second assistant at the hips and legs; and the third assistant on the opposite side to position the backboard.
  - By announced command, the leader directs the procedure and the child is logrolled as a unit onto his or her side. While logrolling, always keep the child's nose in line with the sternum.
  - Slide the backboard against the child's back at a 30 to 45° angle[3] and roll the child onto the backboard. Gently lower the backboard and align the child in the center of the board:
    - For children younger than 8 years of age, the head is disproportionately large. Place padding under the shoulders of the child to maintain the neck in a neutral, aligned position (see Figures 20 and 21).
    - The padding should be in place prior to logrolling the child onto the board.[1,4]
    - The child's shoulder should be in horizontal alignment with the external auditory meatus.[5]

Figure 19
APPLICATION OF A STIFNECK™ COLLAR

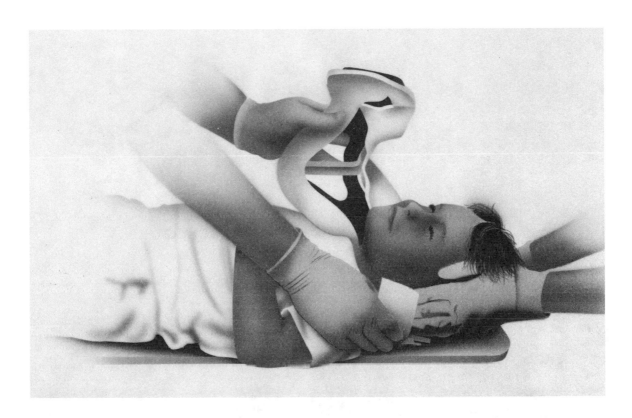

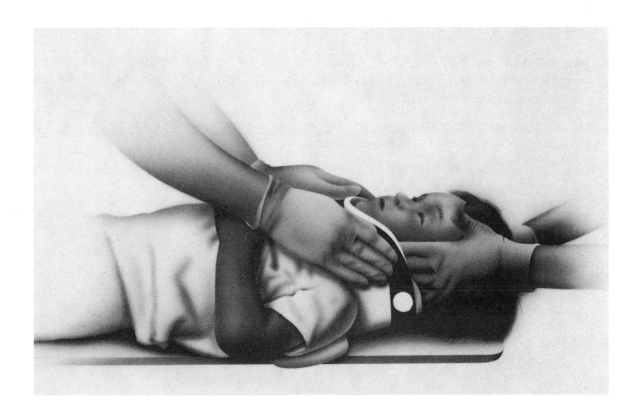

Figure 20
CHILD ON A STANDARD BACKBOARD

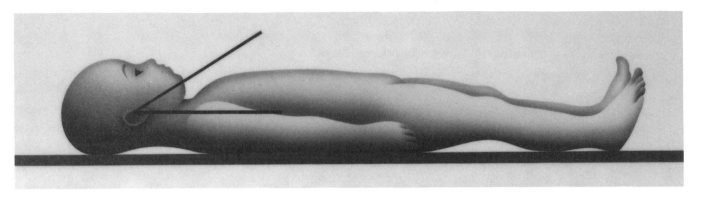

Figure 21
PROPER POSITIONING OF CHILD ON A BACKBOARD

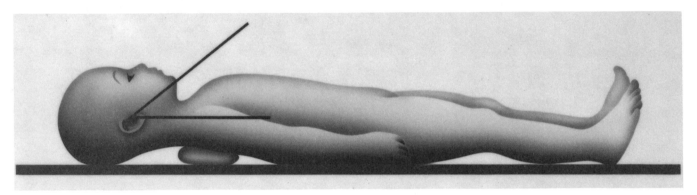

- Secure the child's body to the backboard or immobilization device (see Figure 22). The leader must maintain manual stabilization of the cervical spine until first the body and then the head are secured to the backboard[4]:

  - Place three straps across the child's body. One strap is placed across the chest, one across the hips, and one above the knees.

  - For infants and small children, place towel or blanket rolls along the side of the body to secure the patient and restrict the movement of the hips and knees. If there is a space between the edge of the backboard and the child's body, the child will be able to move beneath the strap. Fill this space with a blanket or towel roll.

- Secure the head to the board after the child's body is secured to the board:

  - Apply a lateral head support device to either side of the head to prevent lateral and anterior movement. Use towels or blanket rolls or a commercially available cervical immobilization device to provide lateral stabilization.[6] For the smaller child, the commercially available foam blocks may be too tall, making it difficult to place the tape securely across the forehead. If lateral stabilization cannot be achieved with available devices, continue manual stabilization.

  - Place a piece of tape across the forehead.

Figure 22
SPINAL IMMOBILIZATION

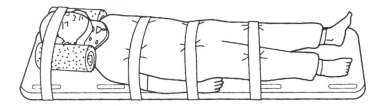

From French JP. Stabilization procedures. In: French JP, ed. *Pediatric Emergency Skills*. St. Louis, Mo: Mosby-Year Book; 1995:141. Reprinted with permission.

Points to Remember:

- The leader must maintain manual stabilization until the head and body are affixed to the backboard.

- Perform a brief evaluation of the child's motor and sensory function before and after logrolling the patient.

- Observe the back for surface injuries and penetrating objects when the child is logrolled. Remove any debris that may cause skin irritation before rolling the child onto the board.

- Do not use a chin strap or tape across the chin. It tends to push the jaw backward, causing occlusion of the airway.

- Never use sandbags as lateral immobilization devices, especially when immobilizing the child in a safety seat. Sandbags place downward pressure on the shoulders and could cause respiratory compromise.[7]

- Observe the child closely for vomiting. If the child vomits, turn the entire backboard as a unit, with the leader controlling the head. Have suction and a tonsil tip suction available.

- Commercially manufactured pediatric immobilization devices are available. Follow the manufacturer's instructions for use.

Spinal Immobilization in a Child Safety Seat

An infant or young child can be immobilized in the child safety seat if the airway, breathing, and circulation are stable[2,7]:

- Immobilize the child's head with a towel roll on each side of the head or place one large towel in a horseshoe shape over the child's head, extending to the shoulders.

- Secure the towel with tape, starting at one side of the child safety seat, and crossing the infant's forehead. Anchor the tape on the other side of the child safety seat. Place a second piece of tape across the chest[2,3] (see Figure 23).

- Ensure that the internal harness strap and clip are properly positioned over the child's body.

- Use additional small towels to fill in any spaces in the child safety seat.

- A small towel can be used as a cervical collar.

Figure 23

IMMOBILIZATION IN A CHILD SAFETY SEAT

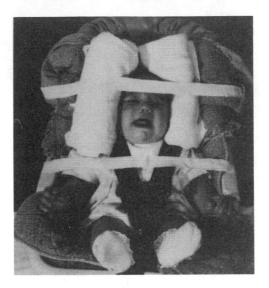

From Lang S. Procedures involving the neurological system. In: Bernardo LM, Bove M, eds. *Pediatric Emergency Nursing Procedures.* Boston, Mass: Jones & Barlett; 1993:148. Reprinted with permission.

Removing a Child from a Child Safety Seat While Maintaining Spinal Immobilization

- While initiating manual control of the head and cervical spine, remove towel rolls if present.

- Remove or cut the shoulder harness and move the safety bar out of the way as much as possible.

- Position the child safety seat at the foot of a backboard. Tip the child safety seat back and lay it down on the backboard.

- Have one person slide his or her hands along each side of the child's head until the hands are behind the child's shoulders. The head and neck are then supported laterally by the person's arms. A second person should take control of the child's body.

- On the instruction of the person controlling the head, slide the child out of the child safety seat to a backboard and immobilize the child as previously described.

- Instruct caregivers to replace the child safety seat when it is involved in a crash. In some areas, auto insurance may cover the cost of replacing the seat.

REFERENCES

1. Silverman BK, ed. *Advanced Pediatric Life Support: The Pediatric Emergency Medicine Course.* Elk Grove Village, Ill: American Academy of Pediatrics and American College of Emergency Physicians; 1993.

2. Bernardo L. Pediatric trauma. In: Newberry L, ed. *Sheehy's Emergency Nursing Principles and Practice.* 4th ed. St. Louis, Mo: Mosby-Year Book; 1998:389-408.

3. Campbell JE, ed. *Basic Trauma Life Support: Advanced Prehospital Care.* 2nd ed. Englewood Cliffs, NJ: Prentice Hall; 1988.

4. Keseg D. Pediatric spinal trauma. In: Dietrich A, Shaner S, eds. *Pediatric Basic Trauma Life Support.* American College of Emergency Physicians. Oakbrook Terrace, Ill: Basic Trauma Life Support International; 1995:50-56.

5. Nypaver M, Treloar DF. Neutral cervical spine positioning in children. *Ann Emerg Med.* 1994;23:208-211.

6. Spinal immobilization/extrication. In: Dietrich A, Shaner S, eds, *Pediatric Basic Trauma Life Support.* American College of Emergency Physicians. Oakbrook Terrace, Ill: Basic Trauma Life Support International; 1995:140-147.

7. Widner-Kolberg M. Immobilizing children in car safety seats – Why, when and how. *J Emerg Nurs.* 1991;17:427-428.

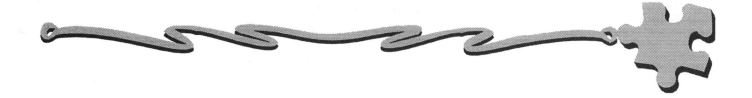

CHAPTER 7

Cardiovascular Emergencies

OBJECTIVES

On completion of this lecture, the learner should be able to:

✦ Identify the anatomic and physiologic characteristics of children as a basis for the signs and symptoms of cardiovascular compromise.

✦ Identify the most frequent causes of shock in children.

✦ Identify the appropriate nursing diagnoses and expected outcomes based on the assessment findings.

✦ Delineate the specific interventions needed to manage the child with cardiovascular compromise.

✦ Evaluate the effectiveness of nursing interventions related to patient outcomes.

✦ Identify health promotion strategies related to the cardiovascular system.

INTRODUCTION

The most common causes of cardiopulmonary arrest in adults are lethal arrhythmias related to heart disease.[1] In the child, however, the most common causes of cardiopulmonary arrest are conditions that lead to shock or respiratory failure.[2,3] Even though cardiopulmonary arrest in children is not common, rates of survival from documented asystole are dismal.[2] This chapter will focus on shock and selected dysrhythmias as these are the most common causes of cardiovascular compromise.

Shock may result from volume loss, most commonly resulting from hypovolemia or sepsis. Some pediatric patients may also suffer cardiogenic shock that results from viral myocarditis, drug ingestion, postoperative complications from cardiac surgery, or cardiac dysrhythmia.[4]

ANATOMIC, PHYSIOLOGIC, AND DEVELOPMENTAL CHARACTERISTICS AS A BASIS FOR SIGNS AND SYMPTOMS

Specific characteristics in the cardiovascular system of the pediatric patient have important clinical significance. These are summarized in Table 18.[5,6]

Table 18

CHARACTERISTICS AND CLINICAL SIGNIFICANCE OF THE CARDIOVASCULAR SYSTEM	
Characteristics	**Clinical Significance**
Myocardium has poor compliance as the myocardial fibers are shorter and less elastic, contractile mass is less, and stroke volume is limited (1.5 ml/kg/beats/minute as compared to 75 to 90 ml/beats/minute in an adult).	Heart rate rather than stroke volume increases to maintain cardiac output, which falls precipitously with bradycardia or heart rates exceeding 200 beats/minute.
Infants have a higher cardiac output (200 ml/kg/minute) than adults (100 ml/kg/minute).	Provides for increased oxygen needs, but leaves little cardiac output reserve. Any stresses such as hypothermia or sepsis can lead to acute deterioration.
Circulating blood volume is 90 ml/kg in the infant; 80 ml/kg in the child; 70 ml/kg in the adult.	Small blood losses can cause circulatory compromise.
Children are capable of maintaining adequate cardiac output for long periods because of strong compensatory mechanisms. Rapid deterioration can occur when compensatory mechanisms are exhausted.	Hypotension is a late sign of circulatory decompensation. Children may remain normotensive until 25% of their blood volume is lost. Assess capillary refill as an indicator of peripheral perfusion; capillary refill should be ≤ 2 seconds.
A greater percent of total body weight is water. Daily water turnover involves more than half of the extracellular fluid; in the adult, one fifth of the extracellular fluid is exchanged daily.	Greater potential for dehydration.

Autonomic Nervous System

Cardiac function is regulated by the hypothalamus, which stimulates the cardiovascular control centers located in the medulla oblongata and the pons. These centers receive impulses from the heart and, by means of a reflex loop, send signals to target organs through the sympathetic and parasympathetic systems.

During the first few weeks of life, there are numerous changes in the autonomic nervous system and the cardiac conduction system. Sympathetic innervation of the heart is incomplete; therefore, the newborn is particularly sensitive to the effects of parasympathetic stimulation. Stimulation of the parasympathetic pathway (e.g., suctioning or defecating) is a common cause of transient bradycardia in the newborn.[3,6] However, as the child matures, sympathetic innervation increases. Older children and adults can also respond to vagal stimulation with the development of bradycardia.

Autoregulation of the Heart

Intrinsic autoregulation of cardiovascular function occurs in response to changes in blood volume. As the heart fills, cardiac muscle fibers stretch. The degree to which these fibers stretch affects the force of contraction and stroke volume.

The neonatal myocardium is less compliant and contains less contractile mass than the myocardium of the older child and adult. In the infant and young child, stroke volume is less than in the adult (1.5 ml/kg/beat; 10-kg child = 15 ml/beat, compared to 75 to 90 ml/beat in the adult). **Because cardiac output is a function of heart rate and stroke volume, the child's principal method of increasing cardiac output during a low-output state is to increase the heart rate.** However, cardiac output will fall: 1) when the heart rate exceeds 180 to 200 beats/minute because ventricular filling time is compromised and 2) during periods of sustained bradycardia because of limited stroke volume. **Bradycardia is considered an ominous sign of impending cardiopulmonary arrest in the pediatric patient.**

DEFINITION OF SHOCK

Shock is the manifestation of cellular metabolic insufficiency. There are multiple causes of shock, but the common denominator of shock, no matter what its etiology, is the reduction in the amount of oxygen consumed by the cells.[7] Shock is commonly referred to as compensated or uncompensated shock. Compensated shock is characterized by tachycardia but a blood pressure within normal limits for age. Uncompensated shock is manifested by tachycardia and hypotension.

Shock Pathway

No matter what the etiology of shock, the body will respond similarly. In early shock, the body will attempt to compensate for the alterations in perfusion and transport that have occurred. Compensatory mechanisms include tachycardia, tachypnea, and restlessness or agitation. The increase in respirations is an attempt to compensate for the resulting metabolic acidosis.

During early shock, the body compensates by increasing the heart rate which increases the cardiac output and maintains perfusion to vital organs (i.e., brain, heart kidneys).[4,7] Poor peripheral perfusion is indicated by delayed capillary refill, cool, pale, mottled skin, and decreasing quality of peripheral pulses until they are no longer palpable. Persistent vasoconstriction causes early renal and gastrointestinal ischemia resulting in decreased urine output and gastrointestinal function.

In an attempt to maintain an adequate circulatory volume, fluid shifts from the interstitial space to the intravascular compartment. If the child remains in shock, fluid will begin to shift out of the vascular compartment into the interstitial and cellular spaces. The cellular ions are also redistributed which contributes to impaired cellular functioning.[8]

As shock progresses and early compensatory mechanisms fail, the body's response becomes more complex and potentially may have lethal consequences. There are systemic as well as cellular-level responses that are initiated to meet the body's oxygen demands (see Figure 24).

Inadequate perfusion leads to cellular ischemia, particularly in those tissues with high metabolic demands or those that have been underperfused for a longer period of time. Cellular ischemia causes the release of vasoactive and inflammatory mediators such as cytokines and arachidonic acid, which can effect the child's microcirculation.[4,7] Alteration in cellular metabolism leads to anaerobic metabolism and the development of acidosis.

Eventually, cardiac output is decreased and hypotension occurs. As systemic perfusion becomes more impaired, the brain is hypoperfused, and the child becomes more irritable, stuporous, and eventually comatose.[8] If left uncorrected, uncompensated shock leads to complete cardiovascular collapse and cardiac arrest.

The consequences of uncompensated shock include:

- Fluid loss from the vascular into the interstitial and cellular compartments, caused by increased vascular permeability and damage to cellular membranes.

- Disseminated intravascular coagulation and the development of other coagulopathies, caused by cellular damage that stimulates the coagulation cascade.[9]

- The continued release of vasoactive and inflammatory mediators.[10]

- Pulmonary tissue hypoxia, which may lead to acute respiratory distress syndrome.

- The development of multiple organ dysfunction and eventually multisystem organ failure and death.[10]

CAUSES OF SHOCK[4-6]

Hypovolemic shock is characterized by an overall decrease in circulating blood or fluid volumes. Hemorrhage, vomiting, and diarrhea are the most common causes of hypovolemic shock in children. Other causes include burns and diabetic ketoacidosis.

Cardiogenic shock is characterized by the inability of the myocardium to maintain an adequate cardiac output, usually due to myocardial ischemia or death. In children, cardiogenic shock is rare but may follow open heart surgery, viral myocarditis, or drug ingestion, or may occur secondary to cardiac dysrhythmia (e.g., asystole, ventricular fibrillation, supraventricular tachycardia).[11]

Distributive shock results from vasodilation and pooling of blood in the peripheral vasculature. Types of distributive shock include:

- Septic shock: One of the most common types of shock in the pediatric patient, it is generally caused by an infectious source. Bacteria most commonly responsible for sepsis include *Escherichia coli, Klebsiella,* and *Staphylococcus.*

- Neurogenic shock: Characterized by a loss of sympathetic tone, it can be caused by spinal cord trauma, brain stem injury, anesthetic agents, or the ingestion of drugs (e.g., barbiturates).

Obstructive shock is caused by an inadequate circulating volume resulting from an obstruction in or compression of the great veins, aorta, pulmonary arteries, or the heart. Obstructive shock may occur from conditions such as pericardial tamponade, tension pneumothorax, mediastinal mass, or congenital abnormality of the great vessels.

Figure 24

THE BODY SYSTEMS' RESPONSE TO SHOCK[7]

Cellular Level

- Alteration in cellular metabolism
- Alteration in the production of adenosine triphosphate
- Failure of the sodium-potassium pump
- Redistribution of cellular ions
- Interstitial fluid shifts
- Development of blisters or blebs on cellular walls
- Damage to the mitochondria
- Rupture of lysosomes with release of its enzymes

Immune System

- Activation of complement cascade system:
  - Factor B: Causes macrophage spreading on cell surface
  - C3b: Immune adherence, enhanced phagoocytosis
  - C5b: Initiates membrane attack; induces neutrophil attachment to the endolethium
  - C6, C7, C8, C9: Attacks cell membrane and lyses cells
- Release of cytokines
- Slow-reacting substance of anaphylaxis

Neurologic System

- Alteration in cerebral perfusion pressure

Cardiac System

- Decrease in cardiac output
- Development of dysrhythmias
- Release of myocardial depressant factor

Pulmonary System

- Acute lung injury
- Acute respiratory distress syndrome

Renal System

- Decrease in urine output
- Decrease in detoxification

Gastrointestinal System

- Priming beds for circulating neutrophils that provoke multiple organ failure

Integumentary System

- Pale, cooler, fragile skin
- Less protection
- Hypothermia

NURSING CARE OF THE CHILD WITH A CARDIOVASCULAR EMERGENCY

Assessment

The child who is suffering from shock requires assessment and the initiation of critical interventions simultaneously.

ADDITIONAL HISTORY

Refer to Chapter 4, "Initial Assessment and Triage," for general questions to obtain a history. Additional or specific history data important in the evaluation of shock include:

- Any obvious bleeding sites or history of blood loss.
- Vomiting and diarrhea.
- Decreased fluid intake.
- Any obvious sites of fluid loss, such as a burn injury.
- Congenital heart disease.
- Potential source or risk factors for infection.

SIGNS AND SYMPTOMS

- Altered level of consciousness. Any alteration in the level of consciousness must be considered a result of decreased cerebral perfusion until proven otherwise:
  - Inability to recognize caregivers.
  - Decreased level of response to environment.
  - Restlessness.
  - Anxiety.
  - Confusion.
  - Irritability.
- Tachypnea.
- Tachycardia or hypotension. In the early stages of shock, the child may be normotensive or demonstrate a slightly increased systolic pressure with a widened pulse pressure. **Hypotension and bradycardia are ominous signs in the pediatric patient in shock.**
- Changes in skin color:
  - Pale.
  - Ashen.
  - Mottled.
  - Cyanotic.

- Changes in the quality of peripheral and central pulses:
  - Weak, thready.
  - Absent.
- Cool, clammy skin.
- Difficulty in obtaining a blood pressure. Because of vasoconstriction and decreased cardiac output, it may be difficult to obtain an accurate blood pressure. Obtain the initial blood pressure by auscultation, palpation, or ultrasonic flow meter. Since there is a potential for an inaccurate reading, correlate noninvasive blood pressure readings with manual measurements.
- Decreased or absent bowel sounds.
- Decreased or absent urine output.

DIAGNOSTIC PROCEDURES

A variety of radiographic and laboratory studies may be indicated, depending on the suspected etiology of the child's condition. Definitive diagnostic testing is performed as the resuscitation effort is in progress or after the child is stabilized. The following procedures or studies may be indicated for the child with shock.

Monitors

- Cardiac monitor.
- 12-lead electrocardiogram.
- Pulse oximeter.
  - Poor perfusion may impede the monitor's ability to obtain an accurate reading.
  - A normal reading does not negate the child's need for supplemental oxygen.
  - Although the saturation reading is within normal limits, shock results in decreased tissue oxygenation.
- Capnography for the intubated patient.

Radiographic Studies

- Chest radiograph to determine the presence of an enlarged heart, pulmonary infection, hemothorax, or pneumothorax.

Other Diagnostic Procedures

- Ultrasound for suspected organ injury or abscess.
- Echocardiogram.

Laboratory Studies

- Complete blood count.
- Serum or whole blood glucose test.
- Electrolytes.

- Blood sample for typing.

- Arterial blood gas. Decreasing pH indicates a worsening of the cellular oxygen debt as metabolic acidosis develops because of anaerobic metabolism and lactic acid production. An elevated $PaCO_2$ indicates respiratory acidosis and impaired ventilation of the alveoli. A low PaO_2 indicates hypoxia.

- Cultures:
  - Blood.
  - Body fluids including cerebrospinal fluid.
  - Wounds.
  - Indwelling devices.

- Urinalysis.

- Other studies, as indicated by the child's condition.

Nursing Diagnoses, Interventions, and Expected Outcomes

NURSING DIAGNOSIS	INTERVENTIONS	EXPECTED OUTCOMES

Gas exchange, impaired, related to:
• Ineffective breathing pattern: Deterioration of ventilatory efforts.
• Ineffective airway clearance.
• Aspiration.
• Impaired tissue perfusion secondary to fluid volume loss or inadequate cardiac rate.
	• Administer oxygen.
	• Consider intubation, as indicated.
	• Place child on monitor and pulse oximeter.
		The child will experience adequate gas exchange, as evidenced by:
		• Oxygen saturation >95% by pulse oximetry.
		• ABG values within normal limits:
		  ■ PaO_2 80 to 100 mm Hg (10.0 to 13.3 KPa).
		  ■ SaO_2 >95%.
		  ■ $PaCO_2$ 35 to 45 mm Hg (4.7 to 6.0 KPa).
		  ■ pH between 7.35 and 7.45.
		• Skin normal color, warm, and dry.
		• Improved level of consciousness.
		• Regular rate, depth, and pattern of breathing.
		• Symmetric chest expansion.
		• Clear and equal breath sounds.

Cardiac output, decreased, related to: • Decreased venous return secondary to blood or fluid volume loss. • Increase in heart rate and decrease in stroke volume. • Massive peripheral vasodilation.	• Control bleeding. • Obtain vascular access and initiate fluid therapy. • Administer blood and colloids. • Initiate drug therapy to manage any dysrhythmia or hypotension. • Initiate cardiopulmonary resuscitation, if needed. • Defibrillate or provide synchronized cardioversion, if needed. • Treat the underlying cause.	The child will maintain adequate circulatory function, as evidenced by: • Strong, palpable peripheral and central pulses. • Adequate blood pressure for age. • Pulse rate appropriate for age. • Absence of dysrhythmias. • Skin normal color, warm, and dry. • Improved level of consciousness. • Urine output of 1 to 2 ml/kg/hour.

NURSING DIAGNOSIS	INTERVENTIONS	EXPECTED OUTCOMES
Fluid volume deficit related to: • Hemorrhage. • Fluid volume loss from injury such as a burn. • Vomiting. • Diarrhea. • Alteration in capillary permeability. • Alteration in vascular tone. • Myocardial compromise.	• Control bleeding. • Obtain vascular access. • Administer fluid bolus. • Initiate volume replacement. • Initiate drug therapy, as indicated by the child's clinical condition. • Place child on monitor and pulse oximeter.	The child will have an effective circulating volume, as evidenced by: • Stable vital signs appropriate for age. • Urine output of 1 to 2 ml/kg/hour. • Urine specific gravity within normal limits. • Strong, palpable peripheral and central pulses. • Improved level of consciousness. • Skin normal color, warm, and dry. • Hematocrit of 30 ml/dl or hemoglobin of 12 to 14 gm/dl or greater. • Moist mucous membranes. • External hemorrhage is controlled. • Management of vomiting and diarrhea. • Management of burn wounds.
Hypothermia related to: • Developmental physiology (i.e., newborn). • Larger total body surface area and increased risk of heat loss in the pediatric patient. • Rapid infusion of resuscitative fluids. • Decreased tissue perfusion. • Exposure.	• Initiate warming measures: ■ Warm blankets. ■ Warm fluids. ■ Overhead lights. ■ Radiant warmer. ■ Warmed humidified oxygen.	The child will maintain a normal core body temperature, as evidenced by: • Core temperature measurement of 36 to 37.5°C (96.8 to 99.5°F). • Absence of shivering, cool skin, pallor. • Skin normal color, warm, and dry.

Triage or Acuity Decisions

EMERGENT Pediatric patient who is pulseless or apneic. Any child with signs and symptoms of compensated or uncompensated shock, such as altered mental status ranging from irritability to coma; pallor; diaphoresis; poor or absent peripheral pulses; increased capillary refill time; marked tachycardia, with or without hypotension; obvious site of uncontrolled bleeding; muffled or distant heart tones; generalized edema; severe respiratory distress; petechial or purpuric rash with fever.

URGENT Pediatric patient with effective perfusion and a history of vomiting or diarrhea or decreased fluid intake; signs and symptoms of mild-to-moderate dehydration.

NONURGENT Pediatric patient with a history of vomiting or diarrhea without signs of dehydration. Minor injury with effective perfusion.

Planning and Implementation

Refer to Chapter 4, "Initial Assessment and Triage," for a description of the general nursing interventions for the pediatric patient. After a patent airway and effective ventilation are assured, the following interventions are initiated, as appropriate, for the child's condition.

ADDITIONAL INTERVENTIONS

- For absent or ineffective pulse, initiate cardiopulmonary resuscitation utilizing the universal pediatric template, when indicated by the child's condition (see Figure 25). (Nursing diagnosis: Decreased cardiac output). See Appendix P for pediatric basic life-support guidelines.

Figure 25
UNIVERSAL PEDIATRIC TEMPLATE

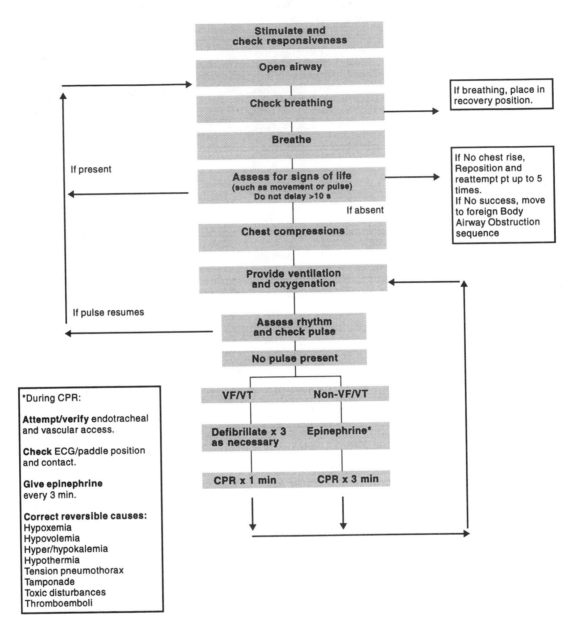

From Nadkarni V, Hazinski MF, Zideman D, Kattwinkel J, Quan L, Bingham R, Zaritsky A, Bland J, Kramer E, Tiballs J. Pediatric resuscitation. *Circulation.*1997;8:2191. Reprinted with permission.

- Perform chest compressions. The technique for the compressions is based on the age and size of the child. The child younger than 1 year of age is considered an infant. Chest compressions can be performed with one hand for the child younger than 8 years of age.

- Initiate chest compressions in all pediatric patients with heart rates too low to adequately perfuse their vital organs. **Profound bradycardia in the infant or child with poor perfusion is usually considered an indication for chest compressions.**[2,3] Chest compressions are initiated if the infant's or child's heart rate is less than 60 beats/minute and signs of poor systemic perfusion are present (see Chapter 10, "The Neonate," for neonatal indicators).

- Control any obvious bleeding. (Nursing diagnoses: Cardiac output, decreased; fluid volume deficit).

- Obtain vascular access. (Nursing diagnoses: Cardiac output, decreased; fluid volume deficit).

  - Peripheral venous access can be difficult and time consuming to obtain once cardio-pulmonary arrest has occurred. Emergent management of the child may require the insertion of an intraosseous needle. Refer to Pediatric Considerations: Vascular Access, Peripheral Access at the end of Chapter 7.

  - If peripheral venous access cannot be established within three attempts or 90 seconds, initiate intraosseous access with a 16-gauge or 18-gauge disposable bone marrow needle. Secure the needle because movement of the needle erodes the entry site, allowing fluid to extravasate into the soft tissues.

  - Insertion of a central line into the subclavian vein in the pediatric patient has inherent risks, such as the development of a pneumothorax. Preferred sites for central line insertion include the external jugular, internal jugular, and femoral veins.

  - Saphenous vein cutdown is not recommended for the emergent patient unless all other methods fail because of the time required for completion of the procedure.

- Defibrillate or provide synchronized cardioversion. (Nursing diagnosis: Decreased cardiac output).

  - For ventricular fibrillation and pulseless ventricular tachycardia, an initial shock of 2 J/kg is recommended followed by two additional shocks at 4 J/kg. If there is no response from the shocks, initiate medications (see Figure 25).

  - Paddle size is chosen by using the largest paddle that will fully contact the child's chest while remaining totally separate from the second paddle.[3]

    - Use infant paddles in infants 1 year of age or younger or weighing 10 kg or less.

    - Adult paddles are generally used for children older than 1 year of age or weighing more than 10 kg.

  - Apply gel or use defibrillation pads. Apply one paddle to the upper right chest below the clavicle. Apply the other paddle to the left side of the chest, lateral to the nipple at the anterior axillary line.

  - Charge the defibrillator and assure safety of all personnel before discharging.

  - Synchronized cardioversion is indicated for the treatment of unstable supraventricular tachycardia and unstable ventricular tachycardia characterized by pallor, decreased perfusion, and altered level of consciousness. An initial dose of 0.5 J/kg is recommended. The subsequent dose is 2 J/kg.[3] Consider sedation in the conscious child.

- Initiate volume replacement. (Nursing diagnosis: Fluid volume deficit).

  - Administer a 20 ml/kg bolus of an isotonic crystalloid solution (0.9% normal saline or lactated Ringer's solution). After each bolus, evaluate the child for clinical improvement. Additional crystalloid fluid boluses, blood, or colloid solutions may be required.

- Because approximately one fourth of the crystalloid solution remains in the vascular compartment, infusion of four to five times the fluid loss may be required to restore plasma volume.[3] Colloids are more efficient volume expanders than crystalloids. However, the child may experience sensitivity reactions or complications with their administration.[3]

- Rapid administration of blood, blood products, crystalloids, colloids, or blood may contribute to the development of hypothermia, metabolic derangements such as hypocalcemia, hypernatremia, and coagulapathies.[3] Blood component therapy may be indicated to correct coagulopathies that can develop from fluid resuscitation.

- Provide supplemental warmth (i.e., overbed warmers, warm blankets, warm intravenous fluids, warm humidified oxygen). (Nursing diagnosis: Hypothermia). In children, the combination of body exposure to the environment, high ratio of body surface area to volume, and the infusion of large amounts of room temperature intravenous fluids can lead to hypothermia. In the hypothermic state, the child may respond poorly to drug and fluid administration. Additionally, hypothermia further depletes compensatory reserves of the already stressed cardiovascular system. Clinically, hypothermia may mimic hypoxia, thus complicating the assessment of the patient.

- Promote and support the family's involvement in the child's care. (Nursing diagnosis: Anticipatory grieving). Assign a health care professional to provide explanations of procedures and the treatment plan to the caregivers. Assign a staff member to provide emotional support interventions and to be with the family during the time in the emergency department.

- Insert gastric tube to reduce gastric distention. (Nursing diagnosis: Impaired gas exchange).

DRUGS AND DRIPS

See Appendix Q for a list of drugs used in resuscitation and Appendix R for a reference on preparing drug infusions during resuscitation.

- Administer antipyretics and analgesics. (Nursing diagnoses: Pain; hyperthermia).

- Correct hypoglycemia. (Nursing diagnosis: Altered tissue perfusion).

  - Infants have limited glycogen stores that are rapidly depleted during periods of stress. A serum or whole blood glucose test is required for any child who is or has been resuscitated. Documented hypoglycemia is treated with intravenous glucose 0.5 to 1 gm/kg:

  - Administer 2 to 4 ml/kg of 25% glucose solution (D_{25}) slowly via intravenous or intraosseous line. If a prepared solution of D_{25} is unavailable, 1 to 2 ml/kg of 50% glucose solution is diluted 1:1 with sterile water and then administered via intravenous or intraosseous access.

  - In *neonates,* 3 to 5 ml/kg of 10% glucose solution (D_{10}) is administered via intravenous or intraosseous access. If D_{10} is unavailable, 1 to 2 ml/kg of a 50% solution is diluted 1:4 with sterile water and then administered via intravenous or intraosseous access.

- Treat the underlying cause of shock. (Nursing diagnosis: Decreased cardiac output).

  - If sepsis is suspected, anticipate the need for antibiotic therapy.

  - If an arrhythmia has resulted from an electrolyte imbalance or a metabolic derangement, administer medications, as prescribed.

- Initiate inotropic agents, as ordered. (Nursing diagnosis: Decreased cardiac output). In the unstable child, continuous infusions of epinephrine hydrochloride, dopamine hydrochloride, or dobutamine hydrochloride may be used to maintain blood pressure and tissue perfusion (see Appendix R for information on preparing the infusions).

- Correct cardiac dysrhythmias. (Nursing diagnosis: Decreased cardiac output).

  - Because children rarely present to the emergency department with primary cardiac dysrhythmia, antidysrhythmic drugs are seldom used.

  - Bradydysrhythmias and asystole are treated with epinephrine hydrochloride. Epinephrine stimulates alpha-adrenergic effects in the vascular bed and beta-adrenergic affects on the heart.

  - Atropine sulfate is used to diminish bradycardia associated with stimulation of the vagus nerve during intubation and symptomatic bradycardia associated with atrioventricular block.[2,3]

  - The initial assessment following administration of epinephrine hydrochloride is palpation of pulses.

  - Hypoxia is a common cause of bradycardia in infants and young children. Administration of atropine sulfate may mask hypothermia-induced bradycardia. The child's oxygen saturation level must be continuously monitored.[2]

- Correct electrolyte and acid-base imbalances. (Nursing diagnosis: Impaired gas exchange).

  - Buffers such as sodium bicarbonate may be administered to the child with documented severe acidosis, but only after the provision of adequate oxygenation and ventilation.[3]

  - A 4.2% solution is used in infants younger than 3 months of age.

- Continually monitor vital signs and the child's response to specific interventions.

- Involve the child's family as soon as possible in the resuscitation process. The majority of pediatric arrests have dismal outcomes; decisions may need to be made about the termination of resuscitative efforts. Involve the caregivers in this decision-making process.[12]

Evaluation and Ongoing Assessment

The child who is in shock requires meticulous and frequent reassessment of a patent airway, breathing effectiveness, perfusion, and mental status. The etiologies of shock and cardiovascular compromise encompass a broad range of disorders. Initial improvements may not be sustained, and additional interventions may be required. The child's response to interventions and trending of the child's condition must be closely monitored. To evaluate the patient's progress, monitor the following:

- Airway patency; endotracheal tube placement.

- Effectiveness of breathing or ventilation.

- Pulse rate and quality.

- Skin color and temperature; capillary refill.

- Blood pressure.

- Core temperature.

- Level of consciousness and pupil reaction.

- Urine output.

- Cardiac rhythm.

- Oxygen saturation.

- End-tidal CO_2, if available.

- Arterial pH, PaO_2, and $PaCO_2$.

SELECTED EMERGENCIES

Rhythm Disturbances

Cardiopulmonary arrest is uncommon in the pediatric population. However, when it does occur, the outcome is generally dismal.[2] The most common cause of cardiac arrest in children is respiratory arrest. In the child, unlike in the adult patient, cardiac arrest is usually not sudden but the end result of respiratory failure or shock.

ASYSTOLE

Asystole is the absence of electrical activity in the heart. It is visualized as the absence of a QRS complex on the monitor and is confirmed by the lack of central pulses (see Appendix S for asystole and pulseless arrest decision tree).

Additional History

- Description of the event prior to arrest, time last seen by the caregiver, last feeding, position in crib, and activities.

- Determine who was the primary caregiver at the time of the event.

- Time the child was found to be pulseless, if known.

- Time basic life support was initiated; by bystander or prehospital personnel.

- Time advanced life support was initiated.

- Caregiver or family support systems.

Signs and Symptoms

- Apnea.

- Poor peripheral perfusion.

- Absent heart tones.

- Absent central and peripheral pulses.

Additional Interventions

- Administer epinephrine hydrochloride per current dosage recommendations. The preferred route of administration is intravenous or intraosseous. If intravenous or intraosseous access is not established, the endotracheal route is used.

- Administer other medications, as appropriate.

- Anticipate the need to decide to terminate resuscitative efforts by considering the following factors[12]:

  - Duration of pulselessness.

  - Use of high-dose epinephrine hydrochloride without restoration of effective rhythm.

  - Etiology of the cardiac arrest.

BRADYCARDIA

Bradycardia is one of the most common terminal rhythms seen in the pediatric population. Bradycardia results from an alteration in function of the sinus node and conduction pathways. Hypoxemia, acidosis, and hypovolemia are the most common factors that may interfere with sinus node function resulting in bradycardia[3] (see Appendix T for bradycardia decision tree).

Additional History

- Description of events prior to onset of bradycardia (i.e., acute fluid volume loss, apnea, hypo-ventilation).

Signs and Symptoms

- Altered level of consciousness.

- Weak or absent peripheral pulses.

- Heart rate less than 60 beats/minute in an infant or child with poor peripheral perfusion.

Additional Interventions

- Cardiac compressions are initiated if heart rate remains less than 60 beats/minute with adequate ventilation and oxygenation.[3]

- Administer epinephrine hydrochloride.

VENTRICULAR FIBRILLATION OR PULSELESS VENTRICULAR TACHYCARDIA

Ventricular fibrillation and pulseless ventricular tachycardia are not common dysrhythmias in the pediatric population. Management is different from that in the adult patient in that defibrillation is administered at much lower energy than in the adult, and appropriate-sized paddles must be available to perform effective defibrillation (see Appendix S for asystole and pulseless arrest decision tree).

Additional History

- Electrocution.

- Recent viral illness.

- History of cardiac surgery or heart transplant.

- Ingestion of toxic substance.

Signs and Symptoms

- Unresponsiveness.

- Absence of a palpable pulse.

- Ventricular fibrillation on the cardiac monitor.

- Presence of ventricular tachycardia on the monitor without palpable pulses.

SUPRAVENTRICULAR TACHYCARDIA

Supraventricular tachycardia is one of the most common dysrhythmias in children. It is characterized by a heart rate greater than 220 beats/minute in infants and greater than 180 beats/minute in children that does not vary with agitation or crying.[3] In the child with supraventricular tachycardia, systemic perfusion may be adequate or compromised with signs of cardiovascular collapse.

Additional History

- History of previous supraventricular tachycardia episode.

- History of *Wolff-Parkinson-White syndrome.*

- History of congenital heart disease.

- Poor feeding.

Signs and Symptoms

- Pallor, mottled skin, or cyanosis.

- Hypotension.

- Faint or absent peripheral pulses.

- Altered mental status.

- Irritability.

Additional Interventions

- Synchronized cardioversion must be used if intravenous access is not available and the child is unstable (i.e., signs of poor perfusion and hypotension are present). The procedure for synchronized cardioversion is similar to defibrillation, with the following modifications[3]:

  - The defibrillator and cardiac monitor must be joined so that the delivery of the countershock can be synchronized to avoid delivery of the energy during the relatively refractory portion of the cardiac electrical activity.

- Initial dose is 0.5 J/kg; repeat doses are delivered at 1 J/kg.

- Discharge buttons must be held until the countershock is delivered.

- Consider administration of analgesics and sedation.

- Adenosine phosphate is the drug of choice for conversion of supraventricular tachycardia in stable children. An antecubital peripheral intravenous line is the preferred site as it is the closest peripheral site to the heart. In the unstable child, cardioversion must not be delayed while venous access is established to administer adenosine phosphate.

  - Adenosine phosphate must be given rapidly at the port closest to the infusion site and flushed with normal saline. It is not uncommon to administer both the drug and the flush at the same time.

  - Adenosine phosphate interrupts the re-entry circuits that involve the atrioventricular node, causing a brief period of asystole. Side effects are rare because the half-life of the drug is 10 seconds.[3]

  - Use with caution in children with heart transplants.[3]

  - Higher doses of the drug may be required in children receiving theophylline or caffeine.[3]

HEALTH PROMOTION

The following preventive measures and recommendations may have an impact on shock-related morbidity and mortality:

- Educate caregivers about the necessity to schedule infants, children, and adolescents for well-child checkups with their primary health care providers.

- Identify strategies to educate and encourage caregivers to assure that infants, children, and adolescents receive vaccinations to prevent illness.

- Develop strategies to educate caregivers, children, and their communities about trauma prevention.

- Develop and implement strategies to decrease the risk of infection in children with indwelling devices such as tracheostomy tubes and long-term intravenous access devices.

SUMMARY

Evaluation of the pediatric patient in shock requires astute assessment of peripheral perfusion, vital signs, level of consciousness, and urine output. Shock and respiratory failure are common pathways to cardiovascular collapse and subsequent cardiac arrest in the pediatric patient. The outcome of cardiac arrest in the child is most frequently death or recovery with poor neurologic outcome.

Early recognition of the signs of shock is critical to the initiation of prompt intervention and the prevention of adverse outcomes. The central piece of the puzzle in the care for the child in shock is the interlocking relationship between early recognition of the life-threatening illnesses and injuries that cause shock and the initiation of the rapid interventions.

REFERENCES

1. Kloeck W. The universal advanced life support algorithm. *Circulation.* 1997;8:2180-2182.

2. Nadkarni V, Hazinski MF, Zideman D, Kattwinkel J, Quan L, Bingham R, Zaritsky A, Bland J, Kramer E, Tiballs J. Pediatric resuscitation. *Circulation.*1997;8:2185-2195.

3. Chameides L, Hazinski MF, eds. *Pediatric Advanced Life Support.* Dallas, Tex: American Heart Association; 1997.

4. Bell L. Shock. In: Fleisher GR, Ludwig S, Silverman BK, eds. *Synopsis of Pediatric Emergency Medicine.* Baltimore, Md: Williams & Wilkins; 1996:27-32.

5. Mott S. Cardiac emergencies. In: Kelley S, ed. *Pediatric Emergencies.* Norwalk, Conn: Appleton & Lange; 1994:199-228.

6. Hazinski MF. Cardiovascular disorders. In: Hazinski MF, ed. *Nursing Care of the Critically Ill Child.* 2nd ed. St. Louis, Mo: Mosby-Year Book; 1992:117-154.

7. Selfridge-Thomas J. Shock. In: Kitt S, Selfridge-Thomas J, Proehl J, Kaiser J, eds. *Emergency Nursing: A Physiological and Clinical Perspective.* Philadelphia, Pa: WB Saunders; 1995:37-53.

8. Britt LD. Priorities in the management of profound shock. *Surg Clin North Am.* 1996;76:645-661.

9. Cohen A. Hematologic emergencies. In: Fleisher GR, Ludwig S, Silverman BK, eds. *Synopsis of Pediatric Emergency Medicine.* Baltimore, Md: Williams & Wilkins; 1996:384-404.

10. Vary TC, Littleton Kearney MT. Pathophysiology of traumatic shock and multiple organ failure. In: Cardona VD, Hurn PD, Mason PJB, Scanlon AM, Veise-Berry SW, eds. *Trauma Nursing: From Resuscitation Through Rehabilitation.* 2nd ed. Philadelphia, Pa: WB Saunders; 1994:114-150.

11. Gewitz MH, Vetter VL. Cardiac emergencies. In: Fleisher GR, Ludwig S, Silverman BK, eds. *Synopsis of Pediatric Emergency Medicine.* Baltimore, Md: Williams & Wilkins; 1996:277-295.

12. Scribano PV, Baker MD, Ludwig S. Factors influencing termination of resuscitative efforts in children: A comparison of pediatric emergency medicine and adult emergency medicine physicians. *Pediatr Emerg Care.* 1997;13:320-324.

Pediatric Considerations: Vascular Access

Vascular access is commonly required for children in the emergency care setting for fluid and/or intravenous medication administration. Access routes include peripheral, intraosseous, and central lines. The technique for rapid fluid administration was discussed in Chapter 3, "Pediatric Considerations: Pain Management and Medication Administration."

Peripheral Vascular Access

- When rapid fluid administration and fluid resuscitation are required, insert the largest catheter that the vessel will accommodate.

- Over-the-needle catheters are preferred because of their stability in the vein. Butterfly needles are rarely used in children, except for simple phlebotomy procedures.

- Preparation of the caregiver and the child prior to the procedure is critically important:

    - Use age-appropriate techniques to prepare the child.

    - Consider the use of dermal anesthetic or iontophoresis.

    - Use distraction and other nonpharmacologic coping and pain management techniques during the procedure.

    - Provide comfort and rewards after the procedure.

- Intravenous sites commonly used in infants and children are the scalp (in infants), hands, feet, and antecubital fossa:

    - In nonemergent situations, attempt distal sites first.

    - For emergent access, the antecubital veins may be the first choice.

    - During cardiopulmonary resuscitation, the preferred site is the largest, most accessible vein that does not require interruption of resuscitation.[1]

    - Contraindications to intravenous insertion include the presence of circumferential burn, infection, marked edema of an extremity from a suspected fracture, or confirmed fracture at the selected site.

    - Superficial scalp veins in the infant are the frontal, superficial temporal, posterior auricular, supraorbital, occipital, and posterior facial veins (see Figure 26):

        ♦ A rubber band can be used as a tourniquet.

        ♦ Insert the needle in the same direction as the venous blood flow to the heart.

        ♦ Contraindications to scalp vein insertion include age greater than 9 months, hydrocephalus, ventricular shunt, anencephaly, and skull fracture.

Figure 26
SCALP VEINS

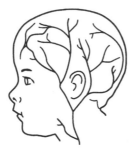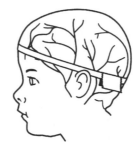

From French JP. Venous access. In: French JP, ed. *Pediatric Emergency Skills*. St. Louis, Mo: Mosby-Year Book; 1995:5. Reprinted with permission.

- Upper extremity veins include the cephalic, median basilic, and antecubital veins in the upper arm. In the dorsum of the hand, the cephalic and basilic veins may be used:

  ♦ The dorsum of the hand is a good site to use in chubby infants.

  ♦ It may be helpful to close the child's hand tightly and flex the wrist.

- Lower extremity veins include the saphenous vein and the veins in the dorsal arch.

Figure 27 illustrates intravenous access sites in the upper and lower extremities. Figure 28 illustrates intravenous access sites in the hand.

- Positioning the child appropriately and securing the selected extremity and insertion site are critical steps of the procedure. Positioning-for-comfort strategies are very effective with intravenous insertion (see Chapter 3, Pediatric Considerations: Pain Management and Medication Administration).

- When inserting a small-gauge catheter, advance the needle slowly. Blood return may be delayed for a few seconds because of the small diameter of the needle.

- When the blood return is observed, advance the catheter off the stylet into the vein.

Figure 27
INTRAVENOUS SITES

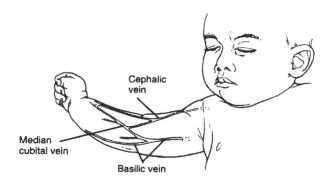

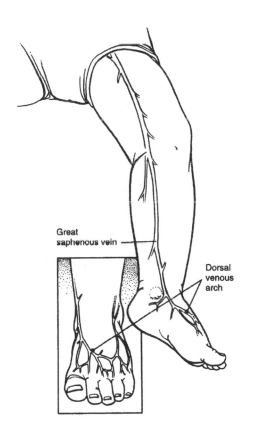

From Chameides L, Hazinski MF, eds. Vascular access. *Textbook of Pediatric Advanced Life Support*. Dallas, Tex: American Heart Association; 1997:5-4. Reprinted with permission.

Figure 28
DORSAL HAND INTRAVENOUS SITES

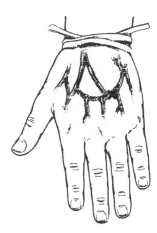

From Schleien CL, Kuluz JW, Shaffner DH. Cardiopulmonary resuscitation. In: Nichols DG, Yaster M, Lappe DG, Haller JA, eds. *Golden Hour: The Handbook of Advanced Pediatric Life Support*. St. Louis, Mo: Mosby-Year Book; 1996:105. Reprinted with permission.

- To avoid shearing the catheter, never reintroduce the stylet into the catheter once it has been withdrawn.

- Blood samples may be drawn prior to initiating fluid therapy. Insert the vacutainer directly into the catheter hub or use a T-connector. If a smaller gauge intravenous needle is used, the suction from the vacutainer may collapse the vessel. If a T-connector is used, withdraw the blood sample before flushing the T-connector with normal saline.

- Attach a T-connector flushed with normal saline to the catheter hub after the stylet is removed. The T-connector provides an access port at the closest point to the site.

- Secure the catheter with tape and gauze or a nonocclusive dressing. Figure 29 illustrates securing of an intravenous catheter in the hand and foot[2]:

    - Tape the catheter securely while maintaining visualization of the site.

    - Use tape to secure the extremity to an appropriate-sized armboard:

        ◆ Position the child's fingers to grasp the armboard rather than outstretched on the board.

        ◆ Use 4 × 4-inch gauze rolls to support the child's extremity in a functional position.

    - Loop the intravenous tubing away from the catheter and secure with tape.

    - Label the site and tubing as per institution policy.

    - Protect the catheter and intravenous site. A commercially available product, such as I.V. HOUSE®, may be applied to protect the site (see Figure 30). A plastic medicine cup cut in half, with the edges taped, may also be used.

- Evaluate the intravenous site periodically for signs of infiltrate.

CHAPTER 7 PEDIATRIC CONSIDERATIONS

Figure 29
METHODS FOR SECURING AN INTRAVENOUS SITE

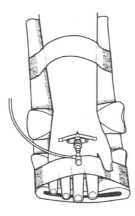

From French JP. Venous access. In: French JP, ed. *Pediatric Emergency Skills*. St. Louis, Mo: Mosby-Year Book; 1995:27. Reprinted with permission.

Figure 30
USE OF I.V. HOUSE®

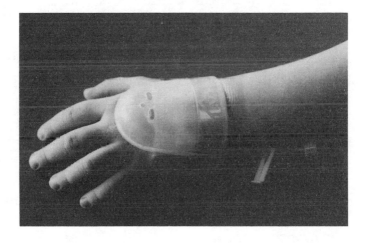

Intraosseous Access

- Intraosseous access is indicated when immediate vascular access is needed for the critically ill or injured child who requires intravenous fluid, medication, and/or blood administration for resuscitation (e.g., cardiopulmonary arrest, decompensated shock).[1,3,4]

- The intraosseous route is a safe and rapid method of accessing the circulatory system and is associated with a low complication rate.

- Intraosseous insertion is a painful procedure. If the child is responding to painful stimuli, use lidocaine hydrochloride for local anesthesia of the tissues and periosteum prior to insertion.

- Obtain intraosseous access by inserting a rigid needle into the medullary cavity of a bone, providing access to a noncollapsible venous plexus:

  - The tibia is the preferred site; the distal femur is an alternative site[4,5]:

    - Anterior medial portion of the tibia: Insert the needle at a 90° angle, 1 to 3 cm below the tibial tuberosity.

    - Anterior, distal portion of the femur: Insert the needle angled down from the growth plate 1 to 2 cm above the upper border of the patella.[5]

  - Limit insertion attempts to one attempt per bone. Multiple sticks in the same bone will result in leaking of fluids and medications into the tissues.

  - A commercially available intraosseous needle or a bone marrow aspiration needle is most commonly used.

  - 18-gauge, 16-gauge, and 15-gauge needles are generally available. The 18-gauge needles are usually used in infants younger than 3 months of age.

Table 19 provides an overview of the principles associated with intraosseous insertion and infusion.

- Intraosseous access is used for the short term, usually for less than 4 hours or until other routes of access are obtained.

- Rapid fluid administration usually requires fluids to be pushed manually. A pressure infusion device or pressure bag is needed to ensure consistent flow. Infusion by gravity flow is inconsistent and unreliable.

- Observe the site closely for extravasation of fluids. Monitor the insertion site and the posterior surface of the extremity (calf or lower thigh) for swelling, tension, or fullness. Discontinue the infusion if extravasation is suspected.

- Tape and secure the intraosseous needle. If the patient becomes responsive, restrain the extremity to prevent movement of the leg or kicking, which may dislodge the intraosseous needle.

- If an intraosseous line is not functional, it may be helpful to keep the needle in place until definitive access is obtained. Keeping the needle in place will alert providers to the fact that an intraosseous line was placed in that bone and further attempts in that bone must be avoided. Mark the intraosseous line as nonfunctional.

- When the intraosseous needle is removed, apply manual pressure for several minutes; then apply a pressure dressing. Label the dressing as an intraosseous site.

Figure 31 illustrates the placement of an intraosseous needle in the tibia and distal femur.

Table 19

INTRAOSSEOUS INFUSION		
Indications	**Contraindications**	**Possible Complications**
Intraosseous insertion is a reliable alternative to venipuncture in children usually younger than 6 years of age who are in shock or cardiopulmonary arrest and peripheral venous access cannot be achieved within a few minutes (usually 90 seconds or two to three vascular attempts, whichever comes first).[1] Usually used only in unconscious children.	• Fracture of the bone selected as the insertion site.[4] • Cellulitis of the overlying skin.[4] • Osteogenesis imperfecta/osteopetrosis.[4] • Previous attempts at intra-osseous insertion in the same bone.[4]	• Tibia fracture.[1] • Compartment syndrome.[1] • Skin necrosis.[1] • Air, fat, or bone embolus.[4]
Preferred Site	**Medication and Fluid Administration**	**Technique**
The flat, anteromedial surface of the tibia, approximately 1 to 3 cm below the tibial tuberosity is the preferred site.[1,3,4] The marrow cavity in this location is very large and the landmark is easily identified.	• Medication administered by the intraosseous route must be followed by a sterile saline flush of at least 5 ml to ensure that the drug is infused into the central circulation.[1] • Fluids must be administered under pressure using a pressure infusion device or manually using a syringe and stopcock.[1]	• Select site and prep skin. • Insert the needle at an angle directed away from the growth plate, or using a 90° angle to the bone.[1,3,4] • Use a to and fro technique with gentle downward pressure.[4] • When the bone marrow is entered, a "pop" or decrease in resistance is felt. • Remove the stylet and attach a 5-ml syringe. • Aspirate bone marrow to con-firm placement. • Flush with normal saline and connect to conventional intra-venous tubing with a pressure bag. • Observe the site closely for extravasation of fluids.

Figure 31
PLACEMENT OF AN INTRAOSSEOUS NEEDLE

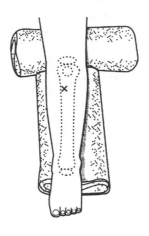

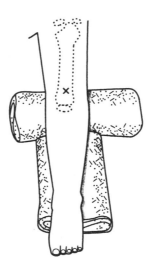

From French JP. Venous access. In: French JP, ed. *Pediatric Emergency Skills*. St. Louis, Mo: Mosby-Year Book; 1995:37. Reprinted with permission.

Central Venous Access

- The advantages of central venous access are rapid delivery of medications and fluids and the ability to measure central venous pressure.

- Central venous access in the pediatric patient is associated with more complications and risks, including infection, hemorrhage, pneumothorax, and cardiac tamponade.

- Central venous access can be obtained in the femoral, internal jugular, or subclavian veins (see Figure 32). The internal jugular site is difficult to access in children with short necks.

Figure 32
CENTRAL VENOUS INSERTION SITES

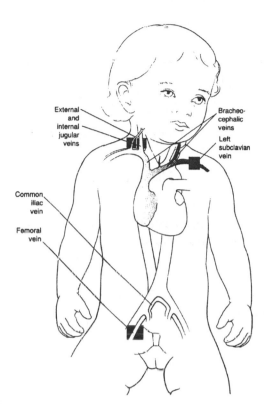

External and internal jugular veins

Bracheo-cephalic veins

Left subclavian vein

Common iliac vein

Femoral vein

Adapted from Lavelle J, Costarino A. Central venous access and central venous pressure monitoring. In: Henretig FM, King C, eds. *Textbook of Pediatric Emergency Procedures*. Philadelphia, Pa: Williams & Wilkins; 1997:252. Used with permission.

- Long-term central venous access devices are inserted when prolonged or frequent venous access is needed and/or peripheral access is not obtainable. The pediatric patient may present to the emergency department with a long-term device in place.

  - Subcutaneous infusion ports, central venous catheters (Broviac, Hickman), and peripheral inserted central catheter (PICC) lines are used in pediatric patients.

  - Follow appropriate procedure to access these devices. Use sterile technique during the access procedure.

  - Noncoring needles (Huber needles) are required to access most subcutaneous infusion ports.

  - Clamping of catheters is dependent on the type of catheter in place. The Hickman and Broviac catheters must be clamped when accessed; the Groshong catheter should not be clamped as it contains a two-way valve.[6]

  - Following collection of blood specimens or the completion of an infusion, the device is typically flushed with heparin sodium solution to maintain patency. The patient's weight and the catheter or device size and type will influence the heparin sodium concentration and volume used.

- Use a sterile technique when replacing central venous catheter dressings.

Points to Remember:

- Always maintain universal precautions when performing any procedure.

- Explain all procedures to the child and family in an age-appropriate and developmentally appropriate manner.

- Use pharmacologic and nonpharmacologic pain management techniques to decrease pain of procedure and facilitate coping.

- Reward and comfort the child after the procedure.

- Ask the child who requires frequent intravenous access (or the caregiver) the preferred site as well as the best location for intravenous access.

- Avoid the dominant hand if possible. If the child sucks his or her thumb, avoid the favored hand if possible.

- Evaluate all potential intravenous sites prior to attempting intravenous access. Avoid the prolonged use of tourniquets and access over bony prominences.

- Obtain assistance if unable to access a vein within two or three attempts.

- Monitor intravenous and intraosseous sites for signs of infiltration at least every hour when administering fluid boluses.

REFERENCES

1. Chameides L, Hazinski MF, eds. Vascular access. *Textbook of Pediatric Life Support.* Dallas, Tex: American Heart Association; 1997:5-1-5-17.

2. Barkin R, Rosen P, eds. *Emergency Pediatrics.* 3rd ed. St. Louis, Mo: Mosby-Year Book; 1990.

3. Guy J, Haley K, Zuspan S. Use of intraosseous infusion in the pediatric trauma patient. *J Pediatr Surg.* 1993;28:158-161.

4. Manley L, Haley K, Dick M. Intraosseous infusion: Rapid vascular access in critically ill or injured infants and children. *J Emerg Nurs.*1988;14:63-69.

5. Hodge D. Intraosseous infusion. In Henretig FM, King C, eds. *Textbook of Pediatric Emergency Procedures.* Baltimore, Md: Williams and Wilkins; 1997:289-298.

6. Wong D, Whaley L, eds. *Clinical Manual of Pediatric Nursing.* 3rd ed. St. Louis, Mo: Mosby-Year Book; 1990.

ADDITIONAL RESOURCES

Seidel J, Henderson D, Brownstein D. *Intraosseous Infusion* (videotape). Washington, DC: National Emergency Medical Services for Children (EMS-C) Alliance; 1994.

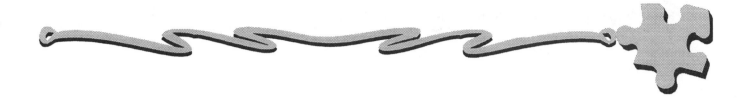

Burns

OBJECTIVES

On completion of this lecture, the learner should be able to:

+ Identify the anatomic and physiologic characteristics of the pediatric patient as a basis for the signs and symptoms of burns.

+ Identify the most frequent causes of burns.

+ Identify the appropriate nursing diagnoses and expected outcomes based on the assessment findings.

+ Delineate the specific interventions needed to manage the child with burns.

+ Evaluate the effectiveness of nursing interventions related to patient outcomes.

+ Identify health promotion strategies related to burns.

INTRODUCTION

In the United States, burn injury is the third leading cause of injury-related death in children 1 to 14 years of age.[1] The majority of burn-related injuries occur at home and are considered preventable. Unfortunately, about 3% of burn injuries are the result of abuse. Health care providers must be alert to the possibility of abuse or neglect when evaluating the pediatric burn patient (see Chapter 9, "Child Maltreatment").

Children younger than 5 years of age have the greatest morbidity and mortality associated with thermal injuries.[1] Developmental level and the ability to avoid or recognize environmental hazards are contributing factors associated with the incidence and type of burn injury among various age groups. Although children may sustain burns from a variety of agents, thermal burns, including scalds, contact with hot objects, and exposure to flame, are most prevalent.

Scalds are a more common cause of burn injury in children younger than 3 years of age. Younger children also suffer burns to the mouth as a result of biting, sucking, or chewing on electrical cords. Thermal burns caused by flames are more common in children 5 years of age and older and account for the majority of burn injuries in these age groups.

Concurrent injuries may also be present in the child who has suffered a burn injury from contact with electricity or an explosive force. Falling or jumping to safety to escape from a burning agent may also result in injury. A comprehensive primary and secondary assessment is essential in identifying other potential injuries.

ANATOMIC, PHYSIOLOGIC, AND DEVELOPMENTAL CHARACTERISTICS AS A BASIS FOR SIGNS AND SYMPTOMS

Anatomy

Burn injury places the pediatric patient at great risk for complications. When evaluating and resuscitating the burn-injured child, consider the following:

- Children have a greater body surface area in proportion to their body weight and will require more fluid during resuscitation. Young children also require maintenance fluids, which are usually not accounted for in most burn resuscitation formulas.[2]

- Children and infants have thinner skin, and infants and young children can suffer significant burn injuries from exposure to lesser amounts of heat:

  - Exposure of tissue to temperatures at or below 44°C (111°F) can be tolerated for extended periods of time by children.

  - Exposure at 54°C (130°F) for 10 seconds produces more severe tissue injury.

  - Exposure at 60°C (140°F) causes tissue destruction in less than 5 seconds.[3]

- Children have immature temperature-regulating centers in the hypothalamus. This places infants and children at greater risk for heat loss associated with burns and the development of hypothermia.

- In the presence of a hypothermic insult, the body resorts to nonshivering thermogenesis. To generate heat, the child's body must catabolize fat. This type of catabolism requires a large amount of oxygen and can result in lactate production and acidosis. Resuscitation of an acidotic, hypothermic infant is very difficult.

- The potential for infection presents some additional risks for the pediatric patient who has suffered a burn injury:

  - The disruption of the integumentary system as a protective barrier predisposes the child to infection or sepsis.

  - In the young infant or the immunocompromised child, the risk for infection is greater.

- The faster respiratory rate in children contributes to greater insensible pulmonary fluid loss.

- In a closed-space fire, the increased respiratory rate in children may lead to increased uptake of toxic gases. Most pediatric victims of closed-space fires die as a result of inhalation of toxic gases such as carbon monoxide and cyanide rather than burns.

- Children have smaller airways. Inhalation of irritants and heated air may cause edema resulting in a decreased airway diameter. This leads to a greater resistance to airflow and more pronounced signs of respiratory distress. Interstitial fluid shifts occurring with major burns may also result in airway edema without inhalation injury.

Pathophysiology

When burns occur, the integument of the body is disrupted. Intravascular capillaries become permeable and, as a result, proteins, electrolytes, and large amounts of fluids shift from the intravascular space to the interstitial space, termed third-spacing. Third-spacing results in edema of the burned area and loss of circulatory volume.

At the burn site, the vessels supplying the area are occluded, decreasing blood flow to the burn. The injured cells release vasoactive substances, causing vasoconstriction and the development of peripheral vessel thrombosis. Tissue necrosis can develop as a consequence of the decreased skin perfusion.

The electrolytes shift following a burn and can produce significant changes in the serum potassium, sodium, calcium, and base bicarbonate levels. For instance, the loss of cell wall integrity allows the extrusion of potassium from the cell into the extracellular fluid. The serum potassium concentration will reflect hyperkalemia, although intracellular potassium is depleted. In addition, the loss of extracellular base bicarbonate and loss of systemic compensatory mechanisms accentuates the development of metabolic acidosis. Young infants are less able to compensate for significant metabolic acidosis because their kidneys are immature and are unable to excrete large amounts of acids or absorb large quantities of bicarbonate.

Approximately 24 to 36 hours after the initial burn trauma, the capillaries are repaired and fluid remobilization begins. Fluid then returns to the intravascular space, the kidneys excrete sodium, and potassium returns to the cells. The child may develop hypernatremia, hypokalemia, and anemia from hemodilution and red blood cell destruction. Fluid administration in this phase must be closely monitored to prevent circulatory overload.[2,4]

Children must be assessed for progressive edema of the soft tissue and mucosa, leading to an airway obstruction. The greater proportion of soft tissue in the child's airway predisposes children to the development of mucosal edema. Approximately 48 to 72 hours after a burn injury, the damaged mucosal layer may slough, producing an acute airway obstruction.

Definitions

MECHANISM OF INJURY

Burn injury can occur through five mechanisms[4]:

- **Inhalation:** Inhalation of product such as carbon monoxide and cyanide, from incomplete combustion, toxic products, or thermal injury to the respiratory tract. Symptoms may not begin until 24 hours after exposure.

- **Thermal:** Dermal exposure to heat or flame.

- **Electrical:** Contact with electrical current (e.g., children biting through an electrical cord). Injuries may include massive tissue necrosis of the muscles, nerves, viscera, and subcutaneous tissue.

- **Chemical:** Dermal exposure to a corrosive agent.

- **Radiation:** Ionizing burns can be seen in children receiving radiation therapy.

DEPTH OF BURN INJURY

Depth of the burn injury may not be completely determined in the emergency department. Burns that initially appear to be partial-thickness burns may be identified as full-thickness burns days after the initial injury.

- Superficial or first-degree burns involve only the dermis and are characterized by:

    - Erythema.

    - Pain.

    - Dry appearance.

    - Blanching.

- Partial-thickness or second-degree burns are characterized by:

    - Moist appearance; blisters are usually present but may be disrupted.

    - Erythema.

    - Pain.

    - Superficial partial-thickness burns involve the upper dermis and deep partial-thickness burns involve deeper portions of the dermis.

- Full-thickness or third-degree burns are characterized by:

    - Dry, leathery appearance.

    - Color ranging from white to brown or black.

    - Decreased sensation to pain in the affected area.

EXTENT OF THE BURN INJURY

● The total burn surface area may be determined by using the rule of nines (see Figure 33) for children 10 years of age and older and the Modified Lund and Browder Chart (see Table 20) for children younger than 10 years of age.

Figure 33

RULE OF NINES

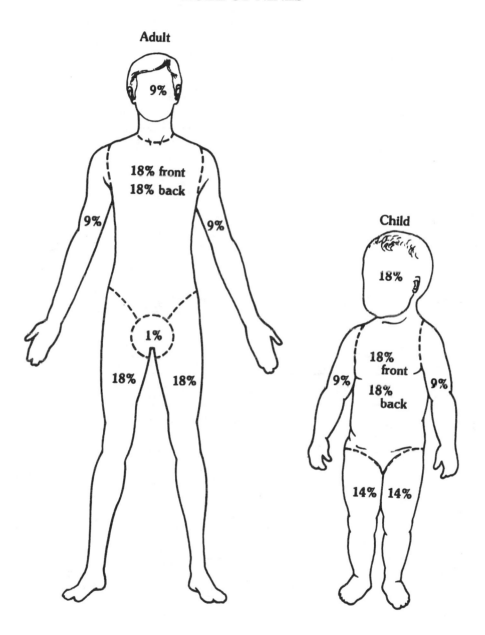

Table 20

Burned Area	MODIFIED LUND AND BROWDER CHART					
	Age (years)					
	1	1 to 4	5 to 9	10 to 14	15 to 18	Adult
	Total Body Surface					
Head	19%	17%	13%	11%	9%	7%
Neck	2	2	2	2	2	2
Anterior trunk	13	13	13	13	13	13
Posterior trunk	13	13	13	13	13	13
Right buttock	2.5	2.5	2.5	2.5	2.5	2.5
Left buttock	2.5	2.5	2.5	2.5	2.5	2.5
Genitalia	1	1	1	1	1	1
Right upper arm	4	4	4	4	4	4
Left upper arm	4	4	4	4	4	4
Right lower arm	3	3	3	3	3	3
Left lower arm	3	3	3	3	3	3
Right hand	2.5	2.5	2.5	2.5	2.5	2.5
Left hand	2.5	2.5	2.5	2.5	2.5	2.5
Right thigh	5.5	6.5	8	8.5	9	9.5
Left thigh	5.5	6.5	8	8.5	9	9.5
Right leg	5	5	5.5	6	6.5	7
Left leg	5	5	5.5	6	6.5	7
Right foot	3.5	3.5	3.5	3.5	3.5	3.5
Left foot	3.5	3.5	3.5	3.5	3.5	3.5

Adapted from Emergency Nurses Association. *Trauma Nursing Core Course (Provider) Manual.* 4th ed. Park Ridge, Ill: Author; 1995:268. Used with permission.

- The Lund and Browder Chart provides a more accurate estimation of the extent of burn injury because it relates the child's age to the proportion of individual body area. The major disadvantage of this chart is the need to have the child physically present because it is difficult to read in an emergency.

- In children younger than 14 years of age, a rapid method to determine the extent of a burn injury is to use the size of the palmar surface of the child's hand including the fingers. This area is approximately 1% of the total body surface area. Adding the number of times the child's palm would fit into the affected area will provide an estimation of the extent of the burn surface area.[3]

NURSING CARE OF THE CHILD WITH A BURN INJURY

Assessment

The child who is suffering from a burn injury requires simultaneous assessment and initiation of critical interventions. Refer to Chapter 4, "Initial Assessment and Triage," for a review of the comprehensive initial assessment and primary assessment interventions. Additional or specific history data and assessment findings important in the evaluation of a burn injury are listed below.

ADDITIONAL HISTORY

- When, where, and how the burn injury occurred.

- Place child was found: Bedroom, closet, contained space.

- Burn injury suggestive of child maltreatment: Inconsistent history, depth of injury, pattern of the burn.

- Type of burn: Thermal, electrical, chemical, or radiation.

- Duration of exposure.

- Treatment prior to ED arrival:

  - Measures taken to stop the burning process:

    - Removal of all clothing, including diapers, which may hold heat, hot liquids.

    - Type of dressing placed on the burn.

  - Removal of jewelry, constricting clothes.

  - Amount of intravenous fluid administered.

  - Wound care.

  - Oxygen administration.

SIGNS AND SYMPTOMS

- Singed nasal hair, facial hair, eyebrows.
- Presence of increased secretions.
- Decreased or absent cough reflexes.
- Changes in voice.
- Burns to face and neck.
- Soot around nose or mouth.
- Respiratory distress.
- Drooling.
- Circumferential burn of chest.
- Hoarse cough.
- Alteration in skin integrity:
  - Depth of the burn.
  - Extent of the burn.
  - Burn location, such as hands, perineum, feet, genitals.
  - Blisters.
- Pain.

DIAGNOSTIC PROCEDURES

Monitors

- Pulse oximetry must be used with caution if carbon monoxide poisoning is suspected. The pulse oximeter cannot differentiate between carboxyhemoglobin and oxyhemoglobin.
- Cardiac monitor, as indicated by severity of burn injury.
- Capnography, as indicated.

Radiographic Studies

Radiographs and other imaging studies are completed, as indicated based on the history of additional injuries related to the burn injury (e.g., explosion, fall).

Laboratory Studies

- Carboxyhemoglobin level.
- Serum cyanide level.
- Urine for specific gravity, myoglobin, protein, and glucose.

Nursing Diagnoses, Interventions, and Expected Outcomes

NURSING DIAGNOSIS	INTERVENTIONS	EXPECTED OUTCOMES
Airway clearance, ineffective, related to: • Edema from burn injury and the smaller size of the child's airway • Inhalation of toxic gases that cause injury to the airway • Inhalation of heat that causes injury to the airway • Pain • Altered level of consciousness secondary to hypoxia • Laryngeal spasm	• Elevate head of bed • Open and clear the airway • Administer oxygen • Suction as needed • Consider airway adjuncts or endotracheal intubation, as indicated	The child will maintain a patent airway, as evidenced by: • Regular rate, depth, and pattern of breathing • Symmetric chest expansion • Absence of signs and symptoms of retained secretions: Fever, tachycardia, and tachypnea • Absence of signs and symptoms of airway obstruction: Stridor, dyspnea, gag reflex, and hoarse voice • Effective cough • Clear sputum of normal amount without abnormal color or odor

Breathing pattern, ineffective, related to:
• Pain
• Circumferential burns to the neck or chest
• Altered mental status resulting from inhalation of toxic gases
	• Elevate head of bed
	• Administer pain medications
	• Prepare for and assist with escharotomy
		The child will have an effective breathing pattern, as evidenced by:
		• Regular rate, depth, and pattern of breathing
		• ABG values within normal limits:
		  ▪ PaO_2 80 to 100 mm Hg (10.0 to 13.3 KPa)
		  ▪ SaO_2 >95%
		  ▪ $PaCO_2$ 35 to 45 mm Hg (4.7 to 6.0 KPa)
		  ▪ pH between 7.35 and 7.45
		• Absence of stridor, dyspnea, and cyanosis
		• Trachea midline
		• Chest radiograph without abnormality
		• Absence of use of accessory muscles or nasal flaring
		• Regular rate, depth, and pattern of breathing
		• Clear and equal breath sounds
		• Symmetric chest expansion
		• Relief of constriction by escharotomy

Gas exchange, impaired, related to:
• Alveolar damage
• Fluid shifts
• Decreased transport, release, and utilization of oxygen secondary to carbon monoxide inhalation
• Ineffective airway clearance
	• Administer oxygen
	• Administer 100% O_2 for closed-space fire
	• Initiate hyperbaric oxygen therapy, when indicated
	• Assist in and maintain endotracheal intubation, as indicated
	• Monitor breath sounds
	• Monitor oxygen saturation and blood gases
	• Insert gastric tube
		The child will maintain adequate gas exchange, as evidenced by:
		• ABG values within normal limits:
		  ▪ PaO_2 80 to 100 mm Hg (10.0 to 13.3 KPa)
		  ▪ SaO_2 >95%
		  ▪ $PaCO_2$ 35 to 45 mm Hg (4.7 to 6.0 KPa)
		  ▪ pH between 7.35 and 7.45
		• Skin normal color, warm, and dry
		• Regular rate, depth, and pattern of breathing
		• Symmetric chest expansion
		• Clear and equal breath sounds
		• Oxygen saturation >95% by pulse oximetry
		• Improved level of consciousness

NURSING DIAGNOSIS	INTERVENTIONS	EXPECTED OUTCOMES
Fluid volume deficit related to: • Abnormal fluid losses • Increased capillary permeability • Protein shifts • Evaporation losses • Third-spacing	• Initiate vascular access • Calculate fluid needs based on burn formula and maintenance needs • Administer intravenous fluids • Monitor urine output	The child will have an effective circulating volume, as evidenced by: • Improved level of consciousness • Urine specific gravity within normal limits • Strong, palpable peripheral and central pulses • Skin normal color, warm, and dry • Hematocrit of 30 ml/dl or hemoglobin of 12 to 14 gm/dl or greater • Moist mucous membranes • Urine output of 1 to 2 ml/kg/hour • Stable vital signs appropriate for age
Tissue integrity, impaired, related to: • Burn injury	• Stop the burning process • Apply moist saline or dry sterile dressings • Absence of signs of infection: Redness, swelling, purulent drainage, odor, and tenderness	The child will experience resolution of impaired tissue integrity, as evidenced by: • Absence of signs of irritation: Redness, ulceration, blanching, and itching • Signs of progressive healing of dermal layer
Hypothermia related to: • Impairment of the child's integumentary system • Fluid resuscitation • Exposure	• Remove any moist dressings • Cover burn sites with sterile, dry dressing • Initiate warming methods	The child will maintain a normal core body temperature, as evidenced by: • Core temperature measurement of 36 to 37.5°C (96.8 to 99.5°F) • Skin normal color, warm, and dry
Infection, risk of, related to: • Impairment of the child's integumentary system • Presence of invasive lines	• Initiate infection control measures • Maintain aseptic technique for all invasive interventions • Culture burn wound • Apply antimicrobial agents, as indicated • Administer tetanus prophylaxis, as indicated	The child will be free from infection, as evidenced by: • Absence of systemic signs of infection: Fever, tachypnea, tachycardia • Core temperature measurement of 36 to 37.5°C (96.8 to 99.5°F) • Wounds free from redness, swelling, purulent drainage, or odor • Urine output of 1 to 2 ml/kg/hour • Negative blood cultures • White blood cell count within normal limits • Improved level of consciousness
Pain related to: • Depth of the burn • Extent of the burn • Wound care	• Assess level of pain • Cover burn site with sterile dressing • Administer pain medication, as indicated • Stop the burning process	The child will experience relief of pain, as evidenced by: • Diminishing or absent level of pain, indicated by patient's self-report using an objective measurement tool in the verbal child • Absence of physiologic indicators of pain: Tachycardia, tachypnea, pallor, diaphoretic skin, and increasing blood pressure • Absence of nonverbal cues of pain: Crying, grimacing, inability to assume position of comfort, and guarding • Ability to cooperate with care, as appropriate

Triage or Acuity Decisions

EMERGENT Pediatric patient with airway compromise or respiratory distress; partial-thickness burn >10% total burn surface area or full-thickness >3% total burn surface area; altered mental status; cardiac dysrhythmia from an electrical injury; severe pain; evidence of inhalation injury; found in a closed space; suspected inflicted burn.

URGENT Pediatric patient with partial-thickness burn <10% total burn surface area or full-thickness burn <3% total burn surface area.

NONURGENT Minor, superficial, localized burn.

Planning and Implementation

Refer to Chapter 4, "Initial Assessment and Triage," for a description of the specific nursing interventions for patients with compromises to airway, breathing, or circulation.

ADDITIONAL INTERVENTIONS

- Stop the burning process. (Nursing diagnoses: Pain; tissue integrity).

    - Remove all clothing and jewelry.

    - If the child has suffered a chemical burn, decontaminate according to the directions dictated by the manufacturer and poison control center.

- Deliver supplemental oxygen by nonrebreather mask if breathing is adequate. Use a humidifier if available. Administer 100% oxygen for all closed-space burn injuries. (Nursing diagnoses: Airway clearance; impaired gas exchange).

- Prepare for intubation and assisted ventilation if the child has a symptomatic inhalation injury with symptoms of airway obstruction, apnea, or respiratory distress. (Nursing diagnoses: Ineffective airway clearance, impaired gas exchange).

- Administer intravenous fluids. A number of fluid administration formulas are available to guide fluid resuscitation in the first 24 hours. The prescribed rate must be adjusted based on patient response. Adequacy of fluid administration is assessed by urine output, vital signs, level of consciousness, and peripheral circulation. Urine output should be maintained at 1 ml/kg/hour in the child weighing less than 30 kg or 30 to 50 ml/hour in the child weighing more than 30 kg. (Nursing diagnosis: Fluid volume deficit).

    - Carvajal formula[2,5]:

        ◆ Uses total body surface area rather than weight to calculate the child's fluid resuscitation. This formula recommends 5,000 ml/m^2/% total burn surface area + 2,000 ml/m^2/day as maintenance. Administer one half in the first 8 hours and the remaining half in the next 16 hours.

        ◆ Solution: Crystalloid with serum albumin.

- Parkland formula[6]:
  - Administer warmed crystalloid solution. As a general guideline, 4 ml × weight in kg × % total burn surface area = total amount of fluid to be infused in 24 hours.
  - Give one half of the 24-hour total fluid amount during the first 8 hours, calculated from the time of injury.
  - The remainder must be given equally over the next 16 hours.
  - The modified Parkland formula includes additional maintenance fluids; 4 ml × kg × % burn surface area + 15 ml/m^2 total burn surface area.

- Apply moist saline or dry sterile dressing to burn area. Because of the risk of hypothermia, moist dressings must not cover greater than 10% total burn surface area. Dry sterile dressings or a sterile sheet must be used with burns that cover more than 10% total body surface area. Consult with the burn center for specific therapy. Air currents flowing across the burn area cause pain; therefore, cover burns as quickly as possible. (Nursing diagnoses: Hypothermia; pain; tissue integrity).

- Administer analgesic medications. The intravenous route is used for pain medication administration in burn patients who require intravenous fluid administration. Morphine sulfate is the preferred medication. (Nursing diagnosis: Pain).

- Initiate warming measures. (Nursing diagnosis: Hypothermia).

- Anticipate antidote therapy for toxic inhalants. This may include administration of 100% oxygen, hyperbaric therapy, and sodium thiosulfate for cyanide inhalation. Contact a poison control center for additional information. (Nursing diagnosis: Impaired gas exchange).

- Administer tetanus prophylaxis, as indicated. (Nursing diagnosis: Infection).

- Insert an indwelling urinary catheter to monitor urine output and assess adequacy of fluid replacement. (Nursing diagnosis: Fluid volume deficit).

- Insert gastric tube for children with moderate and major burns that cover more than 20% of the total burn surface area because of the potential for gastric dilation, ileus formation, and nutritional support. (Nursing diagnosis: Impaired gas exchange).

- Prepare for escharatomies if a full-thickness circumferential burn of the extremity is accompanied by inadequate neurovascular function. A full-thickness burn of the chest has the potential to impair respiratory function; anticipate escharotomy of the chest. (Nursing diagnoses: Ineffective breathing pattern; tissue integrity).

- Treat or assist with burn wound management according to protocol. (Nursing diagnosis: Infection).

- Contact the regional burn center for transfer as per policy or procedure (see Table 21).

Table 21

AMERICAN BURN ASSOCIATION TRANSFER CRITERIA[5]

Patients with these burns must be treated in a specialized burn facility after initial assessment and stabilization at an emergency department.

- Second-degree burns covering more than 10% body surface area in children younger than 10 years of age.
- Second-degree burns covering more than 20% body surface area in other age groups.
- Second-degree and third-degree burns that involve the face, hands, feet, genitalia, perineum, or major joints.
- Third-degree burns covering more than 5% body surface area in any age group.
- Electrical burns, including lightning injury.
- Lightning injuries.
- Chemical burns that pose a serious threat to function or may cause cosmetic impairment.
- Inhalation injury with burn injury.
- Children with pre-existing medical problems that could impair healing or cause further complications from the burn injury.
- Children with associated trauma in which the burn injury poses the greater risk.
- Children with burns that require extensive emotional care or involve suspected maltreatment or substance abuse.
- Circumferential burns of an extremity or the chest.

Evaluation and Ongoing Assessment

The child with a burn injury may require intensive, ongoing intervention. Repeated assessments are necessary to evaluate trends in the child's condition and responses to interventions. Reassessment of the child's airway status, breathing effectiveness, perfusion, and pain management is essential to the evaluation of outcome achievement and the need for further intervention. To evaluate the patient's progress, monitor the following:

- Airway patency; endotracheal tube placement.

- Effectiveness of breathing or ventilation.

- Pulse rate and quality.

- Skin color, temperature, capillary refill.

- Blood pressure.

- Level of consciousness.

- Level of pain.

- Urine output.

- Oxygen saturation.

- Temperature.

SELECTED BURN INJURIES

Inhalation Injuries

Upper airway burns are often associated with facial burns and inhalation of hot gases. Edema produces rapid narrowing and obstruction of the airway. It is important to remember that children are very vulnerable to rapid occlusion of the airway because of their smaller airways and increased proportion of soft tissue.

SIGNS AND SYMPTOMS

- Carbonaceous sputum.

- Singed nasal hair or eyebrows.

- Mucosal redness.

- Tachypnea or alteration in respiratory effort.

- Tachycardia associated with the inhaled toxin.

- Hoarseness, cough, or hoarse cry.

- Decreased ability to handle secretions or swallow.

- Facial burns and swelling.

- Wheezing, crackles, rhonchi, or stridor.

- Oral or facial burns.

ADDITIONAL INTERVENTIONS

- Determine the need for intubation based on the child's level of consciousness, ability to protect airway, and oxygenation.

- Prepare for and assist with fiberoptic bronchoscopy to assess the degree of inhalation injury.

HEALTH PROMOTION

The majority of burn injuries to the pediatric population can be prevented. Stress the following safety measures:

- Install smoke detectors in the home.

- Install carbon monoxide detectors in the home.

- Be sure that hot water heaters are set at safe temperatures.

- Teach the child what to do in case of a fire (e.g., escape routes, drop and roll[7]).

- Teach the child about fire safety:

  - Do not play with matches or lighters.

  - Do not touch potentially hazardous materials.

- Store dangerous chemicals, such as gasoline, out of reach of children or in secure areas.

- Refer caregivers for followup if the child has started a fire.

- Teach the child electrical safety.

SUMMARY

The care and management of the child who has suffered a burn injury requires multidisciplinary collaboration. The central pieces of the puzzle in the care of the child with a burn injury are the interlocking relationship between the recognition of the severity of injury and the need to transfer the child for specialized acute and long-term burn care.

REFERENCES

1. Fingerhut LA, Warner M. *Injury Chartbook. Health, United States, 1996-97*. Hyattville, Md: National Center for Health Statistics; 1997.

2. Joffe MD. Burns. In: Fleisher GR, Ludwig S, Silverman BK, eds. *Synopsis of Pediatric Emergency Medicine*. Baltimore, Md: Williams & Wilkins; 1996:329-333.

3. Nagel TR, Schunk JE. Using the hand to estimate the surface area of a burn in children. *Pediatr Emerg Care*. 1997;13:254-255.

4. Emergency Nurses Association. Burn trauma. *Trauma Nursing Core (Instructor) Course*. 4th ed. Park Ridge, Ill: Author; 1995:253-284.

5. Demuth MW, Dimick AR, Gillespie RW, Gillespie PW, Hunt JL, Miller KL, Mancusi-Ungaro H, Pruitt BA, Robson MC, Smith DJ, Upright JW, Zawacki BE. *Advanced Burn Life Support Instructor Manual*. Lincoln, Neb: Advanced Burn Life Support; 1994.

6. Sadowski DA. Care of the child with burns. In: Hazinski MF, ed. *Nursing Care of the Critically Ill Child*. 2nd ed. St. Louis, Mo: Mosby-Year Book; 1992:875-927.

7. Wade J, Purdue GF, Hunt JL, Childers L. Crawl on your belly like GI Joe. *J Burn Care Rehabil*. 1990;11:261-263.

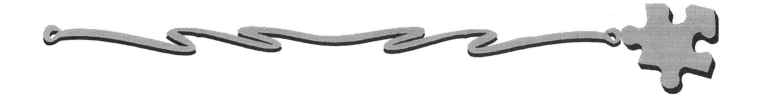

CHAPTER 9

Child Maltreatment

OBJECTIVES

On completion of this lecture, the learner should be able to:

✦ Describe the epidemiology of child maltreatment.

✦ Discuss risk factors for maltreatment and neglect.

✦ Describe the nursing assessment of the maltreated child.

✦ Describe nursing interventions for maltreated children and their families.

INTRODUCTION

The recognition of child maltreatment is of critical importance in the practice of nursing. In 1994, reports of suspected child maltreatment reached 2.9 million in the United States.[1] Although reports of child maltreatment continue to increase each year,[1,2] the actual incidence of maltreatment is difficult to determine. The number of cases not recognized or not reported to authorities is unknown. Fatal and near-fatal child maltreatment is not the rare event many may believe.

In 1995, research from the Centers for Disease Control and Prevention estimated that fatal abuse and neglect occur at a rate of 5.4 of every 100,000 children 4 years of age and younger. Because of misclassification of child deaths, the actual abuse death rate may be as high as 11.6 per 100,000 children 4 years of age and younger.[3] More than five children die every day as a result of child maltreatment.[3] Child maltreatment is the leading cause of injury-related death in children 4 years of age and younger.[3] The tragedy of near-fatal abuse and neglect is even more staggering. In 1990, more than 141,700 children were seriously injured by adult caregivers, and 18,000 sustained injury that resulted in permanent disability.[3]

Nurses are mandated to report suspected cases of maltreatment. State statutes define the conditions for reporting maltreatment in all 50 states. Therefore, it is important to be knowledgeable of child abuse laws in the jurisdiction in which one practices. Failure to report a case of suspected child maltreatment could result in civil or criminal charges.[4]

At times, the maltreated child presents to the emergency department for evaluation with a chief complaint related to potential maltreatment (e.g., possible sexual abuse). However, many maltreated children present to the emergency department for injuries or other health problems without declaration of abuse or neglect. A caregiver's false presentation of the child's history or intentional withholding of information concerning the child's injury or symptoms may contribute to the difficulty in the identification of child maltreatment.[5] The emergency nurse must be knowledgeable and alert to the signs and symptoms suggestive of child maltreatment.

Definitions

Child maltreatment is generally categorized into four major types[6]:

1. Physical abuse: Any inflicted injury to a child by a caregiver.

2. Sexual abuse: Any *sexual contact* between a child and an adult or an older child.

3. Emotional or psychological abuse: A pattern of demeaning behavior toward the child.

4. Neglect: Acts of omission and failure to meet a child's basic needs, including food, clothing, medical care, education affecting cognitive development, a safe environment, or emotional nurturing, affection, and attention.

Predisposing Factors

Multiple dynamics lead to situations that result in the maltreatment of children. There are factors that place the child at risk for maltreatment and the caregiver at increased risk for becoming abusive. These factors are described in Table 22.

Table 22

RISK FACTORS FOR CHILD MALTREATMENT	
CHILD	**ADULT CAREGIVER**
• Prematurity • Prenatal drug exposure • Developmental disability • Physical disability • Chronic illness • Product of multiple births • Product of unwanted pregnancy	• Substance abuse • Childhood history of maltreatment • Unmet emotional needs • Belief in use of corporal punishment • Rigid expectations regarding the child's behavior • Negative perceptions of the child • Unrealistic expectations of the child • Lack of parenting knowledge • Single parent • Social isolation • Psychological distress • Low self-esteem • Extreme poverty • Acute and chronic stressors

NURSING CARE OF THE MALTREATED CHILD

Recognition of Child Maltreatment

The recognition of child maltreatment is often difficult. The observation of child and caregiver interactions and thoughtful evaluation of historical data and physical findings are critical to the identification of the potentially maltreated child. The multidisciplinary team approach to the evaluation and management of these children is essential. Nurses, physicians, social workers, and prehospital personnel all play a role in assessing the child and the family dynamics for indicators of maltreatment.

Evaluating the Child for Indicators of Maltreatment

When a child presents to the emergency department with injury, the historical data and physical findings must be compared and evaluated in terms of congruency. Answering the following questions can assist the emergency team in identifying indicators suggestive of maltreatment.[4,5,7] These questions are not directly asked of the child's caregiver but are used to identify important information that should be collected during the history and physical examination of a child with injury. The interactions among the child, caregivers, and the staff are also important to evaluate.[7]

- Is the caregiver's history congruent with the mechanism of injury and actual injuries?
- Is the caregiver's history congruent with the child's developmental abilities?
- Was there a delay in seeking medical treatment?
- Are there any patterned or unusual marks on the child's body?
- Are there injuries of various ages and multiple types of injuries or multiple injury sites present?
- Does the caregiver deny knowledge of how the injury occurred?
- Is the caregiver's response appropriate to the child's condition?
- Is the caregiver's level of concern appropriate for the child's condition? Overconcern for a minor injury and underconcern or self-concern for a serious or critical injury are important findings.
- Does the child have any pre-existing medical conditions (e.g., bleeding disorder, hemophilia, bone disorder) or family history that could explain the present injuries?
- Who are the caregivers? Has there been recent changes in caregivers for the child?
- Are there any inconsistencies or changes in the history?
- Has the caregiver emphasized unimportant details or unrelated minor problem?
- Has the child been treated before for unexplained or suspicious injuries?
- Has the caregiver sought medical attention for injuries in other area hospitals?
- Has the caregiver bypassed hospitals closer to home to seek care in an emergency department that is farther away?
- Is there tension or hostility between caregivers? Is there hostility or aggression toward the child or staff?

- Is the caregiver uncooperative?

- What are the child's state of cleanliness, nutritional status, and general appearance?

- Could the injury or event have been avoided by closer supervision?

Obtaining a Comprehensive History

It is essential to obtain a comprehensive history when potential maltreatment is identified. The comprehensive history is more rigorous than the history typically obtained during triage or initial assessment and should be elicited in as much detail as possible. It is important to coordinate the collection of the complete history with other health care professionals, including physicians and social workers, who will be involved in the child's care. The following are general guidelines to assist in obtaining a comprehensive history when child maltreatment is suspected:

- Use a nonjudgmental and nonaccusatory approach, even when it is apparent that the caregiver has injured a child. Harsh interrogations can alienate the caregiver.

- Interview the verbal child alone. Use open-ended, nonleading questions. Begin with "What happened?" and follow with more specific questions. Document the child's responses as quotes whenever possible.

- If two caregivers are present, it is useful to interview each separately. Compare their histories and note any inconsistencies. Do not reveal information from one caregiver to the other. Use quotes to document responses.

- Do not reveal information obtained from the child while obtaining history from the caregivers.

- Identify family and child risk factors for maltreatment (see Table 22).

- Complete a diversity assessment, as appropriate.

- If a language barrier is present, it is important to utilize a professional interpreter or member of the staff who is fluent in the language. A family member, friend, or the child should not function as the interpreter.[5]

- Elicit other pertinent history information:

  - Developmental milestones the child has achieved.

  - Social history, including who cares for the child routinely, who lives in the household, and who has cared for the child over the last several days.

  - Family history of chronic disorders. Do not suggest the types of disorders (bleeding disorders or bone disorders); only ask open-ended questions concerning chronic illnesses of immediate and extended family members. If the caregiver provides a history of osteogenesis imperfecta in the family, note the color of the parent's sclera and if teeth are in good or bad repair.

- Obtain pertinent history for the current problem using the CIAMPEDS format.

- The past medical history must include information concerning previous injuries, hospitalizations, and ED visits as well as previous illnesses.

Conditions That Are Confused with Child Maltreatment

The emergency team must maintain an awareness of cultural and religious health practices in the evaluation of potential maltreatment. Southeast Asian groups, for example, use a number of methods that result in patterned lesions or blemishes on the skin. Coining and cupping are two such practices used in the treatment of a variety of ailments (see Appendix E). The resulting superficial cutaneous markings have been mistaken for inflicted injuries.

Prior use of folk remedies should be elicited during the history and diversity assessment. Some folk healing practices are actually dangerous to the child's health. In those situations, the caregivers must be educated regarding the harmful effect of the practice and taught alternative methods of treatment. The decision of whether or not child maltreatment has taken place is formulated by the hospital social worker or child protective agency and the health care team.

In some ethnic groups, normal skin pigmentations have also been frequently confused with bruising. Mongolian spots are bluish gray areas of pigmentation that are present in about 95% of African-American infants and 70 to 80% of Asian, Latino, and Native American infants.[8] These areas of pigmentation are most typically found over the sacral area and buttocks but may also be located on the legs, shoulders, and upper arms. Mongolian spots may persist into adulthood but usually fade during childhood.

Assessment of Specific Types of Maltreatment

NEGLECT

Neglect is the most common form of child maltreatment and accounts for greater than 40% of reported child maltreatment.[1,3]

History

The history of a child who has been neglected may include[3,6,7]:

- Delay in seeking health care for an injury or illness.
- History of previous injuries, ingestions, or exposures to toxic substances.
- Malnourishment or nonorganic failure to thrive, defined as weight below the fifth percentile.
- Excessive absenteeism from school.
- History of being left alone, abandoned, or inadequately supervised.
- Substance abuse in the older child or adolescent.
- Delinquency.

Signs and Symptoms[3,6]

- Based on the type of neglect (e.g., physical or emotional) and history.

- May be inactive or extremely passive.

- Poor hygiene (e.g., dirty clothes, unbathed child).

- Inappropriate attire (e.g., too little clothing in winter).

- Untreated dental caries.

- Developmental delays.

- Bald patches on infant's head (traction alopecia).

PHYSICAL ABUSE

Physical abuse encompasses the full spectrum of injury. Approximately 10% of injuries in children younger than 5 years of age who present to the emergency department are the result of abuse.[9] Inflicted injuries may involve the skin and soft tissues, bones, and all major organ systems. Following physical abuse, the caregiver may bring the child to the emergency department for the injuries sustained or there may be an incidental discovery of the injury by a teacher, relative, or health care provider.[10]

History

The presentation of the history data may reveal descriptions of maladaptive behaviors and indicators of maltreatment. History data may include[6,10]:

- Extreme withdrawal and apathy.

- Depression.

- Acting-out behaviors.

- History inconsistent with developmental milestone achievements or abilities.

- No explanation for the injury.

- Vague, unclear, or changing account of how the injury occurred.

- Discrepancy between the caregiver's and child's account.

- Unreasonable delay in seeking medical attention.

- Unrealistic expectations of the child.

- Family crisis or stress.

- History of previous ED visits or hospitalization for injury.

Signs and Symptoms

General Behaviors[6]

- Inappropriate reactions to procedures (e.g., failure to cry after an injection).
- Appears frightened of caregiver.
- Is withdrawn.
- Goes easily to strangers; uncharacteristic for child's age.
- Expresses extreme apprehension when hearing other children cry.

Bruises[6,9,10]

- Characteristics of noninflicted bruises:
  - Located on the extensor surfaces and bony surfaces, such as the elbows, knees, shins, or forehead.
  - Result from normal childhood activity.
- Characteristics of potentially inflicted bruises:
  - Bruises to the face, neck, chest, abdomen, back, flank, thighs, or genitalia.
  - Bruises in various stages of healing.
  - Bruises suggestive of being struck by an object, such as a looped cord, belt buckle, or open hand. Hand or finger imprints appear as linear bruises alternating with spared areas.
  - Pinch marks; pairs of crescent-shaped bruises.
  - Fingertip or thumb pattern bruises.
  - Bruises suggestive of being kicked. Usually to the lower body, they have a large, irregular shape and may reveal shoe or boot pattern.
  - Bruises to the mouth, gums, or buccal mucosa. A torn frenulum may suggest force feeding.
  - Multiple or symmetric bruises or marks.

Burns[6,9,11]

- An assessment of burn characteristic, depth, extent, and pattern of injury must be completed. Correlation of the severity and pattern of the burn injury with the history provides a basis for the identification of inflicted burns.
- Characteristics of noninflicted burns:
  - Asymmetric.
  - Splash pattern with congruent history.
  - Contact burn not uniform; more intense on one side of the burn.
  - Treatment sought immediately.

- Characteristics of potentially inflicted burns:

    - Immersion burn: Circumferential and often symmetric "stocking" pattern burns to the feet, "glove-like" pattern burns to hands, doughnut pattern burn to buttocks.

    - Burns with sharply demarcated edges without splash burns.

    - Ligature or rope burns on wrists, ankles, torso, or neck.

    - Cigarette or cigar burns, especially on typically concealed surfaces.

    - Contact burns. Dry, uniform imprint may be in configuration of an object used to cause the burn such as an iron, curling iron, register grill.

    - Symmetric burns.

    - Splash patterns in unusual sites (e.g., genitalia) or splash pattern with separated areas; may be from hot liquid being thrown at the child.

    - Burn to the dorsum of the hand.

    - Delays in seeking treatment.

Bites and Other Marks[6,10]

Characteristics of potentially inflicted marks:

- Downturned lesions at the corners of the mouth due to being gagged.

- Human bites: Circular lesion with crescent-shaped bruises; individual tooth marks may be present, and skin may be broken. A distance greater than 3 cm between the third tooth or canine on each side indicates a bite caused by an adult or child older than 8 years of age.

Head Injuries Suggestive of Physical Abuse[6,10]

- Skull fractures: Multiple, complex, or bilateral skull fractures or skull fractures in an infant.

- Cerebral edema and retinal hemorrhage which is common in shaken impact syndrome.

- Subdural hematomas or subarachnoid hemorrhage.

- Traction alopecia and scalp swelling from hair pulling.

Skeletal Fractures Suggestive of Physical Abuse[6,10,12]

- Multiple fractures in different stages of healing or untreated healing fractures.

- Unusual fractures: Ribs, scapula, sternum, vertebra, distal clavicle.

- Metaphyseal injuries that have the appearance of tufts, chips, or "bucket handles" causing arcs of bone. Combination of epiphyseal and metaphyseal fractures.

- Spiral fracture of long bones.

- Transverse fractures.

- Repeated fractures at the same site.

- Multiple, bilateral, or symmetric fractures.

Abdominal Injuries in Physical Abuse

Abdominal injuries result from compression, crushing, or sudden acceleration or deceleration forces to the abdomen. Kicks, punches, or throwing the child against a solid object are typical mechanisms of inflicted abdominal injury.[10] There may be no external signs of injury to the abdomen. Symptoms associated with abdominal injury may include:

- Distended or rigid abdomen.
- Persistent vomiting and abdominal pain.
- Bruising of abdomen.
- Fever.
- Hypovolemic shock from a solid-organ injury.
- Septic shock from a hollow-organ perforation.
- Hematuria.

Eye Injuries in Physical Abuse[6,10]

- Dislocated lens.
- Hyphema.
- Corneal or conjunctival abrasion, laceration, or ulceration.
- Retinal detachment, retinal hemorrhage, or intraocular or vitreous hemorrhage caused by shaking.
- Bruising to eyelid or periorbital tissue; orbital fractures.

Diagnostic Procedures

Laboratory Studies

Laboratory data are obtained, as indicated, for the evaluation of injury or to rule out other disease processes. Examples of studies that may be performed include[7]:

- Rule out bleeding disorders:
    - Complete blood count.
    - Prothrombin time.
    - Partial thromboplastin time.
    - Platelet count.
- Dehydration; suspected water intoxication:
    - Electrolytes.
    - Blood urea nitrogen.
    - Urine specific gravity.

- Suspected poisoning or ingestion:
  - Toxicology screen.
  - Specific drug levels.
- Suspected abdominal solid-organ injury:
  - Amylase.
  - Liver enzymes.
  - Urine for blood.

Radiographic Studies

The role of radiologic imaging in the diagnosis of child maltreatment is to identify the extent and presence of inflicted injury and to document that the injuries observed are the result of nonaccidental trauma.[8] Types of radiologic imaging that may be used in cases of suspected maltreatment are:

- A complete skeletal survey is usually indicated in all infants younger than 2 years of age who have clinical evidence of physical maltreatment or in infants younger than 1 year of age who show evidence of significant neglect. The skeletal survey will detect multiple fractures, old fractures, and bone growth for age.

Other Diagnostic Procedures

- Computerized tomography.
- Magnetic resonance imaging.
- Ultrasonography.
- Radionuclide skeletal scintigraphy or bone scan.

SEXUAL ABUSE

In the United States, the incidence of sexual abuse is estimated to be at least 250,000 to 300,000 cases annually.[13] Victims of sexual abuse can present in a variety of ways. Some children are brought to the emergency department after disclosure of the sexual abuse to a caregiver. Others may present with vague physical or somatic complaints or behavioral changes, or physical signs of sexual abuse may be identified during the child's ED examination.[13] **The interview of children,** when sexual abuse or sexual assault is suspected, **must be conducted by health care professionals who are experienced in the interview techniques for sexual abuse evaluation of children.**[14]

Signs and Symptoms[15]

- There may be an absence of physical signs.
- Trauma to genitals or rectum.
- Abnormal discharge from the vagina or penis.
- Bleeding from the rectum.
- Abnormal bleeding from the vagina.

- Foreign bodies in the vagina, urethra, or rectum.

- Vaginal or rectal pain, discomfort, or itching.

- Sexually transmitted diseases beyond the newborn period, such as gonorrhea, syphilis, trichomonas vaginalis.

- Pregnancy in a young adolescent.

- Psychological symptoms[16]:

    - Low self-esteem.

    - Feelings of detachment, helplessness, and self-blame.

    - Fear of criticism or rejection.

    - Intrusive images.

See Appendix U for additional information regarding interview techniques and diagnostic procedures related to sexual abuse.

Nursing Diagnoses, Interventions, and Expected Outcomes

NURSING DIAGNOSIS	INTERVENTIONS	EXPECTED OUTCOMES
Tissue integrity, impaired, related to: • Physical maltreatment • Sexual abuse • Neglect	• Provide wound care • Provide appropriate treatment for injuries or identified medical needs • Notify social worker or child protective agency • Collect and maintain forensic evidence, as appropriate	The child will experience absence or resolution of impaired tissue integrity, as evidenced by: • Absence of signs of irritation: Redness, ulceration, blanching, and itching. • Signs of progressive healing of dermal layer. • Absence of signs of infection: Redness, swelling, purulent drainage, odor, and tenderness.
Ineffective family coping, disabling, related to: • Lack of support systems • Economic conditions • Lack of role model as a child • High-risk children • High-risk caregivers • Inadequate resources or abilities to meet demands of parenting	• Provide referral for hospital- or community-based resources for parenting skills and high-risk issues (substance abuse, domestic violence). • Provide emotional support.	The caregiver will cope effectively, as evidenced by: • A nonphysical approach to disciplining the child • Appropriate use of family and community support systems • Obtaining assistance to decrease stress and parenting demands • Obtaining assistance for substance abuse, domestic violence, or other factors placing the child at risk for maltreatment
Injury, risk of, related to: • Unsafe environment • Child maltreatment	• Provide a safe environment. • Report suspected child maltreatment.	The child will be free from injury, as evidenced by: • Absence of iatrogenic extension of injury. • Absence of increase in extent of original injury.

NURSING DIAGNOSIS	INTERVENTIONS	EXPECTED OUTCOMES
Knowledge deficit (caregiver) related to: • Normal child development or child's developmental level • Parenting skills • Constructive stress management • Nonphysical methods of discipline	• Provide information regarding normal growth and development • Refer caregiver to hospital or community resources for development of parenting skill • Discuss nonphysical approach to discipline • Explain and prepare child and caregiver for procedures and interventions. • Allow caregiver to remain with the child except during the interview. • Collaboratively plan and implement care • Prepare caregiver for separation if child is admitted or placed in protective custody	The caregiver will experience reduced knowledge deficit, as evidenced by: • Verbalization of understanding of normal expectations for child's behaviors and knowledge of normal child growth and development • Participation in age-appropriate activities • Demonstration of affection and nurturing behaviors toward the child • Use of a nonphysical approach to disciplining the child • Use of stress reduction measures
Fear (child) related to: • Separation from caregiver • Examination and procedures	• Explain procedures and treatment plan • Encourage the child to express feelings	The child will appear less fearful, as evidenced by: • Appearing less anxious, is calm and cooperative
Anxiety (child) related to: • Sexual abuse or abuse experience	• Provide a quiet, safe environment • Develop rapport with the child	The child will appear less anxious, as evidenced by: • Appearing emotionally secure, expressing feelings about the event • Demonstrates coping behaviors
Fear (caregiver) related to: • Possible separation for child's immediate safety	• Provide a safe environment • Comfort the child	The caregiver will appear less fearful, as evidenced by: • Sharing feelings about separation
Infection, risk of, related to: • Possible exposure to sexually transmitted disease	• Administer antibiotic, as ordered • Obtain appropriate cultures and laboratory studies	The child will be free from infection, as evidenced by: • Child/caregiver able to describe medication's purpose, dosage and possible side effects • Patient/caregiver verbalizes understanding of risk of sexually transmitted disease and recommended followup
Powerlessness related to: • Inability to control or prevent situation	• Provides choices whenever possible • Develop rapport with the child • Avoid judgmental approach or attitude	The child/caregiver will experience an increasing feeling of control over the situational crisis, as evidenced by: • Participation in decision-making activities • Verbalization of questions regarding treatment and course of care. • Acceptance of appropriate referrals and resources for support • Use of medical/nursing/allied staff for support and assistance
Rape trauma syndrome related to: • Sexual abuse	• Provide referral for follow-up counseling • Collect and document forensic evidence	The child/caregiver will begin to cope effectively, as evidenced by: • Child/caregiver accepts community agency referral and follow-up plan

Triage or Acuity Decisions

The following guideline may be used for identifying the acuity level of a child who is identified as potentially maltreated.

EMERGENT[6]   Although the child's physiologic status may not reflect an emergent acuity level, the need for psychosocial or medical intervention places all potentially maltreated and neglected children in at least an emergent acuity level.

Planning and Implementation

Refer to Chapter 4, "Initial Assessment and Triage," for a description of the general nursing interventions for the pediatric patient. After a patent airway, breathing, and circulation are assured, the following interventions are initiated, as appropriate, for the child's condition:

- Provide a safe environment. (Nursing diagnosis: Fear; injury).

- Provide appropriate treatment for injuries or identified medical needs. (Nursing diagnosis: Tissue integrity).

- Provide emotional support. Assign one staff member. (Nursing diagnoses: Ineffective family coping; fear).

- Encourage the child to express feelings and develop rapport with the child. (Nursing diagnoses: Fear; powerlessness.)

- Explain and prepare the child and caregiver for all procedures and interventions. (Nursing diagnoses: Knowledge deficit; fear).

- Avoid exhibiting a judgmental approach and attitude toward the caregiver. (Nursing diagnosis: Powerlessness).

- Allow the caregiver to remain with the child except during the interview. (Nursing diagnosis: Knowledge deficit).

- Plan and implement care in collaboration with other members of the health care and child protection teams. (Nursing diagnoses: Knowledge deficit; infection).

- Collect appropriate evidence. (Nursing diagnoses: Impaired tissue integrity; infection):

  - All visible external injuries, such as bruises and burns, should be photographed in color. If a 35-mm camera is being used, an instant, back-up photograph must also be taken. Forensic photographs must include a ruler, standard color chart in the field (if available), and patient data.

  - All injuries must be carefully and consistently documented on the patient's medical record. Document shape, exact size, location, and appearance of all cutaneous injuries.

  - All relevant verbal statements made by the child and caregivers should be documented verbatim, using direct quotations whenever possible.

- Collect appropriate sexual assault and maltreatment forensic evidence. (Nursing diagnoses: Rape trauma syndrome; tissue integrity; infection):

  - In cases of suspected sexual abuse, specific medical and forensic evidence may be collected. Protocols used for collecting and preparing medical evidence may vary from setting to setting. It is important to be familiar with the collection procedures mandated by each state and local jurisdiction.

  - Psychosocial preparation for the examination procedure is essential and increases the likelihood of cooperation:

    - The child must be prepared for the procedure in a manner that is appropriate for the child's developmental level.

    - Children who are unable to cooperate must never be physically restrained for an examination. Forced restraint for examination could further traumatize the child. In such cases, the child may be examined under sedation in the emergency department or general anesthesia in the operating room.

  - The specimens and other evidence collected are determined based on whether the suspected sexual assault occurred within the last 72 hours, and the nature of the sexual acts committed. Specimens for standard comparison and DNA testing may be included.

  - All evidence must be sealed and stored securely in a manner that preserves the evidence (e.g., locked freezer) until released to law enforcement personnel:

    - A written record of *chain of evidence* must be maintained.

    - In cases of criminal prosecution, these specimens will be considered evidence and must be handled by emergency staff accordingly.

- Discuss alternatives to corporal punishment. (Nursing diagnosis: Knowledge deficit).

- Provide information to caregivers regarding normal growth and development. (Nursing diagnosis: Knowledge deficit).

- Refer caregiver to appropriate social and community agencies for support and therapy. (Nursing diagnoses: Ineffective family coping; knowledge deficit; rape trauma syndrome).

- Report suspected child maltreatment in accordance with state or local guidelines. (Nursing diagnosis: Injury).

- Inform caregivers that a report of suspected child maltreatment will be made to proper authorities:

    ◆ It is essential that caregivers be informed whenever child maltreatment is suspected. The disclosure of the suspected maltreatment must be coordinated among the health care team and the child's safety must be assured. The manner in which caregivers are informed will influence their ability to trust health care professionals in the future. The most important approach to this difficult task is to stress concern for the child while being nonjudgmental and caring with caregivers. Caregivers may be told the following:

        > "Based on our assessment of your child's injury, we are concerned that someone may have hurt your child. When we are concerned that someone may have injured a child, the law requires that we report our concerns to Child Protective Services [name of agency may vary geographically]. A child abuse report will be made to Child Protective Services and law enforcement."

    ◆ Always allow the caregiver an opportunity to ask questions regarding the report. If the caregiver responds with anger toward the emergency staff, it is important to be supportive and not defensive. Review with the caregiver specific concerns or findings that are the basis for filing the report. Explain the procedures that will occur subsequent to such a report, services available to the family, and the disposition plan for the child.

- Prepare the caregiver for separation if the child will be admitted to the hospital or placed in protective custody. (Nursing diagnosis: Knowledge deficit):

    - All states in the United States provide a mechanism to protect children in emergencies. Some states give law enforcement agencies and physicians the authority to take a child into temporary protective custody.[4] It is imperative to be knowledgeable about the laws in the state in which one practices.

    - If the caregiver threatens to leave the emergency department before the child has been treated, or before the child's safety on discharge has been determined, it may be necessary to have a police officer present. In some cases, court intervention may be required to admit the child to the hospital without the parent's consent.

Evaluation and Ongoing Assessment

Children who have been maltreated require meticulous and frequent reassessment of airway patency, breathing effectiveness, perfusion, and mental status. Initial improvements may not be sustained, and additional interventions may be needed. The child's response to interventions and trends in the child's condition must be closely monitored for achievement of desired outcomes. The following parameters must be monitored in the child who has been maltreated:

- Airway patency.
- Breathing effectiveness.
- Perfusion.
- Vital signs.
- Level of pain.
- Psychosocial responses.

SELECTED EMERGENCIES

Refer to Chapter 4, "Initial Assessment and Triage," for a review of the comprehensive initial assessment and general interventions. Additional history data, signs and symptoms, and interventions specific to the selected emergency are listed.

Shaken Impact Syndrome

Severe head trauma is the primary cause of death from child maltreatment.[3,6] Inflicted head trauma may result from direct impact, vigorous shaking, or a combination of impact and shaking. Shaken impact syndrome is the result of vigorous shaking of an infant or small child, usually younger than 6 months of age. Injuries sustained are related to the vigorous shaking of the infant or child but may also include impact injury if the child's head is struck against a wall or solid object.

In a study conducted from 1994 to March 1998, there were 523 cases of shaken impact syndrome reported. Of those 523 children, 337 died. In 247 of the cases, the perpetrator was identified as follows[17]:

- 62% of the incidents were caused by parents.

- 20% by live-in boyfriends.

- 14% by nonrelative caregivers.

- 4% by others.

Shaken impact syndrome is the cause of death in 10 to 12% of all abuse-related deaths.[3] About 20 to 25% of shaken impact syndrome victims die, and the majority of survivors sustain brain damage, resulting in lifelong impairment.[3]

At times, the infant is diagnosed as dying from sudden infant death syndrome (SIDS). Health care providers must be careful to obtain an adequate history and be wary of the possibility of shaken impact syndrome as the cause of death. The diagnosis is confirmed on autopsy.

ADDITIONAL HISTORY

The history provided by the caregiver may include:

- Report of a minor fall, seizure activity, or respiratory arrest.

- Altered level of consciousness with no known etiology in the infant younger than 1 year of age.

- Report of minor trauma in a small infant such as a bumped head or fall from a couch.

- Report that the child was well prior to onset of symptoms.

SIGNS AND SYMPTOMS

- Bruising of the upper extremities (grip marks).

- Respiratory distress, decreased respiratory rate, or apnea.

- Irritability.

- Vomiting.

- Altered level of consciousness ranging from lethargy to coma.

- Hypotonia.

- Seizures.

- Full anterior fontanelle.

- Fixed, dilated pupils.

- Retinal hemorrhage.

- Abnormal posturing.

DIAGNOSTIC PROCEDURES

- Head computerized tomography scan.

- Skeletal survey.

ADDITIONAL INTERVENTIONS

- Prepare for definitive airway management, as appropriate.

- Immobilize the spine.

- Continually monitor neurologic status for signs of increased intracranial pressure.

Munchausen Syndrome by Proxy

Munchausen syndrome by proxy is a rare form of child maltreatment in which a caregiver fabricates or produces symptoms of an illness in a child. The deception is usually repeated on numerous occasions, resulting in frequent hospitalizations and considerable morbidity and mortality. Children from infancy to early school age are most typically involved.[6] The mother, who often has some allied health or nursing education, is characteristically the caregiver who fabricates the history or creates the symptoms of the illness. In some circumstances, multiple siblings may be victimized.[18]

ADDITIONAL HISTORY[6]

- Recurrent illnesses for which no medical cause is identified.

- Numerous hospitalizations in different institutions.

- Positive caregiver history of Munchausen syndrome.

- Reports of seizures, apnea episodes, cardiopulmonary arrest, hematuria, or hematemesis.

SIGNS AND SYMPTOMS

- The most common chief complaints or presentations of Munchausen syndrome by proxy include[19]:

  - Bleeding.

  - Seizures.

  - Central nervous system depression.

  - Apnea.

  - Diarrhea.

  - Vomiting.

  - Fever.

  - Rash.

- Signs and symptoms may be present as reported in the history because they were induced by the caregiver.[6]

- Symptoms do not correlate clinically.[6]

- Symptoms are observed only by the caregiver and disappear when the child is separated from the caregiver.

- Drugs used to induce symptoms may be present on toxicologic screening.[6]

ADDITIONAL INTERVENTIONS

- Monitor the caregiver's behavior in the emergency department.

- Prevent the caregiver from having access to any laboratory specimens or tests because he or she may attempt to alter the specimen.

- Document all physical findings and statements.

HEALTH PROMOTION

It is well known that domestic abuse and violence of a spouse also has an impact on children and places them at risk for maltreatment. The emergency nurse should assess the child and his or her family for the risk factors of domestic violence and initiate referral to appropriate social service agencies. Every attempt must be made to assure the child's safety.

- Provide educational and informational materials on parenting techniques, child abuse prevention, and domestic violence. Having information readily available in the ED waiting areas and treatment area provides easy access for families.

- Provide information on community and national resources, agency descriptions, and telephone numbers. Having this information readily available may encourage children and caregivers to call for information and seek assistance.

SUMMARY

Recognizing and reporting child maltreatment is essential to preventing subsequent injury. Most children who die as a result of maltreatment have already experienced some form of maltreatment before the severe or fatal injury is incurred. Emergency nurses play a key role in prevention through the early identification of children at risk and initiation of appropriate referral. Additionally, reporting all cases to the appropriate child protective agency and law enforcement is critical to the prevention of further maltreatment.

Emergency nurses can also participate in the primary prevention of child maltreatment by taking part in community- and school-based prevention programs and in programs targeted to caregivers. All states have chapters of Parents Anonymous, a self-help group whose goal is the prevention of child maltreatment. Parents Anonymous assists caregivers in learning more effective and appropriate parental skills. The National Child Abuse Hotline can also provide information for caregivers. Posting telephone numbers of agencies near patient telephones is one strategy to make caregivers aware of these resources.

REFERENCES

1. Statistical Abstracts of the United States, 1996. 116th ed. *The National Data Book.* Washington, DC: US Bureau of the Census; 1996.

2. Daro D, McCurdy K. *Current Trends in Child Abuse Reporting and Fatalities: Results of the 1990 Annual Fifty State Survey.* Chicago, Ill: National Committee for Prevention of Child Abuse; 1991.

3. US Advisory Board on Child Abuse and Neglect. *A Nation's Shame: Fatal Child Abuse and Neglect in the United States.* Washington, DC: US Department of Health and Human Services; 1995.

4. Myers JEB. *Legal Issues in Child Abuse and Neglect Practice.* Newbury Park, Ca: Sage; 1992.

5. Brucker JM. Child abuse. In: Brucker JM, Wallin KD, eds. *Manual of Pediatric Nursing.* Boston, Mass: Little, Brown, & Co; 1996:351-362.

6. Kelley SJ. Child abuse and neglect. In: Kelley SJ, ed. *Pediatric Emergency Nursing.* 2nd ed. Norwalk, Conn: Appleton & Lange; 1994:87-107.

7. Ludwig S. Child abuse. In: Fleisher GR, Ludwig S, eds. *Textbook of Pediatric Emergency Medicine.* 3rd ed. Baltimore, Md: Williams & Wilkins; 1993:1429-1463.

8. Bays J. Conditions mistaken for child abuse. In: Reece RM, ed. *Child Abuse: Medical Diagnosis and Management.* Philadelphia, Pa: Lea & Febiger; 1994:358-385.

9. Johnson CF, Showers J. *Diagnosis and Management of Physical Abuse of Children: A Self-Instructional Program.* Columbus, Ohio: Children's Hospital; 1987.

10. Hobbs CJ, Hanks HG, Wynne JM. Physical abuse. In: Hobbs CJ, Hanks HG, Wynne JM, eds. *Child Abuse and Neglect: A Clinician's Handbook.* New York, NY: Churchill Livingstone; 1993:47-75.

11. Hobbs CJ, Hanks HG, Wynne JM. Burns and scalds. In: Hobbs CJ, Hanks HG, Wynne JM, eds. *Child Abuse and Neglect: A Clinician's Handbook.* New York, NY: Churchill Livingstone; 1993:77-87.

12. Merten DF, Cooperman DR, Thompson GH. Skeletal manifestations of child abuse. In: Reece RM, ed. *Child Abuse: Medical Diagnosis and Management.* Philadelphia, Pa: Lea & Febiger; 1994:23-53.

13. Finkel MA, DeJong AR. Medical findings in child sexual abuse. In: Reece RM, ed. *Child Abuse: Medical Diagnosis and Management.* Philadelphia, Pa: Lea & Febiger; 1994:185-247.

14. Kelley SJ. Interviewing the sexually abused child: Principles and techniques. *J Emerg Nurs.* 1985;11:234-241.

15. Kelley SJ. Sexual Abuse. In: Kelley SJ, ed. *Pediatric Emergency Nursing.* 2nd ed. Norwalk, Conn: Appleton & Lange; 1994:109-123.

16. Adams JA. Sexual abuse and adolescents. *Pediatr Ann.* 1997;26:299-304.

17. Fitzpatrick D. Shaken baby syndrome fatalities in the United States. *National Information, Support and Referral Service of Shaken Baby Syndrome.* 1998;Autumn:1.

18. Alexander R, Smith W, Stevenson R. Serial Munchausen syndrome by proxy. *Pediatrics.* 1990;86:581-585.

19. Rosenberg DA. Web of deceit: a literature review of Munchausen syndrome by proxy. *Child Abuse Negl Int J.* 1987;11:547-563.

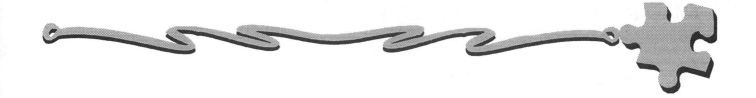

CHAPTER 10

The Neonate

OBJECTIVES

On completion of this lecture, the learner should be able to:

✦ Identify the anatomic and physiologic characteristics of neonates as a basis for their special needs.

✦ Describe normal and abnormal physical findings in the neonate.

✦ Identify the appropriate nursing diagnoses and expected outcomes based on the assessment findings.

✦ Delineate the specific interventions needed to manage the neonate.

✦ Evaluate the effectiveness of nursing interventions related to patient outcome.

✦ Identify health promotion strategies related to the neonate.

INTRODUCTION

Approximately 65% of all deaths in the first year of life occur during the neonatal period.[1] The word neonate is used to describe term infants 37 to 42 weeks' gestation, from birth to 28 days of age.[2] However, the neonatal period for preterm, or premature infants (delivered prior to 37 weeks' gestation) is extended because of delays in or slower progression of development. The premature infant is considered a neonate until the expected due date is reached plus 28 days.

Emergencies in the neonatal period may arise from congenital or acquired conditions. The nurse's systematic examination of the neonate requires knowledge of normal growth and development of the neonate to identify subtle signs of illness or injury. The initial assessment, combined with a comprehensive history, is needed to determine the appropriate nursing diagnoses and needed interventions.

Some information presented in this chapter may also apply throughout infancy. The terms neonate and newborn will be used interchangeably.

ANATOMIC, PHYSIOLOGIC, AND DEVELOPMENTAL CHARACTERISTICS AS A BASIS FOR SIGNS AND SYMPTOMS

Transitional Physiology of the Newborn

The transition from intrauterine life to extrauterine life begins as the newborn takes the first breath and the umbilical cord is cut. As the lungs fill with air and the alveoli fully expand, the partial pressure of oxygen (PaO_2) increases from fetal levels of 25 to 30 mm Hg to a level of 50 to 70 mm Hg. Because oxygen is a potent pulmonary vasodilator, the arterioles in the lungs open. The pulmonary vascular resistance is decreased, and pulmonary blood flow is enhanced. This change from high to low pulmonary vascular resistance must occur in the first few minutes of life to establish normal neonatal circulation. Infants who are unable to elevate their PaO_2 to appropriate levels risk a continuance of fetal circulation, called *persistent pulmonary hypertension of the newborn*.[3]

The majority of newborns will make this transition with minimal assistance, needing only warming, suctioning of the airway, and mild stimulation. Newborns that require intervention usually respond to positive-pressure ventilation with a bag and mask. Approximately 6% of all newborns will require some form of resuscitation. This number increases to 80% for infants who weigh less than 1,500 gm.[4]

Thermoregulation

Neonates are highly susceptible to the development of cold stress, both from increased heat loss and a diminished ability to produce heat. The infant's proportionally large head, body surface area-to-weight ratio, and minimal subcutaneous fat allow rapid heat loss with exposure. A cool ambient environment or a draft blowing across the neonate will increase the neonate's rate of heat loss. Additionally, the neonate or young infant may experience a decrease in core temperature secondary to poor perfusion.[5] These factors, in combination with the neonate's limited ability to produce heat, make this population particularly vulnerable to the development of hypothermia and cold stress.

Infants younger than 6 months of age are unable to shiver and are dependent on nonshivering thermogenesis to produce heat.[6] When the neonate is exposed to a cool environment, the energy-requiring process of nonshivering thermogenesis begins. The consequence is an increase in the neonate's metabolic rate and subsequent increases in oxygen and glucose consumption. The ill neonate's ability to compensate for these additional physiologic demands is limited. As a result, cold stress can lead to hypoxia or accentuate existing hypoxia. Hypoglycemia, increased renal excretion of water and solutes, and metabolic acidosis may also develop. Pulmonary vasoconstriction may also occur, worsening any existing cardiovascular dysfunction and increasing the risk for heart failure.[5,6] Additionally, the presence of cold stress can impede the neonate's ability to respond to resuscitative efforts.

To prevent the deleterious effects of cold stress, a neutral thermal environment that keeps the neonate's core temperature within normal range with minimal heat production must be provided.[7] The use of an *overbed radiant warmer is* critical for the neonate who is already hypothermic or requires significant body exposure for resuscitation or other procedures.

Elevations in body temperature may also be seen in the neonate. Elevation in temperature may result from a number of conditions, including infection, inflammatory process, alteration in heat production, or exposure to extreme heat. Additionally, the neonate is less able to dissipate excess heat than is the older infant; therefore, overbundling in combination with a warm or hot ambient environment may elevate the neonate's body temperature.[7-9] Fever is defined as a rectal temperature greater than 38°C (100.4°F). As with hypothermia, fever increases physiologic demands because of the increase in metabolic rate.

Pulmonary System

Anatomic and physiologic characteristics of the neonate's pulmonary system are described in Chapter 5, "Respiratory Distress and Failure" (see Table 10). The neonate's higher respiratory rate increases with crying and decreases with sleep (see Table 23). The slightly irregular respiratory rate of the newborn is normal and should not be confused with apnea. Apnea is an episode of nonbreathing for 15 to 20 seconds or for less time if accompanied by cyanosis or bradycardia.[7,10]

The small and immature pulmonary system impacts the neonate's ability to respond to increased physiologic demands. Increased oxygen consumption quickly leads to hypoxia in the ill neonate because of the limited ability to increase gas exchange.[6] Because of limited respiratory reserves, increased respiratory demands may precipitate rapid progression from respiratory distress to respiratory failure.[6] Apneic episodes may occur as the neonate in respiratory distress fatigues.

Cardiovascular System

The neonate has a less compliant myocardium and a smaller contractile mass. The limited contractility, in combination with a small stroke volume (1.5 ml/kg), impacts the neonate's ability to maintain cardiac output. Therefore, cardiac output is maintained by increasing the heart rate rather than stroke volume.[5,6] The neonate's resting functional heart rate is higher than in older children and will vary with crying and sleep. Transient bradycardia may occur with sleep or vagal stimulation during suctioning or defecation. However, a sustained bradycardia of less than 100 beats/minute is most commonly a result of hypoxemia.[11]

Blood pressure should be obtained in the ill neonate, although auscultation of the blood pressure may be difficult because of the low systolic blood pressure. With an appropriately sized neonatal cuff, the blood pressure may be assessed by palpation, the use of an ultrasonic flow meter, or automatic blood pressure device. The preferred site for blood pressure measurement is the right arm; however, other sites (forearm, calf, thigh) may be used with an appropriately sized cuff.[7] The thigh is the most uncomfortable site and, if used, may agitate the infant. Additionally, thigh blood pressures may be 4 to 8 mm Hg higher than those of the arm or calf.[7]

The neonate has vasomotor instability and sluggish peripheral circulation that may persist for hours, days, or weeks after birth. This may result in cyanosis of the hands and feet termed acrocyanosis, or mottling, related to transient changes in skin temperature.[2] However, central color should be normal with strong central pulses. Persistent central cyanosis, which does not respond to 100% oxygen and adequate ventilation, may be caused by a congenital defect that interferes with pulmonary or cardiac function.[12]

Table 23

NORMAL NEONATAL VITAL SIGNS[6,7]	
Temperature	Axillary 36.5 to 37°C (97.7 to 98.6°F)
Respiratory rate	30 to 60 breaths/minute
Heart rate	120 to 160 beats/minute
Systolic blood pressure	65 to 86 mm Hg; 60 mm Hg is lower limit of normal

Growth

The newborn normally loses between 5% and 10% of the birth weight by the third or fourth day of life. This is due to the loss of excessive extracellular fluid and the passing of meconium that was present internally at the time of birth. Breast-fed infants may lose slightly more weight than bottle-fed infants because it may take several days for the mother's milk supply to begin. Most newborns have stopped losing weight by day 5 and will again reach their birth weight by day 10.[7] Normal neonatal weight gain is 0.5 to 1.0 oz per day.[6]

Other Characteristics

Other physiologic and anatomic characteristics of the neonate include[6]:

- The presence of primitive or infantile reflexes and uncoordinated movement, which are evidence of the immature neurologic system. Flexion is normal posture.

- An inability to concentrate urine, a higher proportion of extracellular fluid, and increased insensible fluid losses, which contribute to the neonate's higher turnover of extracellular fluid and higher urine output of 2 ml/kg/hour.

- Higher hematocrits and fragile red blood cells with a shorter life span.

- Immature liver function; physiologic jaundice results when the liver's ability to excrete bilirubin from red cell hemolysis is exceeded.

- A relaxed cardiac sphincter and rapid peristalsis, which result in regurgitation or spitting up.

COMMON REASONS FOR NEONATAL ED VISITS

The neonate may be brought to the emergency department for a variety of reasons and caregiver concerns. Common concerns include:

- Irritability.
- Poor feeding.
- Fever.
- Perceived constipation.

- Vomiting.

- Jaundice.

- Increased crying.

More severe concerns include:

- Decreased responsiveness.

- Episodes of apnea with or without cyanosis.

- Obvious respiratory distress.

Although a delivery should preferentially occur in the obstetric department, there are occasions when the emergency department becomes the site for delivery and, potentially, resuscitation of a newborn.

NURSING CARE OF THE NEONATE

Assessment

The initial assessment of the neonate includes the primary and secondary assessments as described in Chapter 4, "Initial Assessment and Triage." The unique developmental characteristics of the neonate dictate adjustments in the approach to the assessment and the incorporation of additional components during the secondary assessment. See Appendix V for a listing of assessment findings and potential causes in the neonate and Appendix W for the care of the premature neonate.

APPROACH TO THE ASSESSMENT OF THE NEONATE

- Make observational assessment prior to touching the infant. The neonate's normal reaction is to cry when disturbed.

- Perform the most intrusive aspects of the assessment last, using a toe-to-head approach to the secondary assessment of the alert, vigorous neonate.

- Protect the neonate against heat loss during the examination.

- Use sensorimotor and tactile comfort measures to soothe the neonate, such as swaddling, rocking, stroking the skin, and a calm and soothing voice.

- Observe the general condition of the neonate:

  - Nutritional status.

  - Quality of cry.

  - Neonate and caregiver interaction.

  - Behaviors and response to comforting measures.

ADDITIONAL HISTORY

Prenatal History

- Mother's health before, during, and after pregnancy.

- Single versus multiple (e.g., twin, triplet) births. If multiple gestation, health status of siblings.

- Drug use during pregnancy.

- Prenatal care.

- Maternal age.

Birth History[13]

- Vaginal or cesarean delivery. If cesarean section, emergent or planned.

- Problems associated with labor.

- Problems at birth.

- Birth weight.

- Gestational age at birth.

- Length of hospital stay.

- Problems or interventions during hospital stay.

Feeding and Sleeping Patterns

- Frequency of feedings.

- Awakens self for feedings or is awakened; changes in this pattern.

- Quality of suck; eagerness to feed.

- Diet:

    - Formula or breast milk.

    - Number of ounces and feedings; length of time infant nurses at each feeding.

    - Typical time required to complete feeding.

    - Interval between feedings.

- Changes in sleeping pattern.

Elimination

- Usual number of wet diapers per day; number of wet diaper in previous 24 hours; last wet diaper.

- Usual number of bowel movements per day; changes in bowel pattern; color, consistency and odor of stools.

PHYSICAL ASSESSMENT

In addition to the head-to-toe assessment components described in Chapter 4, "Initial Assessment and Triage," examine the following:

- Muscle tone and posture:

  - The neonate's normal posture is one of flexion with good muscle tone. The arms are flexed at the elbows, and the hands are usually clenched. The legs are flexed at the knees, the hips are flexed, and the feet are dorsiflexed (see Table 24).

  - Neonates stressed by an acute disease process may have outstretched, limp extremities.

Table 24

Reflex	Response	Duration
Sucking	Exhibits strong movements of the mouth in response to stimulation.	1 year
Rooting	When cheek is touched or stroked along the side of the mouth, neonate turns head toward that side and begins to suck.	1 year
Grasp	Digits flex when palm of hand or sole of the foot is touched.	3 to 8 months
Startle	With sudden, loud noise, arm abducts with flexion of the elbows.	4 months
Babinski	Toes hyperextend and fan when the outer sole of foot is stroked in an upward direction from heel to toes and across the ball of the foot.	1 year

- The umbilicus:

  - Assess the umbilicus for the presence and condition of the umbilical cord stump. The stump should completely separate in 7 to 14 days, and the cord base should be healed by the end of the first month.

  - Until the umbilicus is completely healed, the umbilical vessels are a potential site of entry for infection. Abnormal findings include redness, swelling, drainage, or foul odor.

- The circumcision site:

  - The site will develop a yellowish white scab by the second day after the circumcision. If the Plastibell procedure was used, the plastic ring remains on the penis and will separate in approximately 5 to 8 days.

  - Abnormal findings include bleeding, swelling, exudate, foul odor, or erythema extending down the shaft of the penis.

DIAGNOSTIC PROCEDURES

A variety of radiographic and laboratory studies may be indicated, depending on the suspected etiology of the neonate's condition. In addition to disease-specific studies, the following tests are particularly significant for the neonate.

Radiographic Studies

- Skeletal survey: This film encompasses the torso from the neck to the pelvis and is generally ordered if abdominal distention is present.

- To obtain a good film, the neonate is held on the x-ray plate, maintaining good positioning without rotation. A pacifier may help to calm the neonate during the procedure.

Laboratory Studies

- Glucose: Serum or whole blood glucose test must be performed on all ill neonates. Because of decreased stores of glycogen in the liver, the stressed neonate may be unable to meet metabolic demands and may present with hypoglycemia. A whole blood glucose test must be performed in addition to laboratory specimens. Serial whole blood glucose tests are needed when the ill neonate requires the correction of hypoglycemia.

- Total and direct bilirubin: On neonates who appear jaundiced. The jaundiced coloration of the skin progresses from head to toe as bilirubin levels increase. High levels should be suspected if the neonate's entire body is yellow-orange.[6]

Nursing Diagnoses, Interventions, and Expected Outcomes

NURSING DIAGNOSIS	INTERVENTIONS	EXPECTED OUTCOMES
Airway clearance, ineffective, related to: • Amniotic fluid in airway • Thick secretions • Decreased level of consciousness • Improper positioning • Congenital abnormality	• Suction the airway, using a bulb syringe, immediately after delivery • Position in a neutral position: ▪ Supine, using a shoulder roll if necessary ▪ On side, leaning against a rolled up diaper or blanket • Consider intubation • Consider transfer to a neonatal intensive care unit	The neonate will maintain a patent airway, as evidenced by: • Regular rate, depth, and pattern of breathing • Symmetric chest expansion • Effective cough and gag reflex • Absence of signs and symptoms of airway obstruction: Stridor, dyspnea, and hoarse cry • Absence of signs and symptoms of retained secretions: Fever, tachycardia, and tachypnea
Breathing pattern, ineffective, related to: • Ineffective airway clearance • Pulmonary and neuromuscular immaturity • Decreased respiratory effort resulting from maternal narcotic administration • Aspiration of secretions or amniotic fluid • Presence of a congenital abnormality • Sepsis	• Maintain appropriate positioning • Administer 100% oxygen via infant partial rebreather or head-hood • Administer naloxone, per physician order • Ventilate using a bag-valve-mask device • Prepare for intubation • Obtain vascular access • Consider transfer to a neonatal intensive care unit	The neonate will have an effective breathing pattern, as evidenced by: • Regular rate, depth and pattern of breathing for gestational age • Symmetric chest expansion • Clear and equal bilateral breath sounds • Absence of stridor, dyspnea, and cyanosis • Absence of use of accessory muscles and nasal flaring • Normal skin color • Good muscle tone • Chest radiograph without abnormality

NURSING DIAGNOSIS	INTERVENTIONS	EXPECTED OUTCOMES
Gas exchange, impaired, related to: • Poorly developed lungs secondary to prematurity • Persistence of pulmonary hypertension (fetal circulatory pathways) • Ineffective breathing pattern • Presence of a congenital abnormality	• Maintain appropriate positioning • Administer 100% oxygen via infant partial rebreather or head-hood • Administer naloxone, per physician order • Ventilate using a bag-valve-mask device • Consider intubation • Obtain vascular access • Consider transfer to a neonatal intensive care unit	The newborn will maintain adequate gas exchange, as evidenced by: • Respiratory rate within normal limits for gestational age • Heart rate within normal limits for gestational age • Absence of accessory muscle use with respirations • Normal color centrally • Oxygen saturation >95% by pulse oximetry • Good muscle tone

Fluid volume deficit related to:
• Acute blood loss by the mother prior to delivery
• Acute blood loss by the neonate at time of delivery
• Inadequate oral fluid intake
• Acute fluid losses (vomiting, diarrhea)
• Fluid shifts
• Alteration in capillary permeability
	• Ensure adequate fluid intake, either oral or parenteral
	• Obtain vascular access, as indicated
	• Administer intravenous fluid, as indicated
	• Monitor hydration status:
	  ■ Skin turgor
	  ■ Heart rate
	  ■ Urine output
	• Monitor blood pressure
		The neonate will have an effective circulating volume, as evidenced by:
		• Stable vital signs appropriate for gestational age
		• Urine output of 2 ml/kg/hour
		• Strong, palpable peripheral pulses
		• Skin normal color, warm, and dry
		• Moist mucous membranes

Cardiac output, decreased, related to: • Acute volume loss • Inadequate fluid intake • Myocardial dysfunction	• Obtain vascular access and begin fluid therapy • Administer blood, if necessary • Consider assessment for congenital heart disease • Obtain blood pressure in all extremities • Compare pulse quality between upper and lower extremities	The neonate will maintain adequate circulatory function, as evidenced by: • Adequate blood pressure for gestational age • Urine output of 2 ml/kg/hour • Strong, palpable peripheral and central pulses • Absence of dysrhythmias • Skin normal color, warm, and dry
Thermoregulation, impaired, related to: • Increased rate of heat loss • Immature temperature control mechanisms • Decreased subcutaneous fat • Evaporation of moisture prior to complete drying of amniotic fluid immediately after delivery • Convection losses resulting from movement of cool air past the neonate • Conduction losses resulting from placement of cold items in direct contact with the neonate	• Immediately after delivery, dry newborn thoroughly and place in a prewarmed environment • Monitor axillary temperature • Reassess temperature frequently in unstable infants • Maintain neutral thermal environment; prevent heat loss • Use overbed radiant warmer • Monitor for signs of hyperthermia	The neonate will maintain a normal body temperature, as evidenced by: • Axillary temperature of 36.5 to 37°C (97.7 to 98.6°F) • Warm extremities • Normal color • Normal respiratory rate for gestational age • Normal heart rate for gestational age
Nutrition, altered, related to: • Inability to ingest nutrients because of illness	• Obtain vascular access • Maintain parenteral fluid therapy, as ordered • Provide oral feedings, as appropriate, for neonate's condition • Obtain whole or bedside blood glucose • Correct hypoglycemia • Obtain a weight	The neonate will receive adequate caloric intake, as evidenced by: • Normal blood glucose • Regular weight gain

NURSING DIAGNOSIS	INTERVENTIONS	EXPECTED OUTCOMES
Infection, risk of, related to: ● Deficient immunologic defenses ● Environmental exposure ● Maternal disease ● Presence of cord stump ● Presence of newly circumcised penis	● Use good hand washing techniques prior to each contact with neonate ● Perform eye prophylaxis in the newly born infant ● Assure that staff or caregivers with respiratory infections either wear masks or avoid contact with neonate ● Administer antibiotics ● Keep umbilical stump clean and dry ● Apply or change dressing to circumcision site as needed ● Clean diaper area	The neonate will be free from infection, as evidenced by: ● Core temperature measurement of 37.5 to 38°C (98.7 to 99.6°F) ● White blood cell count and differential within normal limits ● Absence of systemic signs of infection: Fever, tachypnea, and tachycardia ● Clear and infection-free eyes ● Negative blood cultures ● An umbilical stump that is drying and free from redness or drainage ● Healing circumcision site ● Absence of diaper rash ● Wounds free from redness, swelling, purulent drainage, or odor ● Urine output of 2 ml/kg/hour
Trauma, risk of, related to: ● Physical helplessness	● Properly identify newborn with matching identification bands placed securely on neonate and mother ● Administer vitamin K via the intramuscular route, using the vastus lateralis muscle as the injection site ● Avoid use of rectal thermometer in the newborn due to the risk of rectal perforation ● Maintain a safe environment for the neonate	The neonate will be free from trauma, as evidenced by: ● Correct identification of newly born infant with correct mother ● Absence of bleeding ● Absence of physical injury
Pain related to: ● Injury ● Infection ● Invasive procedures	● Assess vital signs for subtle changes that may indicate the presence of pain ● Assess for increasing irritability that may signal that the neonate is in pain ● Provide nonpharmacologic measures to reduce pain and calm the infant, such as providing a pacifier or holding, swaddling, or rocking the neonate ● Encourage caregiver to provide nonpharmacologic measures to reduce pain ● Administer pain medications	The neonate will experience relief of pain, as evidenced by: ● Diminishing or absent pain through assessment of physiologic indicators of pain: Tachycardia, tachypnea, pallor, diaphoretic skin, and increasing blood pressure. ● Absence of nonverbal cues of pain: Crying, grimacing, and guarding. ● Restful state of neonate.
Family process, altered, related to: ● Maturational crisis ● Birth of infant ● Change in family unit	● Encourage caregivers to see and hold the infant ● Encourage interaction between the new mother or family and neonate	The family will exhibit behaviors that indicate an attachment between neonate and mother or other primary caregivers: ● Touching newborn ● Calling newborn by name ● Talking to newborn in "cooing" tone ● Participating in care of newborn
Breast-feeding, interrupted, related to: ● Neonatal illness and inability to feed	● Provide a private area for the mother to use a breast pump ● Provide access to a breast pump ● Provide bottles and refrigeration for the storage of the pumped milk	The mother will not experience discomfort from engorgement and will be able to comfortably express milk for storage and later feeding to her neonate.

NURSING DIAGNOSIS	INTERVENTIONS	EXPECTED OUTCOMES
Anxiety and fear (caregiver) related to: • Unfamiliar environment • Unpredictable nature of condition • Invasive procedures • Unpredictable outcome	• Keep family informed • Encourage family to stay with and hold the neonate if possible • Provide psychosocial support • Prepare the caregiver for admission or transfer	The caregiver will experience decreasing anxiety and fear, as evidenced by: • Orientation to surroundings • Ability to describe reasons for equipment and procedures used in treatment • Ability to verbalize concerns and ask questions of the health care team • Use of effective coping skills
Knowledge deficit (caregiver) related to: • Treatment plans or discharge instructions	• Keep family informed • Encourage family to stay with and hold the infant if possible • Provide psychosocial support • Review discharge instructions and assure caregiver understanding of procedures and medications	The caregiver will experience reduced knowledge deficit, as evidenced by: • Ability to verbalize understanding of nursing and medical management • Ability to identify signs and symptoms requiring medical intervention as related to newborn's diagnosis • Ability to demonstrate the necessary skills to provide illness-related care for newborn at home • Verbalization of understanding of normal expectations for neonate's behavior and knowledge of normal growth and development • Participation in age-appropriate activities. • Demonstration of affection and nurturing behaviors toward the neonate

Triage or Acuity Decisions

EMERGENT A neonate experiencing cardiopulmonary arrest; respiratory distress; heart rate <100 beats/minute or >200 beats/minute; absent or slow respirations; grunting respirations; persistent central cyanosis; signs of decreased perfusion; fever; hypothermia; decreased reflexes such as suck, or startle; poor muscle tone; history of apnea, cyanosis, diarrhea, vomiting, poor feeding, decreased temperature, or fever.

URGENT A neonate's condition can deteriorate quickly, therefore few situations exist where the symptomatic neonate should be categorized as urgent.

NONURGENT A full-term neonate with vital signs within normal limits, with regular, nonlabored spontaneous respirations, normal skin color and temperature, good muscle tone, good cry and suck, no fever; and no history of apnea, cyanosis, vomiting, diarrhea, fever, or poor feeding.

Planning and Implementation

Refer to Chapter 4, "Initial Assessment and Triage," for a description of interventions performed during the primary assessment and general nursing interventions.

ADDITIONAL INTERVENTIONS

- Prepare the caregiver for admission or transfer of the neonate to a newborn intensive care unit, pediatric intensive care unit, or pediatric floor equipped to care for neonates. (Nursing diagnoses: Anxiety/fear; ineffective airway clearance; ineffective breathing pattern; impaired gas exchange).

- Prevent heat loss and correct hypothermia. Use overbed radiant warmer or heat lamps for the neonate who requires invasive procedures, resuscitation, or exposure for close observation. Cover the neonate's head and wrap the neonate in a blanket when exposure is not required for procedures or observation. Monitor temperature. Immediately after delivery, dry the newborn thoroughly and place in a prewarmed environment. (Nursing diagnosis: Altered thermoregulation).

- Completely undress the neonate and obtain a weight. (Nursing diagnosis: Altered nutrition).

- Cleanse around the umbilical cord stump with alcohol as needed. Reapply a diaper, folding it down so that the umbilical stump is exposed. (Nursing diagnosis: Infection).

- Apply a petroleum gauze dressing over the unhealed circumcision site and apply a diaper loosely to prevent friction against the penis. (Nursing diagnosis: Infection).

- Encourage caregivers to remain with the neonate and to hold and comfort the neonate. Promote sensory soothing interventions such as rocking, stroking the skin, or sucking on pacifier. (Nursing diagnoses: Pain; family process altered).

- Provide the mother access to a breast pump with disposable fittings and privacy, as needed. (Nursing diagnosis: Breast-feeding interrupted).

- Treat hypoglycemia.[12] (Nursing diagnosis: Altered nutrition):

  - Administer 15 to 30 ml of 5% dextrose orally to the stable newborn older than 34 weeks' gestation with no respiratory distress.

  - Administer 3 to 5 ml/kg of 10% dextrose/water intravenously over 1 minute to the unstable or stressed newborn. Follow the bolus with a continuous infusion of 10% dextrose/water at 4 ml/kg/hour.[6] Administer 10% dextrose and 0.2% normal saline if older than 24 hours.

  - Reassess serum glucose 15 to 20 minutes after the dextrose bolus and hourly until glucose level is stable.

- Monitor hydration status and provide oral feedings or deliver maintenance intravenous fluids, as indicated by patient condition. (Nursing diagnoses: Fluid volume deficit; decreased cardiac output; altered nutrition).

- Explain all procedures and treatment plan to caregivers. (Nursing diagnosis: Anxiety/fear).

Evaluation and Ongoing Assessment

The care of the neonate is challenging and requires knowledge of transitional and immature physiology. The neonate requires meticulous and frequent reassessment. Subtle signs and symptoms of illness may be indicative of critical illness in the neonate. Ongoing evaluation of airway patency, breathing effectiveness, circulation, temperature, and urine output is essential to evaluating progress toward expected outcomes.

SELECTED EMERGENCIES

Delivery of a Baby in the Emergency Department

Although the obstetric suite is the ideal location for delivery, many births will occur either in the emergency department or prior to arrival at the hospital. The ED staff must be prepared to care for both the mother and the newborn and must have an understanding of the neonate's special needs in the first few minutes of life. Any neonate born prior to arrival in the emergency department must receive the same serial assessment and care as outlined for the neonate born in the hospital.

The assessment and resuscitation of the newly born infant should occur simultaneously. The inverted pyramid (see Figure 34) indicates the order of assessment as well as the relative frequencies of resuscitative efforts. The most frequently performed interventions are at the top of the pyramid and the least frequent are at the bottom. Resuscitation should be done rapidly and progresses sequentially down the steps in the pyramid, with continuous re-evaluation occurring before each step. Figure 35 provides an algorithm to summarize the interventions for neonatal resuscitation.

There are many conditions that place the newborn at risk for complications at the time of or immediately following delivery. Examples of these conditions are listed in Table 25.[14]

Table 25

RISK FACTORS FOR COMPLICATION[14]		
Maternal Factors	**Environmental Factors**	**Fetal Factors**
• Maternal age younger than 15 or greater than 35 years of age • Maternal prepregnant weight <45.5 kg (100 lbs) • Anemia • *Cephalopelvic disproportion* • Maternal obesity • Hypertension • Maternal nutritional deficiencies • Maternal drug use (alcohol, cocaine, narcotics) • Maternal chronic disease (renal disease, diabetes, heart disease)	• Poverty (related to poor nutrition and health care) • Exposure to environmental toxins	• Multiple gestation • Abnormal fetal heart rate • Meconium-stained amniotic fluid • Low birth weight • Large for gestational age

ADDITIONAL HISTORY

Although a maternal history can alert the health care team to potential neonatal problems, it may be impractical to obtain a detailed history in the emergency department when delivery is imminent. Should a delivery be necessary in the emergency department, the following may aid in preparing for the birth:

- Asses for the presence of meconium in the amniotic fluid. Ask "What color was your water when it broke?" Neonates who have meconium-stained fluid require more treatment.

- Estimate gestational age of the fetus. Ask "When is your baby due?" Premature infants may require ventilatory support more frequently than term infants.

- Determine the anticipated number of fetuses. Ask "How many babies are there?" A multiple birth will require more personnel and equipment at the time of delivery.

- Assess the drug history. Ask "Have you taken any medications or drugs?" A history of narcotic use in the 4 hours prior to delivery may result in a newborn with depressed respiratory effort.

ADDITIONAL INTERVENTIONS

Figure 34

INITIAL STEPS IN THE CARE OF THE NEWBORN AT DELIVERY

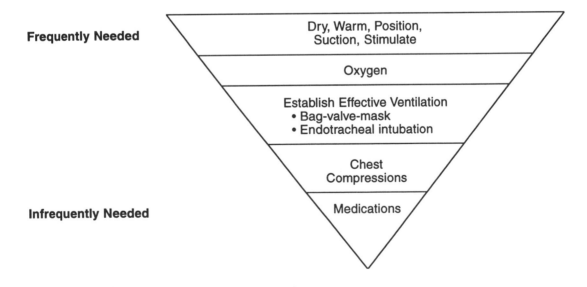

Assess and Support: Temperature (warm and dry)
Airway (position and suction)
Breathing (stimulate to cry)
Circulation (heart rate and color)

Frequently Needed — Dry, Warm, Position, Suction, Stimulate

Oxygen

Establish Effective Ventilation
• Bag-valve-mask
• Endotracheal intubation

Chest Compressions

Medications

Infrequently Needed

Adapted from Chameides L, Hazinski, MF, eds. *Pediatric Advanced Life Support.* Dallas, Tx: American Heart Association; 1997:9-1. Used with permission.

- Assemble equipment:
  - All personnel participating in the delivery and care of the newborn must observe universal precautions. Wear gloves, gowns, masks, and protective eyewear or face shields.
  - Mouth-to-mouth resuscitation must not be performed. Therefore, a bag-valve-mask device must be available at the bedside for every delivery.
  - See Appendix X for recommended equipment list.
- Following the clamping and cutting of the umbilical cord, dry and warm the newborn:
  - Place the newborn in a warm area and dry thoroughly:
    - ◆ A radiant warmer, heat lamps, or an examination light may be used as a heat source.
    - ◆ Quick removal of amniotic fluid from the head and body helps to prevent evaporative heat loss.
- Remove wet towels and wrap the newborn with prewarmed towels or blankets; cover the newborn's head with a blanket or hat.

Airway (see Figure 35)

- Position the newborn in a neutral position. A rolled washcloth or cloth diaper may be used under the shoulders to facilitate maintenance of correct airway position.
- With a bulb syringe, suction the mouth and then the nose:
  - Always suction the mouth first because nasal suctioning may cause gasping or crying, resulting in the aspiration of oral secretions.
  - The bulb syringe is usually adequate; however, an 8-French or 10-French suction catheter connected to mechanical suction may be used. The negative pressure must not exceed -100 mm Hg.
  - Perform repeated suctioning of the mouth, as necessary.
  - Avoid deep suctioning of the posterior pharynx, as this may cause a vagal response, resulting in bradycardia.

Breathing (see Figure 35)

- The majority of newborns will begin effective respirations in response to the stimulation provided with drying and suctioning. If not, two additional methods may be tried for 5 to 10 seconds to stimulate breathing:
  - Rub the newborn's back with firm pressure up and down the spine.
  - Tap or flick the soles of the feet.
- Assess the respiratory rate, effort, and effectiveness of respiration. Positive-pressure ventilation with 100% oxygen is required if the infant is not able to establish effective respiration after these interventions.

- Perform positive-pressure ventilation with a bag-valve-mask and 100% oxygen immediately for any newborn exhibiting the following:
  - Persistent cyanosis after delivery of 100% oxygen.
  - Gasping respirations.
  - Apnea.
  - Bradycardia: Heart rate less than 100 beats/minute.
- Assess effectiveness of bag-valve-mask ventilation by observing chest wall rise and fall and auscultating bilateral breath sounds laterally:
  - Ventilate the newborn at 40 to 60 breaths/minute.
  - Insert an 8-French or 10-French gastric tube, orally, to prevent gastric distention secondary to ventilation.
- Anticipate intubation:
  - For infants with meconium-stained amniotic fluid.
  - To facilitate prolonged ventilation.
  - When bag-valve-mask ventilation is not effective (rare).

Circulation (see Figure 35)

- Assess the heart rate and quality of pulses:
  - Auscultate heart tones.
  - Palpate central pulse, either femoral or umbilical. The heart rate must be greater than 100 beats/minute:
    - If the infant's heart rate is less than 100 beats/minute, initiate positive-pressure ventilation with 100% oxygen.
    - If the heart rate is below 60 or between 60 and 80 beats/minute and not increasing after 15 to 30 seconds of positive-pressure ventilation with 100% oxygen, begin cardiac compressions.
    - To perform compressions: Use two fingers or two thumbs placed one finger breadth below the nipple line.
    - Use a compression rate of 120 beats/minute.
    - The ratio of compressions to ventilations is 3:1.
    - Re-evaluate the heart rate after 30 seconds of chest compressions.
    - Stop compressions when the heart rate is 80 beats/minute or greater.

- Assess the newborn's color:

  - The newborn may be dusky at the time of delivery but should rapidly turn normal with the establishment of effective respirations.

  - Deliver 100% oxygen if the newborn remains centrally dusky with effective respirations and an adequate heart rate.

  - A simple face mask, held firmly on the face, with an oxygen flow rate of 5 liters/minute is the preferred method.

  - An alternative method is to cup your hand over the mouth and nose of the newborn and place standard oxygen tubing with a flow rate of 5 liters/minute through your fingers so that your hand becomes a "reservoir" for oxygen buildup.

- Once the newborn's color is normal, gradually withdraw the oxygen, continually assessing the color. If at any time the infant again becomes cyanotic, reapply the oxygen and do not attempt further weaning.

- Obtain vascular access:

  - The umbilical vein is the most common and accessible route for administering drugs and fluids in the newborn:

    - Umbilical catheter insertion is a sterile procedure performed only by trained individuals.

    - There are one umbilical vein and two umbilical arteries. The umbilical vein is the larger, thin-walled vessel.

    - Prior to insertion, flush the catheter with saline and attach a 3-way stopcock.

    - An abdominal radiograph is obtained following insertion to confirm placement.

  - Veins in the scalp and extremities can be used; however, these sites can be difficult in the newborn with poor perfusion.

  - Intraosseous routes can also be used in the newborn using an 18-gauge intraosseous needle.

- Administer medications (see Appendix Y for medications used during neonatal resuscitation):

  - Medications are indicated when the heart rate is less than 80 beats/minute after 30 seconds of chest compressions and positive-pressure ventilation with 100% oxygen.

  - Epinephrine is the drug of choice for bradycardia or asystole.

  - If the neonate has poor respiratory effort, it may be secondary to narcotics taken by the mother in the 4 hours prior to delivery.

    - Administer naloxone per protocol. It can induce a withdrawal reaction and seizure activity in an infant of a narcotic-addicted mother; use with caution if addiction is suspected.

    - Narcotic duration may exceed that of naloxone; repeated doses may be needed.

- Give volume expanders when there is evidence of hypovolemia, such as profound pallor, weak pulses with a normal or rapid heart rate, and a poor response to resuscitation:

  - Administer 10 ml/kg intravenously over 5 to 10 minutes:

    - 0.9% normal saline or lactated Ringer's solution.

    - 5% albumin or other plasma substitute.

    - O-negative blood crossmatched with the mother.

See Appendix Z for neonatal resuscitation guidelines.

- Assign an Apgar score (see Table 26).

  - The Apgar score is a standardized rating system that describes the condition of a newborn. The infant should be assessed at 1 and 5 minutes of age.

  - Although the score is seen as an indicator of the need for resuscitation at birth, resuscitative efforts should not be withheld to obtain the Apgar score.[11,12]

Table 26

APGAR SCORE			
	Score		
Sign	0	1	2
Heart rate	• Absent	• Less than 100 beats/minute	• Greater than 100 beats/minute
Respiratory effort	• Absent	• Slow, irregular	• Good, crying
Muscle tone	• Limp	• Some flexion	• Active motion
Reflex irritability	• No response	• Grimace	• Cough or sneeze
Color	• Blue or pale	• Normal color body with blue extremities	• Normal over entire body

- Prevent hypothermia which is defined as a core temperature less than 36.5°C (97.7°F) by maintaining a neutral thermal environment using the most appropriate method for the situation:

  - Place in an open crib with radiant warmer or in a prewarmed isolette.

  - Bundle the neonate in prewarmed blankets and keep the head covered.

  - Place the neonate under a heat lamp, away from drafts.

- Assess whole blood glucose at the bedside.

  - Hypoglycemia in the newborn is defined as a blood glucose level less than 30 mg/dl.[12]

  - Some newborns may be symptomatic with blood glucose levels between 30 and 40 mg/dl. Any newborn with a blood glucose less than 40 mg/dl should be carefully evaluated and treated.[3]

- Apply matching identification bands to mother and newborn that are available in many disposable delivery packs.

ADDITIONAL INTERVENTIONS: DELIVERY OF THE NEONATE WITH MECONIUM-STAINED AMNIOTIC FLUID

- Meconium is the first stool passed by the newborn. If passed by the fetus prior to delivery, meconium will appear in the amniotic fluid and can be described as thin or thick:

  - When small amounts of meconium discolor the amniotic fluid but no particles are noted, this fluid is described as thin or watery meconium-stained fluid.

  - With larger amounts of meconium passed, the amniotic fluid will contain actual pieces of meconium. The descriptor in this case is "pea soup" amniotic fluid. If aspirated by the newborn, the particulate matter will interfere with the normal expansion of alveoli. This begins a cascade of events that prevent the transition from intrauterine to extrauterine ventilation and circulation.

- If any meconium is present in the amniotic fluid, the mouth and nose of the newborn must be suctioned on the perineum as soon as the head is delivered:

  - Use a bulb syringe.

  - Mechanical or wall suction with negative pressure no greater than –100 mm Hg and a 10-French or larger suction catheter can be used.

- If the meconium is thin and the newborn is active, continue as for the delivery of the neonate with clear amniotic fluid.

- Thin meconium in a depressed infant or thick meconium in any infant:

  - Suction the hypopharynx under direct vision.

  - Intubate the trachea and suction any meconium present in the lower airway:

    - Use a meconium aspirator device and the appropriately sized endotracheal tube.

    - Intubate the newborn, attach the meconium aspirator, and apply continuous suction as the endotracheal tube is removed. Reintubation may be necessary if a large amount of meconium was obtained or if the infant is depressed.

  - The remainder of the care is the same as for the neonate with clear amniotic fluid.

Figure 35
INTERVENTIONS AT DELIVERY

NEONATAL RESUSCITATION

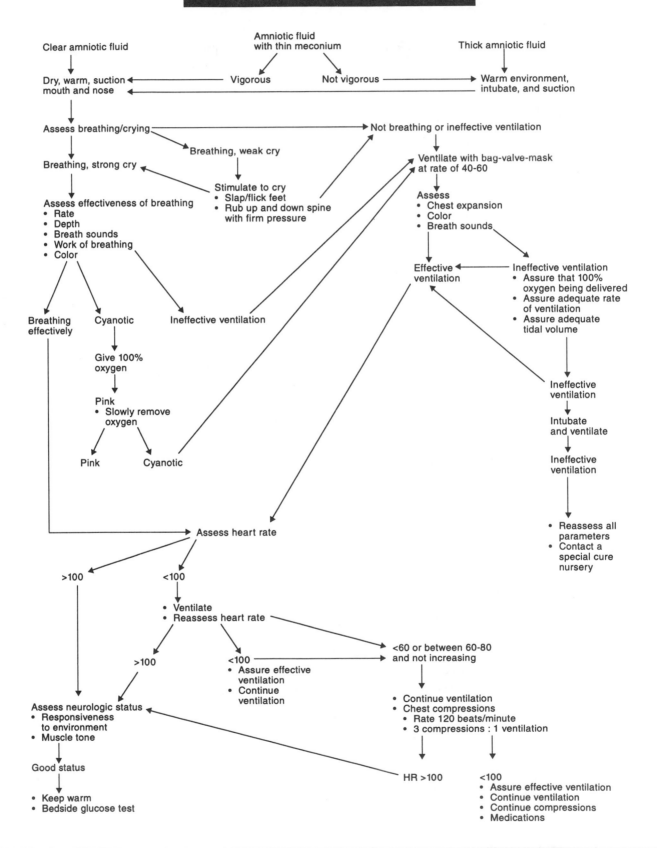

Neonatal Sepsis

The neonate is at risk for infection and sepsis because of its immature immune system due to decreased production of immunoglobulin G and complement and poor phagocytosis. Other contributing factors include exposure to infectious agents in the birth canal and environmental exposures. Because of the newborn's poor response to pathogens, the reaction is frequently not localized, and symptoms are vague and generalized.[2,3,5]

ADDITIONAL HISTORY[16]

- Increased crying.
- Increased sleeping; not awakening for feeding.
- Change in behavior pattern; "not acting right."
- Poor feeding; lack of interest in feeding.
- Fever.
- Seizure activity (e.g., smacking, eye deviation and fluttering, bicycling).

SIGNS AND SYMPTOMS

- Episodes of apnea.
- Respiratory distress, including tachypnea.
- Central cyanosis or pallor.
- Tachycardia.
- Mottled extremities despite warming measures.
- Decreased or altered level of consciousness:
  - Does not focus; will not track objects; does not maintain eye contact.
  - Decreased muscle tone; decreased resistance to extension of extremities.
  - Posture: Extremities extended; may be limp or flaccid rather than flexed.
  - Weak or absent reflexes.
  - Inconsolable; *paradoxical irritability.*
  - Decreased or no response to procedures.
- Temperature instability; fever or hypothermia may be present.
- Seizure.
- Jaundice.
- Vomiting.

DIAGNOSTIC PROCEDURES

- Prepare for and assist with sepsis workup.[2,15]

  - Complete blood count with differential and platelets.

  - Serum or whole blood glucose test.

  - Blood culture.

  - Urine culture.

  - Cerebrospinal fluid analysis: Culture and gram stain.

  - Chest radiograph.

- Laboratory tests, including:

  - Surface cultures from eyes, umbilical cord, nares, and culture from any obvious infected or draining site.

  - Prothrombin time; partial thromboplastin time.

  - Electrolytes.

  - Arterial or capillary blood gas.

  - Bilirubin.

ADDITIONAL INTERVENTIONS

In addition to standard airway, breathing, and circulation interventions described in Chapter 4, "Initial Assessment and Triage," and those previously listed in this chapter, the following interventions may be required:

- Administer 100% oxygen if respiratory distress or signs of shock are present.

- Ventilate with bag-valve-mask and 100% oxygen, if there are signs of respiratory distress and a poor neurologic response, or if there is a slower than expected respiratory rate and signs of poor neurologic response.

- Prepare for intubation.

- Obtain vascular access.

- Administer a fluid bolus of 10 ml/kg of 0.9% normal saline or 5% albumin/saline solution, as ordered for poor perfusion.

- Give nothing by mouth if any respiratory distress is noted or if neurologic status is depressed.

- Initiate cardiac and pulse oximetry monitoring.

- Administer antipyretics and medications, per protocol.

- Defer lumbar puncture until the neonate is stabilized. Pulse oximetry monitoring during the procedure is recommended if not already initiated.[6]

- Start continuous infusion of 10% dextrose at 4 ml/kg/hour to maintain serum glucose.[17]

Congenital Heart Disease

Some neonates with congenital heart defects may exhibit signs and symptoms at birth, but others may not for days, weeks, or months. The majority of infants with significant congenital heart lesions do, however, exhibit symptoms by 3 months of age. Congenital heart lesions may include a single structural anomaly or a combination of anomalies. The broad terms often used to classify congenital heart defects are *cyanotic* and *acyanotic*. Hemodynamics, the ratio of pulmonary to systemic blood flow and the direction of blood flow through the lesion, is also used to describe the defect.[18] Defects resulting in left-to-right shunts, right-to-left shunts, or obstruction may be present (see Table 27).

Table 27

SUMMARY OF CONGENITAL CARDIAC DEFECTS
• Left-to-right shunts (acyanotic):   ■ Patent ductus arteriosius   ■ Atrial septal defect   ■ Ventricular septal defect   ■ Complete atrioventricular canal defect
• Right-to-left shunts (cyanotic):   ■ Transposition of the great arteries   ■ Tetralogy of Fallot   ■ Total anomalous pulmonary venous return   ■ Truncus arteriosus   ■ Tricuspid atresia   ■ Hypoplastic left-heart syndrome
• Obstructive lesions: ■ Aortic stenosis   ■ Pulmonary stenosis   ■ Coarctation of the aorta

Adapted from Redfearn S. Cardiovascular system. In Soud TE, Roger JS, eds. *Manual of Pediatric Emergency Nursing*. St. Louis, Mo: Mosby-Year Book; 1998:238. Used with permission.

Defects that produce left-to-right shunts result in increased pulmonary blood flow. These include patent ductus arteriosus, atrial septal defect, ventricular septal defect, and atrioventricular canal defect. In the heart, the blood is shunted from the left (systemic) side of the heart to the right (pulmonary) side; therefore these defects are also termed acyanotic.[18] The increased pulmonary blood flow may lead to congestive heart failure, if significant. Cyanotic defects are those in which blood is shunted from the right side of the heart to the left side, bypassing the pulmonary circulation and mixing with blood being pumped to the systemic circulation. Obstructive defects may occur on either side of the heart and, when combined with other anomalies, shunting of blood may occur. Some obstructive and right-to-left shunting congenital heart defects would not be compatible with life except for the presence of other anomalies or a patent ductus arteriosus.

The ductus arteriosus is a fetal circulation structure connecting the pulmonary artery to the aorta. The rising arterial PaO_2 after birth stimulates constriction and closure of the ductus arteriosus. However, infants with congenital heart disease may have a delayed closure of the ductus arteriosus, in part because of a lower PaO_2. Infants with defects dependent on the patent ductus to maintain pulmonary blood flow will exhibit symptoms within the first weeks of life as the ductus arteriosus begins to close. Congestive heart failure, pulmonary edema, or shock occurs.[18] If the circulation to the lower extremities is dependent on the patent ductus arteriosus, the infant will show signs of profound deterioration as the ductus closes. A prostaglandin E_1 (PGE_1) infusion which has a direct dilatory effect on the ductus, is used to re-establish the patency of the ductus arteriosus.

Infants with right-to-left shunting will exhibit a lower arterial PaO_2 and saturation in their left arm and lower extremities. Measurements that are preductal (before the patent ductus arteriosus, through which blood shunts) may be higher than those that are postductal. For this reason, the pulse oximeter should be placed on the right arm. If a second pulse oximeter is available, it can be placed on a lower extremity and concurrent readings can be recorded. Always record the location of the pulse oximeter probe along with the actual reading.[19] An *oxygen challenge test* may be performed to differentiate between a cardiac and pulmonary origin for cyanosis in the neonate.[18]

ADDITIONAL HISTORY

Infants with congenital heart disease may exhibit any or all of the following signs and symptoms. Because the caregivers may not recognize all of these as a problem, specific behavioral information must be elicited:

- Cyanosis during crying or feeding.

- Dyspnea during crying or feeding.

- Easily fatigued.

- Does not cry much or for long ("such a good baby").

- Does not feed well or for as long as would be expected; falls asleep early in feeding.

- Poor weight gain.

- Excessive sweating.

- Respiratory distress.

SIGNS AND SYMPTOMS

- Clear breath sounds in a tachypneic, cyanotic infant is highly suspicious of congenital heart disease.

- Diminished lower extremity pulses. Some cardiac defects may result in diminished pulses in the lower extremities (e.g., coarctation of the aorta).

- Lower blood pressure reading in lower extremities. This may be as much as 20 mm Hg difference with some defects.[18]

- Murmur may or may not be present.

- Cyanosis.

- Profound pallor.

- Dyspnea.

- Increased work of breathing.

- Decreased level of consciousness.

DIAGNOSTIC PROCEDURES

Monitors

- 12-lead electrocardiogram.

Radiographic Studies

- Chest radiograph.

Other Diagnostic Procedures

- Echocardiogram.

Laboratory Studies

- Arterial blood gas.

- Complete blood count with differential.

- Blood cultures.

- Serum or whole blood glucose test.

ADDITIONAL INTERVENTIONS

- Ensure that a neutral thermal environment is maintained because neonates with congenital heart disease are especially vulnerable to hypothermia.[5]

- Administer oxygen. Concentration recommendations vary; 40 to 50% is commonly prescribed.[20,21]

- Initiate pulse oximetry and cardiac monitoring.

- Obtain vascular access for maintenance fluids and medication administration.

- Give nothing by mouth.

- Administer PGE_1 via continuous intravenous infusion, as indicated, to re-establish patent ductus arteriosus[20,21]:

    - May be given via a peripheral intravenous line or an umbilical arterial or venous line but must be given directly into the hub of the infant's vascular access; it cannot be piggybacked several inches up the intravenous tubing.

    - PGE_1 also causes vasodilation of all arterioles, inhibits platelet aggregation, and stimulates intestinal smooth muscle.

    - Maximal drug effect is usually seen in 30 minutes, but the immediate effects of an increase in oxygen saturation and decreasing cyanosis are noted within minutes.

- Prepare to intubate, if it has not already been done. The infant must be intubated for transport to another facility.[21]

- Monitor for side effects of PGE_1:

  - Apnea; hypoventilation.

  - Hypotension.

  - Edema.

  - Cutaneous vasodilation.

  - Fever.

  - Hypoglycemia.

  - Hypocalcemia.

  - Diarrhea.

  - Hemorrhage.

  - Thrombocytopenia.

  - Irritability.

  - Seizures.

HEALTH PROMOTION

The first few weeks of life require major adjustments from both the infant and the caregivers. A new mother is experiencing hormonal changes, body image changes, and sleep deprivation. Although the caregivers may have attended prenatal classes and received educational information after the birth of the child, the overwhelming responsibilities of the newborn may cause frustration and exhaustion. Information previously learned may be forgotten. The following information is a sample of what can be shared both verbally and via written materials.

Illness Prevention

- Educate the caregiver concerning immunizations and immunization schedules. Provide referral to community immunization resources, as needed.

- Review with the caregiver the importance of well-baby checks and establishing a relationship with a primary care provider for the infant. Provide primary care provider referral or resources for obtaining or selecting a primary care provider.

- Review with the caregiver:

  - When to call the primary care health professional.

  - When to go to the emergency department.

- Advise the caregiver to keep the newborn's environments, including the home and car, smoke free.

- Teach the caregiver the early signs of illness in the neonate and infant: Fever, poor feeding, vomiting, diarrhea, unusual irritability, decreased activity, decreased responsiveness, extended posture.

- Encourage the caregiver to learn infant cardiopulmonary resuscitation. Provide information on hospital-based or community-based classes.

- Review feeding information, as appropriate:

  - Stress the need for good maternal diet when breast-feeding.

  - Refer the mother to a lactation consultant if experiencing difficulties with breast-feeding.

  - Review formula preparation and mixing.

  - Review the risk of infant botulism if honey is given to an infant.

  - Review safe bottle-feeding practices. Do not prop the bottle or put the infant to bed with a bottle.

Injury and Abuse Prevention

- Review the use of an infant car seat. Stress the importance of using a rear-facing car seat, properly secured in the rear seat, with the infant strapped into the car seat at all times.

- Discuss the infant's sleeping position with the caregiver. Current recommendations state that newborns should be positioned on the back or side with the head elevated, not prone.

- Review and discuss general infant safety measures with the caregiver:

  - Set the hot water heater thermostat at less than 48.9°C (120°F).

  - Always test the water temperature with a bath thermometer or at your wrist to make sure it is not too hot before bathing the infant. Never leave the baby alone in a tub of water.

  - Assure that crib slats are no more than 2⅜ inches apart with a snug-fitting mattress. Keep the sides of the crib raised.

  - Do not put the infant on soft surfaces such as a water bed, couch, or pillow.

  - Do not leave the infant on high places, such as changing tables, beds, sofas, or chairs. Always keep one hand on the infant.

  - Never leave the baby alone or with a young sibling or pet.

  - Do not drink hot liquids while holding the infant or pour hot liquids while reaching over the infant.

  - Avoid overexposure to the sun.

  - Install smoke detectors if not already in place.

- Review the dangers of shaking an infant.

- Provide referral or information, as appropriate, for community resources to assist with financial concerns, parenting skills, inadequate housing, limited food resources, lack of transportation, lack of appropriate car seat, domestic violence and child abuse prevention, or other such issues.

SUMMARY

Neonates are our smallest patients, and often our scariest. They cannot speak for themselves so the nurse must be their advocate. Signs of illness are often subtle, challenging the nurse to look for the pieces of the puzzle to obtain the whole picture. It is important not to forget the incredible miracle of this small being. The ability to fine tune the assessment, discover and treat a problem, provide educational information to the caregiver, and offer support and encouragement to the family can make a difference in the life of the neonate.

REFERENCES

1. Anderson K. *Mosby's Medical, Nursing and Allied Health Dictionary*. 4th ed. St. Louis, Mo: Mosby-Year Book; 1994:1055.

2. Kliegman RM. The high-risk infant. In: Nelson WE, Behrman RE, Kliegman RM, Arvin AM, eds. *Nelson Textbook of Pediatrics*. 15th ed. Philadelphia, Pa: WB Saunders; 1996:451-462.

3. Cloherty JP, Stark AR, eds. *Manual of Neonatal Care*. 3rd ed. Boston, Mass: Little, Brown; 1992.

4. Leuthner SR, Jansen RD, Hageman JR. Cardiopulmonary resuscitation of the newborn: An update. *Pediatr Clin North Am*. 1994;41:893-907.

5. Hazinski MF. Children are different. In: Hazinski MF, ed. *Nursing Care of the Critically Ill Child*. 2nd ed. St. Louis, Mo: Mosby-Year Book; 1992:1-17.

6. Burke SS. Neonatal topics. In: Soud TE, Rogers JS, eds. *Manual of Pediatric Emergency Nursing*. St. Louis, Mo: Mosby-Year Book; 1998:660-685.

7. Wong DL, ed. Health promotion of the newborn and family. *Whaley & Wong's Essentials of Pediatric Nursing*. 5th ed. St. Louis, Mo: Mosby-Year Book; 1997:179-220.

8. Cheng TL, Partridge JC. Effect of bundling and high environmental temperature on neonatal body temperature. *Pediatrics*. 1993;92:238-240.

9. Grover G, Berkowitz CD, Lewis RJ, Thompson M, Berry L, Seidel J. The effects of bundling on infant temperatures. *Pediatrics*. 1994;94:669-673.

10. Barone MA, ed. *The Harriet Lane Handbook*. 14th ed. St. Louis, Mo: Mosby-Year Book; 1996:380.

11. Bloom R, Cropley C. *Textbook of Neonatal Resuscitation*. Dallas, Tx: American Heart Association; 1995.

12. Chameides L, Hazinski MF. *Pediatric Advanced Life Support*. Dallas, Tx: American Heart Association; 1997.

13. Bailey C, Boyle R, Kattwinkel J, Ferguson J. *Outpatient Perinatal Education Program, Book Two: The Infant at Risk After Discharge*. Charlottesville, Va: Division of Neonatal Medicine, University of Virginia Health Sciences Center; 1997.

14. Bailey C, Boyle R, Kattwinkel J, Ferguson J. *Outpatient Perinatal Education Program, Book One: The High Risk Mother and Fetus*. Charlottesville, Va: Division of Neonatal Medicine, University of Virginia Health Sciences Center; 1997.

15. Kelnar CJH, Harvey D, Simpson C. *The Sick Newborn Baby*. 3rd ed. London, England: Baillicrc Tindall; 1995.

16. Schulte EB, Price DL, James SR. *Thompson's Pediatric Nursing: An Introductory Text*. 7th ed. Philadelphia, Pa: WB Saunders; 1997.

17. Burchfield DJ. Acute distress in the neonate and postnatal period. In: Barkin RM, ed. *Pediatric Emergency Medicine*. 2nd ed. St. Louis, Mo: Mosby-Year Book; 1997.

18. Redfearn S. Cardiovascular system. In: Soud TE, Rogers JS, eds. *Manual of Pediatric Emergency Nursing*. St. Louis, Mo: Mosby-Year Book; 1998:233-265.

19. Moss MM. Cardiovascular system. In: McCloskey K, Orr R, eds. *Pediatric Transport Medicine*. St. Louis, Mo: Mosby-Year Book; 1995:218-237.

20. Children's Memorial Hospital. *Transport Team Protocols*. Chicago, Ill: Author; 1998.

21. Buser-Gills M. Neonatal transport: Congenital heart disease. In: McCloskey K, Orr RA, eds. *Pediatric Transport Medicine*. St. Louis, Mo: Mosby-Year Book; 1995:424-426.

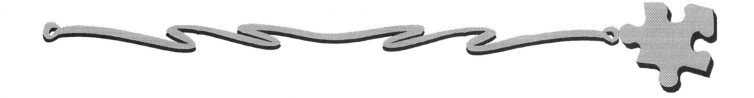

CHAPTER 11

Medical Emergencies

OBJECTIVES

On completion of this lecture, the learner should be able to:

✦ Identify the physiologic characteristics of children as a basis for the signs and symptoms of medical illness.

✦ Identify common causes of medical emergencies in children.

✦ Identify the appropriate nursing diagnoses and expected outcomes based on the assessment findings.

✦ Delineate interventions for the management of the child with selected medical emergencies.

✦ Evaluate the effectiveness of nursing interventions.

✦ Identify health promotion strategies related to illness prevention.

INTRODUCTION

Children visiting the emergency department for a medical illness encompass the entire spectrum of acuity. The most common illness-related chief complaints include fever, ear pain, respiratory symptoms, vomiting, diarrhea, sore throat, rash, urinary tract symptoms, and abdominal pain.[1] Medical emergencies comprise a variety of illnesses and disorders. This chapter will provide an overview of selected medical emergencies, including infectious diseases, as well as neurologic, metabolic, hematologic, and immune system disorders.

ANATOMIC, PHYSIOLOGIC, AND DEVELOPMENTAL CHARACTERISTICS AS A BASIS FOR SIGNS AND SYMPTOMS

Fever

Fever is a nonspecific symptom of an underlying infectious or inflammatory process and is one of the most common symptoms encountered in pediatrics. The public readily recognizes fever as a symptom of illness, and approximately 20% of all ED visits by children are attributable to fever.[2]

Fever is a rise in the core body temperature that follows a resetting of the body's thermostat, located in the hypothalamus. A child is generally considered febrile when the rectal temperature is over 38°C (100.4°F).[3]

The duration and degree of fever may provide some clues to the underlying illness, although the degree of fever does not reflect the severity of illness. Seriously ill infants and children may be normothermic or hypothermic rather than febrile. The presence of fever, or a history of fever at home, may impact triage and treatment decisions in children who are at increased risk for sepsis or other serious illness, including infants younger than 8 weeks of age, *immunocompromised patients*, patients with chronic illnesses, and children younger than 2 years of age without an identified source of infection.[4]

Although fever in itself is not an emergency, a febrile state does impact physiologic function. Fever can contribute to increases in insensible fluid loss, metabolic rate, oxygen consumption, caloric consumption, heart rate, and respiratory rate.[4] Control of fever with cooling measures and antipyretics often helps the child feel better and, more importantly, may decrease some physiologic demands in the seriously or critically ill child.

Dehydration

Total body water is comprised of extracellular and intracellular fluid. Extracellular fluid is composed of the interstitial fluid and the circulating blood plasma. The following are characteristics of fluid and electrolyte balance unique to the pediatric population:

- Essential and insensible fluid losses occur through the skin, respiratory system, gastrointestinal tract, and urinary systems:

    - The child's higher metabolic rate increases heat production, which in turn increases insensible fluid loss.

    - The immature kidney function of young infants results in a limited ability to concentrate and dilute urine. Consequently, the infant also lacks the ability to conserve or secrete sodium.[5]

    - The transport of sodium and potassium occurs as the result of fluid shifts between the intracellular and extracellular compartments.

- A greater body surface area-to-mass ratio results in a larger quantity of water loss per unit of mass. For example, in young infants with no intake, fluid losses will equal 7.5% of body weight per day. This is five times greater than the loss that would occur in the adult for the same period.[6]

- Although infants and young children have a larger extracellular fluid-to-intracellular fluid volume ratio, dehydration occurs more rapidly because of their large body surface area, increased metabolic rate, and a smaller absolute volume of extracellular fluid.

In the otherwise healthy child, dehydration is most often caused by gastrointestinal losses from vomiting or diarrhea coupled with inadequate fluid intake.[1,3,4] Other causes of dehydration include increased insensible fluid loss resulting from respiratory illness or fever; excessive renal fluid loss such as diabetes insipidus or diabetes mellitus; skin loss such as burns, cystic fibrosis, third-spacing of fluids; and incorrect formula preparation.[7]

There are three types of dehydration which reflect the proportion of sodium-to-water losses: Isotonic (serum sodium = 130 to 150 mEq/L), hyponatremic (serum sodium <130 mEq/L), and hypernatremic (serum sodium >150 mEq/L).[4,8] The most common type of dehydration in children is isotonic dehydration, where sodium and fluid losses are equal.

Hyponatremic or hypotonic dehydration is less common but may develop from excessive water intake causing water intoxication or excessive salt loss where sodium loss exceeds water loss. Hypernatremic or hypertonic dehydration usually results from a deficit of free water where water is lost in excess of sodium. Improper formula dilution, as well as gastrointestinal losses coupled with high fever or decreased intake, can result in hypernatremic dehydration.

The degree of dehydration is based on clinical signs and symptoms. Dehydration is usually classified as mild, moderate, or severe. Table 28 correlates the signs and symptoms with the degree of dehydration.[3] In moderate and severe levels of dehydration, urine output decreases and alterations in mental status become apparent.

Table 28

SIGNS AND SYMPTOMS OF DEGREES OF DEHYDRATION			
Degrees of Dehydration			
	Mild	**Moderate**	**Severe**
Percentage of loss of body weight	5%	10%	15%
Signs and Symptoms			
Mucous membranes and lips	Dry	Very dry, cracked	Parched
Skin turgor	Normal	Slightly decreased	Tenting
Anterior fontanelle	Normal	Sunken	Sunken
Eyeballs	Normal	Sunken	Sunken
Tearing	Normal	Decreased	Absent
Heart rate	Normal or slightly increased	Increased	Increased
Respiratory rate	Normal or slightly increased	Increased	Increased
Blood pressure	Normal	Normal	Decreased
Skin perfusion	Normal, pale	Mottled, cool	Slow capillary refill time, cold, cyanotic

Adapted from Barkin RM, Rosen P. *Emergency Pediatrics*. 3rd ed. St. Louis, Mo: Mosby-Year Book; 1994:52-59. Used with permission.

Rashes

Rashes are one of the most common symptoms of children presenting to the emergency department. The etiology of the rash can be related to acute or chronic conditions and can include systemic or localized bacterial, viral, or fungal infections; hypersensitivity reactions from environmental allergens, medications, bites and stings, or products such as latex; or infestation of lice, or scabies. The evaluation of the lesion must include:

- Pattern of distribution.

- Appearance of the lesions.

- Presence or absence of fever.

- History related to the eruption and evolution of the rash (chronic versus acute).

Table 29 lists types of lesions, their description, and possible diagnoses associated with the presence of that lesion type.[9,10] Figures 36 to 39 are illustrations of selected lesions.

NURSING CARE OF THE CHILD WITH A MEDICAL EMERGENCY

Assessment

Refer to Chapter 4, "Initial Assessment and Triage," for a review of the initial assessment of the pediatric patient. Additional assessment data, signs and symptoms, and additional interventions are discussed with each selected emergency.

DIAGNOSTIC PROCEDURES

Monitors

The use of cardiac and pulse oximetry monitoring is based on the child's condition. Indications for initiating monitoring are described in the selected emergencies section.

Laboratory Studies

Specific laboratory studies will be ordered depending on the appearance of the child, the history, signs and symptoms, and the absence of an identifiable source of infection. Specific laboratory studies are discussed in the additional interventions for each selected emergency.

Radiographs and Imaging Studies

Radiographs and imaging studies may be indicated based on clinical status and evaluation. Specific studies are discussed in the additional interventions for the selected emergency, as appropriate.

Table 29

CORRELATION OF SKIN LESIONS AND CAUSES

TYPE OF LESION	LESION DESCRIPTION	POTENTIAL DIAGNOSIS OR ETIOLOGY
MACULE (see Figure 36 on next page)	Flat, nonpalpable lesion with altered color, <1 cm in diameter.	• Freckles • Nevi • Mongolian spot • Kawasaki disease • Fifth disease • Scarlatina • Rubella • Roseola • Measles
PAPULE (see Figure 37 on next page)	Raised, discolored lesion above the skin surface, <1 cm in diameter.	• Lyme disease • Acne • Folliculitis • Insect bites • Urticaria • Contact dermatitis • Scarlatina
NODULE (see Figure 38 on next page)	Deep in skin, epidermis moves over the top of the nodule, soft or solid mass above or below the skin.	• Lipoma • Cyst • Rheumatoid nodules • Lymphadenitis
PUSTULE	Raised lesion containing exudate, which gives a yellow appearance.	• Folliculitis • Impetigo • Candidiasis
WHEAL (see Figure 39 on next page)	Edematous, circumscribed, elevated lesion; flat topped, >1 cm.	• Insect bites • Drug reaction • Urticaria • Erythema multiforme • Stevens-Johnson syndrome
VESICLE AND BULLA	Vesicle: <0.5 cm blister containing transparent fluid. Bulla >0.5 cm blister.	• Burns • Insect bites • Herpes simplex • Chickenpox • Varicella zoster • Scabies • Bullous impetigo staphylococcal • Scalded skin syndrome or toxic epidermal necrolysis • Hand-foot-mouth disease from the coxsackievirus • Contact dermatitis (i.e., poison ivy)
PETECHIA AND PURPURA	Petechia <1 cm flat, nonpalpable lesion. Purpura >1 cm flat, nonpalpable lesion. May vary in color from dark red to purple. Does not blanch when pressed. Bruising is a form of purpura. May be macular or papular.	• Henoch-Schönlein purpura • Rocky Mountain spotted fever • Meningococcemia • Sepsis • Idiopathic thrombocytopenic purpura

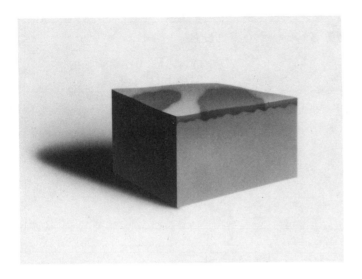

Figure 36

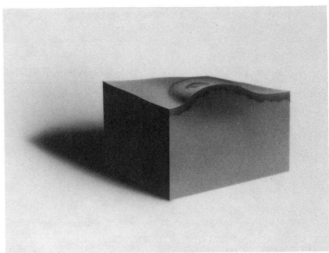

Figure 37

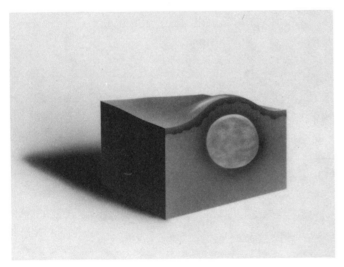

Figure 38

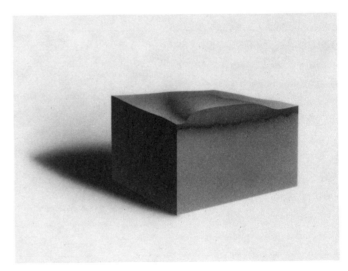

Figure 39

Nursing Diagnoses, Interventions, and Expected Outcomes

NURSING DIAGNOSIS	INTERVENTIONS	EXPECTED OUTCOMES
Airway clearance, ineffective, related to: • Inability to remove excess secretions • Seizure activity • Increased production of oropharyngeal secretions • Decreased level of consciousness	• Position to maintain open airway • Administer oxygen • Suction as needed • Prepare for endotracheal intubation, as indicated	The child will maintain a patent airway, as evidenced by: • Regular rate, depth, and pattern of breathing • Symmetric chest expansion • Effective cough and gag reflex • Absence of signs and symptoms of airway obstruction: Stridor, dyspnea, and hoarse voice • Clear sputum of normal amount without abnormal color or odor • Absence of signs and symptoms of retained secretions: Fever, tachycardia, and tachypnea.

Breathing pattern, ineffective, related to:
• Prolonged seizure activity
• Decreased energy and fatigue
• Decreased level of consciousness
• Pharmacologic agents
	• Position supine, elevate head of bed
	• Administer oxygen
	• Assist ventilation, if needed
	• Consider endotracheal intubation
	• Initiate cardiopulmonary resuscitation, as indicated
		The child will have an effective breathing pattern, as evidenced by:
		• Regular rate, depth, and pattern of breathing
		• Clear and equal bilateral breath sounds
		• Symmetric chest expansion
		• ABG values within normal limits:
		  ■ PaO_2 80 to 100 mm Hg (10.0 to 13.3 KPa)
		  ■ SaO_2 >95%
		  ■ $PaCO_2$ 35 to 45 mm Hg (4.7 to 6.0 KPa)
		  ■ pH between 7.35 and 7.45
		• Absence of stridor, dyspnea, and cyanosis
		• Absence of use of accessory muscles or nasal flaring
		• Trachea midline
		• Chest radiograph without abnormality

Gas exchange, impaired, related to:
• Ineffective breathing pattern
• Ineffective airway clearance
• Aspiration
• Prolonged seizure activity
• Decreased oxygen-carrying capacity of blood
	• Administer oxygen
	• Assist ventilation, as indicated
	• Consider endotracheal intubation
	• Monitor oxygen saturation with pulse oximeter
		The child will maintain adequate gas exchange, as evidenced by:
		• Oxygen saturation >95% by pulse oximetry
		• ABG values within normal limits:
		  ■ PaO_2 80 to 100 mm Hg (10.0 to 13.3 KPa)
		  ■ SaO_2 >95%
		  ■ $PaCO_2$ 35 to 45 mm Hg (4.7 to 6.0 KPa)
		  ■ pH between 7.35 and 7.45
		• Skin normal color, warm, and dry
		• Improved level of consciousness
		• Regular rate, depth, and pattern of breathing

NURSING DIAGNOSIS	INTERVENTIONS	EXPECTED OUTCOMES
Fluid volume deficit related to: • Alteration in capillary permeability and fluid shifts • Inadequate fluid intake • Diarrhea or vomiting and inadequate intake • Sickling of red blood cells • Defective, deficient, or absent clotting factors • Increased metabolic needs • Diabetic ketoacidosis	• Control bleeding • Obtain vascular access • Initiate intravenous fluids, as indicated • Consider intravenous bolus of 20 ml/kg of normal saline or lactated Ringer's solution • Initiate oral rehydration, as appropriate • Insert indwelling urinary catheter, as indicated • Prepare for administration of blood or blood products, as indicated	The child's will have an effective circulating volume, as evidenced by: • Stable vital signs appropriate for age • Moist mucous membranes • Urine output of 1 to 2 ml/kg/hour • Urine specific gravity within normal limits • Serum electrolyte values within normal range • Strong, palpable peripheral pulses • External hemorrhage is controlled • Improved level of consciousness • Skin normal color, warm, and dry • Hematocrit of 30 ml/dl or hemoglobin of 12 to 14 gm/dl or greater
Tissue perfusion, altered cardiopulmonary, renal, gastrointestinal, and peripheral, related to: • Interrupted blood flow secondary to sickling of red blood cells • Bleeding caused by deficient or absent clotting factors • Increased viscosity of blood caused by hyperglycemia or dehydration	• Control external bleeding • Obtain vascular access • Initiate intravenous fluids • Consider intravenous bolus of 20 ml/kg of normal saline or lactated Ringer's solution • Consider blood replacement or blood product administration, as indicated • Administer medications, as ordered to support blood pressure and perfusion	The child will maintain adequate tissue perfusion, as evidenced by: • Improved level of consciousness • Urine output of 1 to 2 ml/kg/hour • Adequate blood pressure for age • Pulse rate appropriate for age • Strong, palpable peripheral pulses • Skin normal color, warm, and dry
Cardiac output, decreased, related to: • Decreased venous return • Acute blood loss • Massive vasodilation • Myocardial compromise • Sepsis, septic shock	• Control bleeding • Obtain vascular access • Initiate intravenous fluid replacement • Administer blood or blood products, as indicated • Administer medication to support blood pressure, as indicated • Initiate cardiopulmonary resuscitation, as indicated	The child will maintain adequate circulatory function, as evidenced by: • Improved level of consciousness • Strong, palpable peripheral and central pulses • Pulse rate appropriate for age • Absence of dysrhythmias • Skin normal color, warm, and dry • Urine output of 1 to 2 ml/kg/hour • Adequate blood pressure for age
Pain, related to: • Disease process • Decreased tissue perfusion secondary to vasoocclusive event • Hemorrhage into joints and muscles • Invasive procedures	• Administer pain medications, as indicated • Initiate nonpharmacologic pain management techniques • Immobilize affected joint; support position of comfort • Apply ice or cold packs, as appropriate • Transport via wheelchair or stretcher to decrease movement	The child will experience relief of pain, as evidenced by: • Absence of nonverbal cues of pain: Crying, grimacing, inability to assume a position of comfort, and guarding • Ability to cooperate with care, as appropriate • Diminishing or absent level of pain, indicated by patient's self-report using an objective measurement tool in the verbal child • Absence of physiologic indicators of pain: Tachycardia, tachypnea, pallor, diaphoretic skin, and increasing blood pressure
Hypothermia related to: • Decreased tissue perfusion • Exposure • Rapid infusion of intravenous fluids	• Initiate measures to prevent heat loss • Initiate warming measures	The child will maintain a normal core body temperature, as evidenced by: • Absence of shivering, cool skin, pallor • Skin normal color, warm, and dry • Core temperature measurement of 36 to 37.5°C (96.8 to 99.5°F)

NURSING DIAGNOSIS	INTERVENTIONS	EXPECTED OUTCOMES
Hyperthermia related to: • Infection	• Administer antipyretics • Unbundle, undress • Provide oral fluids, as appropriate	The child will maintain a normal core body temperature, as evidenced by: • Skin normal color, warm, and dry • Core temperature measurement of 36 to 37.5°C (96.8 to 99.5°F)
Infection, risk of, related to: • Impaired skin integrity • Immunocompromised state • Decreased host defenses secondary to protein depletion caused by hyperglycemia	• Administer antibiotics, as ordered • Initiate isolation precaution to protect patient from exposures • Monitor for signs of infection • Ensure good hand washing techniques • Avoid rectal temperature and rectal suppositories in immunocompromised child • Maintain universal precautions	The child will be free from infection, as evidenced by: • Core temperature measurement of 36 to 37.5°C (96.8 to 99.5°F) • Absence of systemic signs of infection: Fever, tachypnea, and tachycardia • Wounds free from redness, swelling, purulent drainage, or odor • Urine output of 1 to 2 ml/kg/hour • Negative blood cultures • White blood cell count and differential within normal limits • Improved level of consciousness
Anxiety and fear (child and caregiver) related to: • Unfamiliar environment • Unpredictable nature of condition • Invasive procedures	• Keep family informed of treatment plan • Facilitate family participation in care and presence • Provide explanations of procedures • Provide psychosocial support	The child/caregiver will experience decreasing anxiety and fear, as evidenced by: • Orientation to surroundings • Ability to describe reasons for equipment and procedures used in treatment • Ability to verbalize concerns and ask questions of health care team • Use of effective coping skills • Vital signs returning to within normal limits

Triage or Acuity Decisions

EMERGENT Any infant or child currently exhibiting seizure activity; with hemophiliac who sustained blunt abdominal or head trauma or penetrating trauma; who is actually or potentially immunocompromised with a fever; who is younger than 30 days of age and febrile; with a generalized petechial or purpuric rash; with moderate-to-severe pain related to sickle cell crisis.

URGENT Pediatric patient with mild-to-moderate dehydration; who had a seizure prior to arrival but is now awake and alert; with syncopal episode before arrival; with moderate abdominal cramping or pain; who has hemophilia with acute muscle or joint bleed.

NONURGENT Pediatric patient with sore throat without dysphagia; with vomiting or diarrhea without dehydration; who is older than 3 months of age and febrile but is active, alert, and without other symptoms; with cold symptoms (rhinhorrea, cough); with nonpetechial rash with generalized or localized distribution.

Planning and Implementation

Refer to Chapter 4, "Initial Assessment and Triage," for airway, breathing, and circulation interventions appropriate during the primary assessment. General interventions are also listed in Chapter 4. Refer to Chapter 5, "Respiratory Distress and Failure" and Chapter 7, "Cardiovascular Emergencies" for additional interventions related to respiratory compromise and shock, respectively.

- Avoid rectal temperatures and rectal suppositories in a child who is immunocompromised. (Nursing diagnoses: Infection; injury).

- Maintain universal precautions. (Nursing diagnosis: Infection).

- Initiate appropriate isolation measures. (Nursing diagnosis: Infection).

- Administer antipyretics per protocol. (Nursing diagnosis: Hyperthermia).

Evaluation and Ongoing Assessment

The pediatric patient with a serious or life-threatening illness requires frequent reassessment and evaluation of progress toward desired outcomes. Improvements in airway, breathing, circulation, or neurologic status may not be sustained, and additional intervention may be required. To evaluate the patient's response and progress, monitor the following:

- Airway patency.

- Effectiveness of breathing.

- Pulse rate and quality of peripheral and central perfusion.

- Vital signs.

- Level of consciousness and activity level.

- Urine output.

- Level of pain.

- Cardiac rhythm, as indicated.

- Oxygen saturation, as indicated.

SELECTED MEDICAL EMERGENCIES

The following selected medical emergencies are common in the pediatric population. Additional history, signs and symptoms, and additional interventions specific to the selected medical emergency are listed. Standard assessment data and interventions outlined in Chapter 4, "Initial Assessment and Triage," and previously in this chapter are not repeated with each disorder but should also be applied, as appropriate.

Infectious Disorders

SEPSIS

Infants younger than 3 months of age lack the immunocompetence of older infants and children and are reliant on maternal antibodies for protection from infection.[1] These factors place this age group at higher risk for serious bacterial infection. A rectal temperature >38°C (100.4°F) typically necessitates a septic workup in these infants. Other children at high risk for bacterial infections of the bloodstream, termed bacteremia or sepsis, include those with the following conditions:

- Younger than 2 years of age with high fever.

- On current immunosuppressive chemotherapy (e.g., chronic steroids, antirejection medications following transplant, oncology treatment).

- Compromised or absent splenic function (e.g., sickle cell disease, postsurgical removal of spleen).

- Human immunodeficiency virus or acquired immunodeficiency syndrome.

- Long-term central venous catheters.

Although fever is often associated with sepsis, many seriously ill infants and children are normothermic or hypothermic rather than febrile. Additionally, temperatures greater than 42°C (107.6°F) are not usually infectious in origin but are related to central nervous system disturbances or heat stroke.[2]

Additional History

- History of pre-existing disease.

- Prior exposure to illness (day care, home, school).

- Immunization status.

- Characteristics of illness onset and progression.

- Changes in feeding pattern or poor feeding.

Signs and Symptoms

- Rectal temperature greater than 38°C (100.4°F) for infants younger than 3 months of age.[3]

- Tachycardia.

- Tachypnea.

- Decreased activity level or lethargy.

- Paradoxical irritability.

- Dry mucous membranes or decreased tear production resulting from increased insensible fluid loss.

- Mottled skin.

- Decreased peripheral perfusion.

Diagnostic Procedures

Laboratory Studies

- Complete blood count with differential and platelets.

- Serum or whole blood glucose test.

- Blood culture.

- Urine for urinalysis and culture.

- Cerebrospinal fluid analysis, culture, and gram stain; may need to be deferred in unstable children.

- Electrolytes.

Radiographic Studies

- Chest radiograph.

Monitors

- Cardiac monitor.

- Pulse oximeter.

Additional Interventions

- Administer oxygen. Anticipate the need for early, elective intubation to optimize and maintain oxygen delivery.

- Administer antipyretics, per protocol.

- Anticipate and prepare for full or modified sepsis workup.

- Administer fluids orally or intravenously, depending on the child's condition.

MENINGITIS

Meningitis is an inflammation of the meninges of the brain and spinal cord caused by a variety of bacterial or viral agents. The most common causative organisms are *Haemophilus influenzae* (H-flu), *Neisseria meningitidis,* and *Streptococcus pneumoniae.* Viral meningitis is more common in children and is associated with a lower morbidity and mortality rate. **Mortality rates are as high as 30% for bacterial meningitis.**[11] The outcome varies depending on the infectious organism, the child's age, and state of immune competence. Long-term effects may include deafness, epilepsy, hydrocephalus, and learning and motor disorders.[11]

Complications of meningitis include cerebral edema and increased intracranial pressure, seizures, septic shock, disseminated intravascular coagulation, subdural effusions, and anemia. One of the most common complications of bacterial meningitis is *Syndrome of Inappropriate Antidiuretic Hormone,* which results in hyponatremia and water intoxication.

Additional History

- Poor feeding; decrease in appetite.

- Vomiting.

- Fever.

- Recent ear infection or upper respiratory tract infection.

- Presence of rash, petechia, or purpura.

- Photophobia.

- Seizure.

- Headache or neck pain.

- Decreased activity level, irritability, decreased level of consciousness.

Signs and Symptoms

The signs and symptoms of meningitis based on the child's age are summarized in Table 30.

Table 30

SIGNS AND SYMPTOMS OF MENINGITIS BY AGE[12]		
Younger than 2 Months of Age	**3 Months of Age to 2 Years of Age**	**Older Than 2 Years of Age**
• Fever • Apnea, cyanosis • Temperature instability • Altered level of consciousness • Seizures • Vomiting or diarrhea • Bulging fontanelle • Jitteryness; irritability • Petechiae or purpura (bacterial infection) • Poor feedings	• Fever • Scizures • Bulging fontanelle • Ataxia • Vomiting • Stiff neck • Altered mental status • Petechiae or purpura (bacterial infection) • Bulging fontanelle (late sign)	• Fever • Headache • Altered mental status or irritability • Seizures • Stiff neck • Petechiae or purpura (bacterial infection) • Vomiting • Photophobia • Positive *Brudzinski's sign* • Positive Kernig's sign

Diagnostic Procedures

Laboratory Studies

- Sepsis workup. Obtain laboratory specimens as outlined under Sepsis. Anticipate additional laboratory studies based on clinical condition.

Other Diagnostic Procedures

- Computerized tomography scan, as indicated. A computerized tomography scan may be obtained when the patient has experienced a focal seizure and is typically completed prior to the lumbar puncture.

Additional Interventions (in addition to those listed under Sepsis)

- Obtain vascular access and administer intravenous fluids. If signs and symptoms of shock exist, administer a 20 ml/kg bolus of warmed crystalloid fluid. Repeat the bolus as necessary.

- Evaluate neurologic status and vital signs for increased intracranial pressure. Trend neurologic status.

- Administer medications:

    - Intravenous antibiotic therapy. In suspected bacterial meningitis, **do not delay antibiotic administration while awaiting laboratory specimen collection or results.**

    - Antipyretics.

    - Inotropic agents or vasoactive agent to support blood pressure, as indicated.

    - The use of corticosteroids remains somewhat controversial for reducing inflammation.[11] Dexamethasone is recommended in the treatment of children older than 6 weeks of age with *Haemophilus influenzae* type b meningitis.[13] Administration of the initial dose must occur shortly before or at the time antibiotics are given. Its efficacy in pneumococcal and meningococcal meningitis has not been proven.[13]

- Initiate respiratory isolation *(droplet precautions)*.[14]

MENINGOCOCCEMIA

Meningococcemia is a potentially life-threatening clinical entity in which *Neisseria meningitidis* gains access to the bloodstream. The incubation period is 2 to 10 days, and the bacterium is usually spread via the oral or nasal route. The disease course can be fulminating, with a rapid onset of symptoms. Death may occur in several hours if treatment is not provided. Most cases occur in younger children; the peak age group is 6 months to 1 year of age. Survival may be determined in the first 12 hours after treatment has been initiated. With the use of antibiotics and supportive measures, the fatality rate is near 10%.[2] The ultimate prognosis and outcome depends on the child's immune status, splenic function, fulminance of the infection, and prompt medical intervention. Complications include meningitis, shock, septic arthritis, pneumonia, pericarditis, myocarditis, disseminated intravascular coagulation, and death.[2]

Additional History

- Recent exposure to known infected person.

- Fever.

- Nausea or vomiting.

- Irritability, lethargy, or poor feeding in infants.

- Malaise or joint pain.

- Rash.

Signs and Symptoms

- Fever or temperature instability.
- Decreased level of consciousness.
- Vomiting.
- Petechiae or purpura.
- Irritability.
- Weakness.
- Headache.
- Hypotension.

Diagnostic Procedures (in addition to those listed under Sepsis)

Laboratory Studies

- Coagulation studies.
- Fibrinogen split products.

Monitors

- Cardiac monitor.
- Pulse oximetry.

Additional Interventions (in addition to those listed under Sepsis)

- Initiate respiratory isolation (droplet precautions).[14]
- Monitor for signs of meningitis and increased intracranial pressure.
- Monitor for signs of disseminated intravascular coagulation.
- Administer inotropic or vasoactive agents (e.g., epinephrine drip) to maintain blood pressure.
- Administer antibiotic prophylaxis for household contact or health care providers who experience intimate contact with the child's respiratory secretions through the mucous membranes or non-intact skin or blood.

Neurologic Disorders

SEIZURES

Seizures are one of the most frequently encountered pediatric medical emergencies. Approximately 5% of all children experience one or more seizures.[15] The most common causes of seizures include febrile illness, infections, and metabolic disturbances, but seizures may also be caused by toxins, trauma, tumors, and noncompliance with seizure medications.[16,17] The clinical manifestations of the seizure depends on several factors. These include the part of the cortex involved, the rate and direction of electrical discharge of neurons within the cortex, and the age of the child. Newborns often have subtle manifestations of seizure activity (e.g., eye deviation and fluttering, lip smacking, bicycling) because of their cortical immaturity.[16]

The two categories of seizures are partial and generalized.[3,15]

- Partial seizures include:

    - Simple: No loss of consciousness. Includes motor and autonomic symptoms.

    - Complex: Impairment of consciousness. Aura often present.

- Generalized seizures are categorized by their specific patterns of movement and include:

    - Petit mal: Absence of movement. Brief lapses in awareness.

    - Grand mal: Tonic-clonic. Sustained muscle contraction, rhythmic jerking, and spasms of the extremities.

    - Minor motor: Myoclonic. Brief muscle contractions occur unilaterally or bilaterally, tonic, or clonic.

    - Atonic: Abrupt loss of muscle tone, usually causing the child to collapse.

Most childhood seizures are single, generalized, tonic-clonic events lasting only a few minutes. A seizure lasting more than 15 minutes is considered a prolonged seizure. Status epilepticus is defined as continuous seizure activity that exceeds 30 minutes duration or recurrent seizures without an intervening period of recovery.[17,18]

Febrile seizures are common in infants and young children, constituting 30% of all childhood seizures,[16] and are usually associated with changes in body temperature from an acute minor illness. Febrile seizures usually occur in children between 3 months and 5 years of age, peaking at 9 to 30 months of age. Most are benign and self-limiting.[16] The exact mechanism of febrile seizures is unknown. Frequently, there is a positive family history for similar febrile seizures in childhood, but a negative history for other types of seizure disorders. Children with one simple febrile seizure have a 30% chance of having one or more reoccurrences.[16]

Prolonged seizure activity results in airway obstruction, hypoxia, acidosis, increased intracranial pressure, hypoglycemia, and hyperthermia. If not abated, hypotension can develop, along with respiratory, cardiovascular, and renal failure. A single, brief (less than 30 seconds) seizure is usually not associated with permanent sequelae.[18]

Additional History

- Past history of seizures.

- History of neurologic disorder.

- Presence of ventricular-peritoneal shunt.

- Family history of seizure disorder or febrile seizures.

- Description of seizure activity prior to arrival to the emergency department to include length of seizure, type of movements, and color change.

- Head trauma; may be immediate or delayed.

- Possibility of toxic exposure.

- Amnesia.

Signs and Symptoms

- Tonic or clonic muscle activity. Infants may exhibit rigid posturing and fine motor tremors.

- Dilated pupils or eyes deviated upward or outward.

- Incontinence of urine or stool.

- Decreased level of consciousness during and following the seizure, termed the postictal state.

- Blank stare or slight tremors of the extremities, termed a petit mal seizure.

- Presence of pallor, cyanosis.

- Headache.

Diagnostic Procedures

Laboratory Studies

- Serum or whole blood glucose test.

- Toxicology screen.

- Anticonvulsant levels (if on current therapy).

- Electrolytes.

- Magnesium.

- Calcium.

- Carboxyhemoglobin.

Additional Interventions

- Administer medications:

  - Anticonvulsant therapy, as indicated.

  - Antipyretics, as indicated.

- Immobilize the spine if trauma is suspected.

- Initiate seizure precautions according to protocol to protect against self-injury.

- Evaluate neurologic status and vital signs for increased intracranial pressure.

- Initiate cardiac or pulse oximetry monitoring for patients with status epilepticus, prolonged seizure, receiving intravenous anticonvulsant therapy, or as indicated by patient condition.

Fluid, Electrolyte, and Metabolic Disorders

GASTROENTERITIS

Worldwide, gastroenteritis is second only to respiratory illness as a cause of morbidity from complications of dehydration, electrolyte imbalance, and malnutrition. It is responsible for up to 10% of all hospitalizations in children younger than 5 years of age.[19] Gastroenteritis is an inflammation of the gastrointestinal tract caused by a bacterial, viral, or parasitic agent. Viral diarrhea is the most common and accounts for 80% of all infections in children.[19,20] Rotavirus is the most common form, followed by adenovirus and enterovirus. Diarrhea may also be caused by antibiotic therapy, cystic fibrosis, milk allergy, and lactose deficiency.[19]

Identification of risk factors can assist the caregiver in identifying the transmission of the causative agent. Table 31 identifies risk factors and their associated pathogens.

Table 31

CAUSES OF GASTROENTERITIS	
Risk Factors	**Associated Pathogens**
Day care centers	• Rotavirus • *Giardiasis* • *Shigella*
Household pets • Iguanas, turtles, and snakes • Puppies, kittens • Birds, reptiles	• *Salmonella* • *Campylobaciter* • *Cryptosporidium*
Foods • Raw hamburger • Raw eggs, poultry	• *Escherichia coli* • *Salmonella*
Antibiotic use	*Clostridium difficile*
International travel	Enterotoxigenic *Escherichia coli*

Adapted from Belamarich P. Gastrointestinal emergencies. In: Crain EF, Gershel JC, eds. *Clinical Manual of Emergency Pediatrics*. 3rd ed. New York, NY: McGraw-Hill; 1997:191-248. Used with permission.

Additional History

- Recent travel.
- Pets in the home.
- Duration of symptoms.
- Description of diarrhea stool, frequency, number, and onset.
- Number of wet diapers in last 8 hours; last urination.
- Use of antibiotics.
- Attendance at day care.

Signs and Symptoms

- Vomiting.
- Diarrhea: Mucoid, bloody, watery.
- Fever.
- Abdominal pain.
- Sunken fontanelle.
- Sticky or dry mucous membranes.
- Lack of tears.
- Poor skin turgor.
- Tachycardia.
- Tachypnea.
- Orthostatic vital sign changes.

Additional Interventions

- Initiate rehydration via intravenous or oral route, as indicated:
    - Oral rehydration is usually adequate for the child who has mild dehydration and can tolerate fluids.
    - Moderate-to-severe dehydration usually requires intravenous fluids and an initial bolus of crystalloid solution.
- Monitor fluid intake and output.
- Administer antidiarrheal agents, as ordered. This is rarely indicated.
- Obtain hemoccult of stool.
- Obtain stool for culture, ova, and parasites, rapid enzyme immunoassay for rotavirus.
- Provide caregivers with proper home care instructions to prevent transmission of disease.

DIABETIC KETOACIDOSIS

Insulin-dependent diabetes mellitus is a disease resulting from an inadequate or absolute deficiency of the hormone insulin. It is one of the most common chronic diseases starting in childhood. Insulin is responsible for glucose transport, protein synthesis, and storage and synthesis of lipids. Thus, diabetes mellitus is a disorder of energy metabolism. It is estimated that diabetes affects one of every 400 to 600 children younger than 18 years of age.[21]

Diabetic ketoacidosis is a condition caused by an insulin deficiency that results in hyperglycemia. It is commonly seen in both adult and pediatric emergency departments. Diabetic ketoacidosis can be life threatening and is the most common cause of death in diabetic children.[22,23] The manifestations of diabetic ketoacidosis mimics signs and symptoms associated with gastroenteritis with dehydration. Additionally, 20 to 40% of children with a new onset of diabetes present to the emergency department with diabetic keto-acidosis. Diabetic ketoacidosis is defined as the following[22]:

- Hyperglycemia with a serum glucose concentration >300 mg/dl.
- Ketonemia.
- Serum pH of 7.30 or less.
- Bicarbonate level of 14 mEq/L or less.

Additional History

- Frequent urination or nocturia.
- Excessive thirst or fluid intake.
- Fatigue.
- Recent weight loss.
- History of diabetes or family history of diabetes.
- History of recent viral illness.

Signs and Symptoms

- Abdominal pain and tenderness.
- Nausea and vomiting.
- *Kussmaul* respirations or deep, rapid respirations.
- Decreased level of consciousness.
- Tachycardia.
- *Orthostatic vital sign changes.*
- Dry mucous membranes or absence of tears.
- Acetone or "fruity" odor on breath.
- Flushed dry skin.

Diagnostic Procedures

Laboratory Studies

- Arterial or capillary blood gas.

- Serum or whole blood glucose test.

- Electrolytes: Potassium level is important as well as blood urea nitrogen and creatinine.

- Urine for urinalysis, ketones, and glucose.

Additional Interventions

- Obtain vascular access and initiate intravenous fluids:

  - Administer a 20 ml/kg bolus of 0.9% normal saline.

  - Repeat the bolus as necessary.

- Administer regular insulin intravenously. Verify dose and volume before administering.

- Anticipate the need to further correct acidosis with an intravenous buffer solution when pH is less than 7 (controversial).

- Correct electrolyte deficits. This is usually calculated and carefully replaced over 24 hours.

- Evaluate neurologic status and vital signs for increased intracranial pressure.

- Monitor fluid intake and output.

Hematologic Disorders

SICKLE CELL CRISIS

Sickle cell disease is an inherited disorder of the hemoglobin structure characterized by the presence of an abnormal type of hemoglobin in the red blood cell, termed hemoglobin S. It occurs in approximately 1 of every 500 African-Americans. However, it may be seen in individuals of Mediterranean, Middle Eastern, and Indian descent.[24] When the cell becomes hypoxic, these red blood cells assume an irregular shape, causing an increase in blood viscosity that results in stasis, sludging, and further deoxygenation. This causes microvascular obstruction and tissue ischemia, and may result in necrosis. The resulting ischemia causes the painful sickle cell crisis.[25] The sickling process occurs with local tissue hypoxia, dehydration, acidosis, and hypertonicity.[5] The sites most commonly involved are the joints, mesenteric vessels, liver, spleen, brain, lungs, and penis.[25]

Sickle cell crisis may be precipitated by an infection, physical exertion, exposure to cold, or emotional stress.[26] Vasoocclusive crisis, the most common type of crisis, is produced by stasis of red blood cells in small capillaries. Aplastic crisis normally follows a viral infection causing an impairment of red cell production in the bone marrow that results in bone marrow suppression, and presents with worsening anemia and reticulocytopenia. Splenic sequestration crisis occurs from pooling of red blood cells in an enlarged spleen, causing organ failure. If untreated, this can be fatal.[27]

Aplastic crisis and splenic sequestration are potentially life-threatening complications of sickle cell disease. Additionally, children with sickle cell disease are at higher risk for serious bacterial infections (e.g., meningitis, pneumonia, sepsis) related to *functional asplenia*.[24] Infection remains the leading cause of death in early childhood for these patients. Causative agents include *Streptococcus pneumoniae* and *Haemophilus influenzae* type b.[27]

Other complications of sickle cell disease include impaired growth and delayed puberty, stroke, and acute chest syndrome. Acute chest syndrome is a painful crisis accompanied by symptoms clinically similar to those of pneumonia. Chest pain, cough, dyspnea, fever, tachypnea, hypoxia, leukocytosis, and pleural effusions characterize this syndrome. It is important to differentiate between pneumonia and pulmonary infarction.[28]

Additional History

- Pain or swelling of hands or feet which may be accompanied by warmth and tenderness, known as dactylitis or hand-foot syndrome.

- Frequent infections, failure to thrive, jaundice, or anemia in an infant.

- Family members with sickle cell anemia.

- Fever.

- Previous hospitalizations.

- Known presence of sickle cell disease or trait.

- Current medications:

    - Prophylactic penicillin.

    - Immunizations, specifically the pneumococcol vaccine.

    - Home pain regimens.

    - Folic acid.

Signs and Symptoms

- Soft tissue swelling and tenderness over the affected site.

- Joint, abdominal, or back pain.

- Nausea or vomiting.

- Headache.

- Fever.

- Chest pain or dyspnea.

- Priapism.

- Visual changes.

- Right upper quadrant pain, particularly in children older than 10 years of age. This is usually associated with cholelithiasis.

- Left upper quadrant mass. This is usually associated with splenic sequestration crisis.

- Jaundice.

Diagnostic Procedures

Laboratory Studies

- Complete blood count.

- Blood cultures, as indicated.

- Reticulocyte count.

- Urine for urinalysis and culture.

- Cerebrospinal fluid for culture and gram stain, if meningitis is suspected.

- Type and crossmatch if transfusion is needed (e.g., stroke, sequestration crisis).

- Arterial blood gas for acute chest syndrome or hypoxia.

Radiographic Studies

- Chest radiograph if pneumonia or acute chest syndrome is suspected.

Additional Interventions

- Administer oxygen if evidence of hypoxia is present. Oxygen delivery concentration is controversial, as it may cause rebound crisis after discontinuation.

- Obtain vascular access and administer intravenous fluids to maintain hydration or rehydrate the child.

- Administer medications:

  - Analgesic medications to control pain; morphine sulphate is the drug of choice.

  - Antipyretics for fever control.

  - Antibiotics, as indicated, for infection.

- Promote rest.

- Anticipate need for transfusion in selected situations.

HEMOPHILIA

Hemophilia is a genetic disorder of coagulation characterized by a clotting factor deficiency. Hemophilia primarily affects males, but females carry the trait. Hemophilia most commonly results from a factor VIII deficiency, occurring in 1/7,500 male births, or a factor IX or Christmas deficiency, occurring in 1/30,000 male births.[29] The prognosis and severity of bleeding can be predicted by the level of factor coagulant activity.

Additional History

- Frequent bleeding episodes.

- Family member with hemophilia.

Signs and Symptoms

- Pain.

- Joint bleeding. This is common in large joints, such as the knees and elbows.

- Limitation of range of motion in the involved joint.

- Muscle bleeding.

- Subcutaneous bleeding.

- Oral bleeding.

- Epistaxis.

- Hematuria.

- Headache, vomiting, altered mental status, or seizures related to intracranial or intra-abdominal hemorrhage.

- Hematemesis, melena, abdominal pain, tenderness, and distention related to upper and lower gastrointestinal bleeding.

Additional Interventions

- Apply direct pressure to areas of external bleeding.

- Anticipate replacement of missing coagulation factors, such as cryoprecipitate, fresh-frozen plasma, or factor concentrates. Initiate treatment as quickly as possible and continue until healing occurs.

- Provide pain management measures:

  - Splint and immobilize the affected extremity for 12 to 24 hours.

  - Administer analgesic medications.

- Avoid invasive procedures because of tissue friability:

  - Rectal temperature.

  - Urinary catheter.

  - Intramuscular injections because of muscle bleeding.

- Anticipate the need for laboratory specimens if there is significant injury or evidence of intra-abdominal or intracranial bleeding.

- Prepare for computerized tomography scan if head trauma is present.

Immune System Disorders

HUMAN IMMUNODEFICIENCY VIRUS AND ACQUIRED IMMUNODEFICIENCY SYNDROME

As of December 1994, the World Health Organization estimated that more than 1 million children world-wide had acquired the human immunodeficiency virus (HIV).[30] By 1993, approximately 4,000 cases of acquired immunodeficiency syndrome in children 13 years of age and younger had been reported. Children can acquire the disease by several modes. However, 90% of children younger than 12 years of age have acquired the human immunodeficiency virus perinatally.[2] Sexual abuse, breast-feeding, and unprotected sex and intravenous drug use in adolescents are also modes of transmitting the human immunodeficiency virus. Children, especially hemophiliacs who received blood transfusions before 1985 are at high risk of being HIV positive.

First recognized as a disease entity in 1981, the first pediatric case of acquired immunodeficiency syndrome was reported in 1982. It is a progressively debilitating, multisystem, viral infection that most commonly attacks the immune and nervous system. It has become the eighth leading cause of death in children 1 to 4 years of age, and the sixth in adolescents 15 to 24 years of age.[31,32]

The etiologic agent of acquired immunodeficiency syndrome is the retrovirus known as the human immunodeficiency virus. Because the pathology of this disease involves the immune system, children are at high risk for developing bacterial, viral, parasitic, and fungal infections, eventually leading to death.[2] Pneumonia is the most common infection acquired. The incubation period and disease course are shorter for children than adults. Eighty percent of all children infected with the human immunodeficiency virus are symptomatic by 2 years of age.[32]

The diagnosis of the human immunodeficiency virus may not be known at presentation to the emergency department. Testing may be completed as part of the ED workup or at an alternative site if the child is not ill but has risk factors for the human immunodeficiency virus.

An enzyme-linked immunosorbent assay which is a human immunodeficiency virus antibody test, is the test performed on children older than 18 months of age. If the enzyme-linked immunosorbent assay is positive, confirmation of the disease is usually done by a Western blot. Children who are younger than 18 months of age may carry maternal antibodies. Therefore, the polymerase chain reaction test is usually done.[32]

Additional History

- If acquired in the perinatal period, history may include failure to thrive, recurrent infections, and lymphadenopathy.

- Frequent or recurrent infections (e.g., candidiasis).

- Progressive regression from developmental achievements.

- Persistent weight loss.

- Mother is positive for the human immunodeficiency virus or has developed acquired immunodeficiency syndrome.

- Child has a history of hemophilia.

- Child is sexually active or has been sexually abused.

- History of substance abuse or sharing needles.

- History of blood transfusion prior to 1985.

- Current medication regimen.

Signs and Symptoms

- Most of the presenting signs and symptoms of human immunodeficiency virus infection are nonspecific.

- Chronic diarrhea.

- Recurrent fever.

- Generalized lymphadenopathy.

- Chronic encephalopathy (e.g., generalized weakness, ataxia).

- Vomiting.

- Dental infections.

- Visual disturbances.

- Other signs and symptoms may vary and are associated with opportunistic infections.

Additional Interventions

- As with all patients, use universal precautions for protection of both the patient and emergency care team. Initiate protective or reverse isolation measures to protect the patient from exposures in the emergency department.

- Provide psychological support for the family and patient.

- Obtain laboratory work, as appropriate, for the patient's condition. Obtain consent according to policy or procedure prior to drawing specimens.

- Provide referral for counseling and followup if the human immunodeficiency virus test is obtained in the emergency department or if the human immunodeficiency virus is suspected and testing at an alternate site is preferred.

HEALTH PROMOTION

The following prevention measures and recommendation have an impact on medical illness:

- Educate caregivers and patient about disease processes and prevention strategies:

    - Positioning of infants on their back or side with the head elevated to decrease the risk of aspiration. Infants should not be positioned prone.

    - Fever control measures.

    - Immunizations and resources to obtain them, if needed.

- Educate caregivers on methods to give medications, including using droppers or syringes.

- Encourage safe practices and safe-sex strategies to reduce risk of sexually transmitted disease, including the human immunodeficiency virus.

- Provide referrals to available support groups in the area for children with chronic conditions (e.g., hemophilia, human immunodeficiency virus, diabetes).

- Educate patient and caregivers on how to obtain a primary care provider and the importance of care continuity. Provide referral to a primary care provider or referral resource and encourage the caregiver to obtain a primary care provider.

- Provide caregivers with written information identifying common prevention strategies for each developmental stage.

SUMMARY

Medical emergencies encompass a vast array of disorders. Knowledge of the unique characteristics of the pediatric patient is essential for the interpretation of assessment data and the formulation of nursing diagnoses and interventions. Early recognition of shock, respiratory compromise, and neurologic alterations is fundamental to the prompt identification of and intervention for medical emergencies. The interlocking relationship between early recognition of life-threatening illness and the initiation of rapid interventions is the central piece to the puzzle of care for the pediatric patient.

REFERENCES

1. Soud TE. The febrile child. In: Soud TE, Rogers JS, eds. *Manual of Pediatric Emergency Nursing.* St. Louis, Mo: Mosby-Year Book; 1998:606-621.

2. Felter RA, Bower JR. Infectious disorders. In: Barkin RM, ed. *Pediatric Emergency Medicine: Concepts and Clinical Practice.* 2nd ed. St. Louis, Mo: Mosby-Year Book; 1997:926-971.

3. Barkin RM, Rosen P, eds. *Emergency Pediatrics.* 4th ed. St. Louis, Mo: Mosby-Year Book; 1994.

4. Noble MN. Fluid and electrolyte imbalances. In: Soud TE, Rogers JS, eds. *Manual of Pediatric Emergency Nursing.* St. Louis, Mo: Mosby-Year Book; 1998:313-331.

5. Wong DL, ed. The child with gastrointestinal dysfunction. *Whaley and Wong's Essentials of Pediatric Nursing.* 5th ed. St. Louis, Mo: Mosby-Year Book; 1997:802-899.

6. Finberg L. Fluid and electrolytes. In: Finberg L, ed. *Saunder's Manual of Pediatric Practice.* Philadelphia, Pa: WB Saunders; 1998:32-35.

7. Sacchetti A, Brilli RJ. Fluids and electrolyte balance. In: Barkin RM, ed. *Pediatric Emergency Medicine: Concepts and Clinical Practice.* 2nd ed. St. Louis, Mo: Mosby-Year Book; 1997:166-189.

8. Watkins SL. The basics of fluid and electrolyte therapy. *Pediatr Ann.* 1995;24:16-22.

9. Bank DE. Dermatologic emergencies. In: Crain EF, Gershel JC, eds. *Clinical Manual of Emergency Pediatrics.* 3rd ed. New York, NY: McGraw-Hill; 1997:69-114.

10. Weston WL, Lane AT, Morelli JG. *Color Textbook of Pediatric Dermatology.* 2nd ed. St. Louis, Mo: Mosby-Year Book; 1996.

11. Strauser D. Pediatric bacterial meningitis in the emergency department. *J Emerg Nurs.* 1997;23:310-315.

12. Nozicka CA. Pediatric meningitis: clinical guidelines, issues, update. *Pediatr Emerg Med Rep.* 1997;2:47-56.

13. American Academy of Pediatrics. Dexamethasone therapy for bacterial meningitis in infants and children. In Peter G, ed. *1997 Red Book: Report of the Committee on Infectious Diseases.* 24th ed. Elk Grove Village, Ill: Author; 1997:620-622.

14. American Academy of Pediatrics. Infection control for hospitalized children. In: Peter G, ed. *1997 Red Book: Report of the Committee on Infectious Diseases.* 24th ed. Elk Grove Village, Ill: Author; 1997:100-107.

15. Bunch B, Avner JR. Neurologic emergencies. In: Crain EF, Gershel JC, eds. *Clinical Manual of Emergency Pediatrics.* 3rd ed. New York, NY: McGraw-Hill; 1997:437-476.

16. Fuchs SM. Neurologic emergencies. In: Barkin RM, ed. *Pediatric Emergency Medicine: Concepts and Clinical Practice.* 2nd ed. St. Louis, Mo: Mosby-Year Book; 1997:972-1024.

17. Dannenbery BW. Pediatric seizure disorders: prompt assessment and emergency management. *Pediatr Emerg Med Rep.* 1996:1:41-52.

18. Segeleon JE, Haun SE. Status epilepticus in children. *Pediatr Ann.* 1996;25:380-386.

19. Belamarich P. Gastrointestinal emergencies. In: Crain EF, Gershel JC, eds. *Clinical Manual of Emergency Pediatrics.* 3rd ed. New York, NY: McGraw-Hill; 1997:191-248.

20. Horton M, Soud TE, Inman C, Standifer P. Gastrointestinal system. In: Soud TE, Rogers JS, eds. *Manual of Pediatric Emergency Nursing.* St. Louis, Mo: Mosby-Year Book; 1998:332-343.

21. White NH. Diabetes mellitus in children. In: Rudolph AM, Hoffman JIE, Rudolph CD, eds. *Rudolph's Pediatrics.* Stanford, Conn: Appleton & Lange; 1996:1804.

22. Rosenblum AL, Hanas R. Diabetic ketoacidosis (DKA): treatment guidelines. *Clin Pediatr.* 1996;35:261-266.

---

23. Klemkamp J, Churchwell KB. Diabetic ketoacidosis in children: initial clinical assessment and treatment. *Pediatr Ann.* 1996;25:387-393.

24. Bachman DT, Barkin RM, Brennan SA, Recht M. Hematologic and oncologic disorders. In: Barkin RM, ed. *Pediatric Emergency Medicine: Concepts and Clinical Practice.* 2nd ed. St. Louis, Mo: Mosby-Year Book; 1997:907-911.

25. Mason SK, Hatfield SL. Hematologic emergencies. In: Newberry L, ed. *Sheehy's Emergency Nursing: Principles and Practice.* 4th ed. St. Louis, Mo: Mosby-Year Book; 1998:639-646.

26. Drake EE. Hematologic system. In: Fox JA, ed. *Primary Health Care of Children.* St. Louis, Mo: Mosby-Year Book; 1997:455-464.

27. Weinblatt M. Hematologic emergencies. In: Crain EF, Gershel JC, eds. *Clinical Manual of Emergency Pediatrics.* 3rd ed. New York, NY: McGraw-Hill; 1997:314-319.

28. Raghuram N, Pettignano R, Gal A, Harsch AA, Adamkicwicz TV. Plastic bronchitis: an unusual complication associated with sickle cell disease and the acute chest syndrome. *Pediatrics.* 1997;100:139-142.

29. Bush MT, Roy N. Hemophilia emergencies. *J Emerg Nurs.* 1995;21:531-537.

30. Rothrock SG. Management of infants and children with HIV infection in the ED. *Pediatr Emerg Med Rep.* 1997;2:27-38.

31. Manley L, Bechtel NM. Hematologic and immune systems. In: Soud TE, Rogers JS, eds. *Manual of Pediatric Emergency Nursing.* St. Louis, Mo: Mosby-Year Book; 1998:390-416.

32. Shea KA. Human immunodeficiency virus/acquired immunodeficiency syndrome. In: Fox JA, ed. *Primary Health Care of Children.* St. Louis, Mo: Mosby-Year Book; 1997:878 892.

Pediatric Considerations:
Positioning for Medical Procedures

Lumbar Puncture

A lumbar puncture involves the placement of a spinal needle in the subarachnoid space of the lumbar area to obtain a cerebrospinal fluid sample. This diagnostic test is most often performed on children with a suspected or potential central nervous system infection, such as meningitis. The lumbar puncture is a standard component of a sepsis workup. Universal and appropriate isolation precautions are also initiated. See Chapter 3, "Pediatric Considerations: Pain Management and Medication Administration," for a review of pharmacologic and nonpharmacologic pain management techniques.

- Place the child in the lateral decubitus position on the stretcher or examination table. The child's knees are drawn up to the abdomen, and the head is flexed forward[1] (see Figure 40).

  - Place the child's shoulders and hips perpendicular to the stretcher or examination table.[1]

  - Secure the child throughout the procedure by placing one arm over the child's neck and the other behind the child's knees.[2]

- Place the infant in an upright position, if desired:

  - Seat the infant upright with the thighs against the abdomen and the neck flexed forward; the assistant holds the infant's arm and leg with one hand[1,2] (see Figure 41).

  - The upright position may also be used for children in respiratory distress or when access to the lumbar region is difficult.[1,2] Have the child dangle his or her legs over the side of the stretcher or examination table, bending slightly forward at the waist.[1]

Figure 40
LATERAL DECUBITUS POSITIONING FOR LUMBAR PUNCTURE

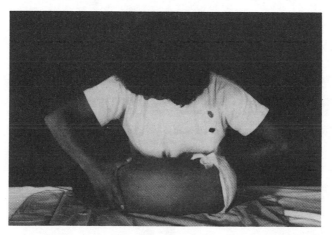

From Lang S. Procedures involving the neurological system. In: Bernardo LM, Bove M, eds. *Pediatric Emergency Nursing Procedures.* Boston, Mass: Jones & Barlett; 1993:154. Reprinted with permission.

Figure 41
SITTING POSITION FOR LUMBAR PUNCTURE

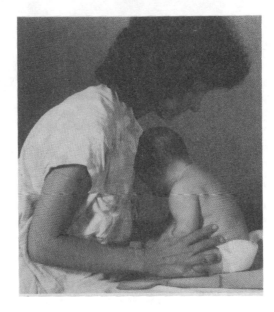

From Lang S. Procedures involving the neurological system. In: Bernardo LM, Bove M, eds. *Pediatric Emergency Nursing Procedures.* Boston, Mass: Jones and Barlett; 1993:155. Reprinted with permission.

Points to Remember:

- If a urine specimen is needed, place a urine collection bag on the child or perform catherization prior to the procedure.

- Plan the use of the topical anesthetic to allow adequate time for the application to take effect.

- Avoid hyperflexion of the neck and vigorous holding in infants because these may lead to respiratory compromise.

- Observe the infant's color, respiratory pattern, and muscle tone during the procedure. Place the child on a pulse oximeter for the procedure to monitor respiratory status.

- Have older children and adolescents lie flat after the procedure to avoid the risk of a postlumbar puncture headache. Younger children and infants may be held by their caregivers in a position of comfort.

Gastric Tube Insertion

Gastric tubes are inserted via the nasal or oral routes to decompress the stomach, perform gastric lavage, or administer medications or nutrition. Single-lumen tubes are used for gavage feedings. Double-lumen or vented tubes are used for decompression. Special vented tubes are available for gastric lavage.

The oral route for gastric tube insertion is used in young infants who are obligatory nose breathers, in patients with facial trauma or suspected basilar skull fracture, and for gastric lavage when a large tube is needed to effectively evacuate the stomach. The procedure for gastric tube insertion is:

- Determine the appropriate-sized tube:

  - The child's age group may be used to estimate the correct tube size[3]:

    - Infant: 8-French to 10-French.

    - Toddler to preschooler: 10-French.

    - School-aged: 12-French.

    - Adolescent: 14-French to 16-French.

  - A length-based tape, such as the Broselow™ tape, may also be used to estimate appropriate tube size.

  - A larger gastric lavage tube (22-French to 36-French) may be selected when gastric lavage is needed. These larger tubes are placed orally, rather than nasally, because of their size.

- Determine the length of tube to be inserted (see Figure 42):

  - Using the appropriate-sized nasogastric tube, measure from the tip of the child's nose to the earlobe, and then from the earlobe to the tip of the xiphoid process. Mark this point on the tube with a piece of tape.

  - Using the appropriate-sized orogastric tube, measure from the corner of the mouth to the earlobe, and then from the earlobe to the tip of the xiphoid process. Mark the point on the tube with a piece of tape.

- Position the awake child in a high-Fowler's position with the head slightly flexed.[3]

Figure 42

MEASUREMENT OF A NASOGASTRIC TUBE

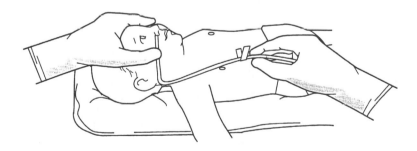

From French JP. Stabilization procedures. In: French JP, ed. *Pediatric Emergency Skills*. St. Louis, Mo: Mosby-Year Book; 1995:163. Reprinted with permission.

- Either hug the child or hold the child's arms securely:

  - A caregiver may assist with the hugging hold.

  - A young infant may be swaddled and held in an upright position in the caregiver's or staff member's arms.

  - Additional staff assistance is required to assist with controlling head movement and to suction the patient if vomiting occurs or if excessive secretions are present.

- Consider placing the unresponsive child in a head-down, decubitus position. To reduce the risk of aspiration prior to gastric tube insertion, consider endotracheal intubation.[4]

- If permitted, have the child swallow or sip water; an infant can suck on a pacifier. Blowing a puff of air in the infant's face may cause reflex swallowing.

- Lubricate the distal end of the gastric tube with water-soluble lubricant. Topical 2% lidocaine jelly may be placed in the nares prior to insertion of the nasogastric tube.[4]

- Direct the tube straight back during insertion, not upward, along the floor of the nose (see Figure 43). Insert the orogastric tube through the mouth following the contour of the tongue:

  - Never force the tube if resistance or obstruction is met.

  - If the child develops signs of respiratory distress, color change, and/or is unable to cry or speak, remove the tube immediately.[3]

- Ensure the tube's placement by aspirating the stomach contents. Then instill 3 to 10 ml of air while auscultating over the epigastric region.[4] The amount of air instilled is dependent on the size of the child.

- Tape the tube securely, anchoring the tape across the upper lip (nasogastric tube) or side of the face (orogastric tube) (see Figure 44). A clear, occlusive dressing may be used to secure the tube to the child's cheek.

Figure 43

INSERTION OF A NASOGASTRIC TUBE

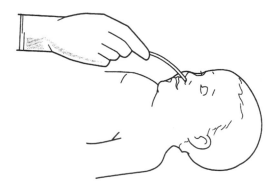

From French JP. Stabilization procedures. In: French JP, ed. *Pediatric Emergency Skills*. St. Louis, Mo: Mosby-Year Book; 1995:164. Reprinted with permission.

Figure 44

SECURING A GASTRIC TUBE

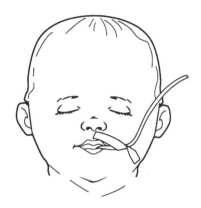

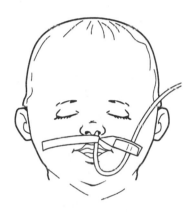

From French JP. Stabilization procedures. In: French JP, ed. *Pediatric Emergency Skills*. St. Louis, Mo: Mosby-Year Book; 1995:167-168. Reprinted with permission.

Points to Remember:

- Nasogastric tube placement is contraindicated in patients with major facial and/or head trauma. The oral route is used in these patients.

- Have all equipment and assistants prepared prior to beginning the procedure. Have the suction turned on and a rigid tonsil tip suction ready.

- Explain the procedure using age-appropriate terms. Use age-appropriate distraction and relaxation techniques to facilitate the child's cooperation and coping during the procedure. Encourage the caregiver to comfort the child and assist with distraction techniques.

- After the procedure, protect the tube from dislodgment by applying hand mitts or soft wrist restraints, holding the child's hands, or giving the child something to hold, such as a security object.

- When performing gastric lavage in infants and young children, use a 20-ml or 50-ml syringe to instill and withdraw the lavage fluid. Keep an accurate record of intake and output.

- Reconfirm placement of the tube prior to instillation of any fluids or medications.

- Use universal precautions during gastric tube insertion and/or gastric lavage, including goggles or face shield.

Urinary Catheterization

Urinary catheterization is performed to obtain a sterile urine specimen, relieve urine retention, and/or monitor urine output.

- Position the child. Place the female child in the frogleg position. Place the male child supine, and lift the penis perpendicular to the child's body.

- Assure adequate lighting and privacy.

- Select an appropriate-sized catheter.

- If an indwelling catheter is being placed, inspect and test the balloon before insertion using sterile technique:

  - Note the volume of the balloon prior to insertion. Smaller catheters typically have a 3-ml balloon.

  - Use sterile water to test the balloon and remove all of the water prior to insertion.

  - Fill the balloon with the appropriate amount of sterile water after insertion.

- Using sterile technique, lubricate and insert the catheter slowly. If resistance is met, select a smaller catheter.

  - If the catheter is inadvertently inserted into the vagina, obtain a new sterile catheter to insert into the bladder.

  - The first catheter may be left in the vagina during the second attempt to assist in identifying the vaginal opening.

- Tape an indwelling catheter to the thigh in the female or the abdomen in the male (see Figure 45).

- Cleanse the perineal area with warm water after the procedure.

Points to Remember:

- Urinary catheter insertion is contraindicated if there is blood present at the urethral meatus, perineal or scrotal hematoma or ecchymosis, or other evidence of urethral trauma.[3]

- Explain the procedure using age-appropriate terms:

  - Young children have fantasies about their bodies, and they may misinterpret what is happening to them during this procedure.[3]

  - Older children and adolescents are very modest about their bodies, and they may have questions about the experience (e.g., can the health care professional look at them and tell if they have had sexual relations).

  - Use age-appropriate distraction and relaxation techniques to facilitate the child's cooperation during the procedure.

- Encourage the caregiver to comfort the child and assist with distraction techniques.

- Indwelling catheters cause the child to have the sensation of needing to void:

    - Explain to the child that he or she may feel like they have to urinate but the catheter or tube will let the urine drain into the bag.

    - Encourage the child to relax and remind him or her that the catheter is in place as needed. The child may fear wetting the bed.

    - Continue to use distraction techniques as needed.

Figure 45
SECURING AN INDWELLING URINARY CATHETER

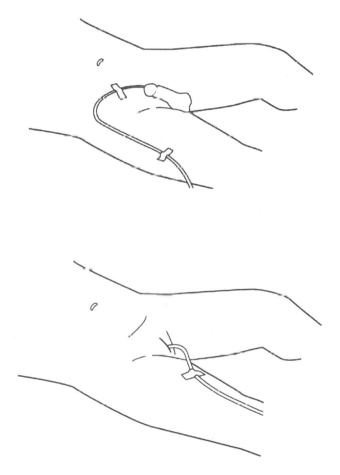

From French JP. Stabilization procedures. In: French JP, ed. *Pediatric Emergency Skills*. St. Louis, Mo: Mosby-Year Book; 1995:174-175. Reprinted with permission.

REFERENCES

1. Lang S. Procedures involving the neurological system. In: Bernardo LM, Bove MA, eds. *Pediatric Emergency Nursing Procedures.* Boston, Mass: Jones & Bartlett; 1993:143-162.

2. Cronan KM, Wiley JF III. Lumbar puncture. In: Henretig FM, King C, eds. *Textbook of Pediatric Emergency Procedures.* Baltimore, Md: Williams & Wilkins; 1997:541-551.

3. Clemence B. Procedures involving the gastrointestinal and genitourinary systems. In: Bernardo LM, Bove MA, eds. *Pediatric Emergency Nursing Procedures.* Boston, Mass: Jones & Bartlett; 1993:125-142.

4. Simon HK, Lewander W. Gastric intubation. In: Henretig FM, King C, eds. *Textbook of Pediatric Emergency Procedures.* Baltimore, Md: Williams & Wilkins; 1997:909-914.

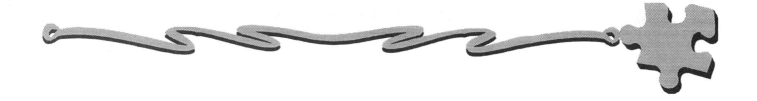

CHAPTER 12

Toxicologic Emergencies

OBJECTIVES

On completion of this lecture, the learner should be able to:

✦ Identify the most common causes of pediatric toxicologic emergencies.

✦ Identify the appropriate nursing diagnoses and expected outcomes based on the assessment findings.

✦ Delineate the specific interventions needed to manage the child who has suffered a toxicologic emergency.

✦ Evaluate the effectiveness of nursing interventions related to patient outcomes.

✦ Identify health promotion strategies related to preventing toxicologic emergencies.

INTRODUCTION

The term *poisoning* implies that a chemical injury has occurred to a body system. In 1996, about 53% of human poison exposures occurred in children younger than 6 years of age.[1] Because of the weight and size of children, they are more susceptible to injury and potentially death from a toxicologic exposure.

Children are at risk for toxic exposures, particularly through ingestion, because of developmental and environmental factors. Factors that put toddlers and younger children at risk include greater mobility, curiosity, a tendency to put things in their mouths, an inability to differentiate a toxic substance from a nontoxic one, and the improper storage or availability of toxic substances in their immediate environment.

Poisonings may be either unintentional or intentional. The majority of poisonings are unintentional and occur most frequently in children younger than 5 years of age.[1,2] In 1994, the Centers for Disease Control and Injury Prevention (CDC) reported that 255 children between 0 and 19 years of age died from unintentional poisoning.[3] Intentional poisonings may occur by self-poisoning (e.g., suicide attempt) or when an adult knowingly administers an overdose of medication or a toxic substance to a child. Intentional self-poisoning is the leading cause of death in Australian adolescents.

ANATOMIC, PHYSIOLOGIC, AND DEVELOPMENTAL CHARACTERISTICS AS A BASIS FOR SIGNS AND SYMPTOMS

Exposure and Absorption

Poisoning results when an exogenous substance exerts a toxic effect on one or more body systems. The body's absorption of the substance typically occurs through one of six routes of entry: Oral ingestion, dermal, ocular, inhalation, *envenomation*, or parenteral. The distribution of the substance within the child's body, the child's metabolic rate, and the rate of excretion determine the amount of active toxin that is available in the body.

Although the properties of the substance affect absorption rate, distribution in the body, and elimination, pediatric physiologic immaturity also influences these factors in infants and young children. Most ingested substances are absorbed through the small intestine by passive diffusion, although they can be absorbed along the length of the gastrointestinal tract.[4] Variability in gastric emptying, rapid peristalsis, higher gastric pH in infants younger than 9 months of age, and a high milk diet influence absorption of drugs and other substances from the gastrointestinal tract in infants and younger children.[4] Additionally, substances absorbed by a lactating mother may be excreted in breast milk and consequently ingested by the breast-fed infant. A variety of over-the-counter, illicit, and therapeutic medications as well as environmental and occupational chemicals may be excreted at varying levels in breast milk.[5]

Absorption of topical agents varies with age as well. The skin acts as a protective barrier in most instances. However, substances that are both water and lipid soluble may pass through the epidermal layers and be absorbed. In infants, the outer layer of the epidermis is thinner, which may allow increased absorption from dermal exposure.[6]

Factors such as increased metabolic rate, decreased renal clearance in infants younger than 1 year of age, and fluctuations in metabolic rate resulting from variable temperature regulation affect the half-life of drugs and duration of effect. Lower serum albumin concentrations in infants results in fewer binding sites for drugs and increases the potential for toxicity.[6] However, more rapid elimination of drugs can occur because of the rapid exchange of extracellular fluid and the higher ratio of total body fluid to body weight in children.[6]

The inhalation of gases, fumes, or mist may effect the upper or lower airways. Irritation, increased mucous production, or inhalation of insoluble particles which can act as foreign bodies, can occur. The rate of absorption is determined by the child's metabolic rate, ventilation, and pulmonary blood flow.

Causes of Poisonings

Of all pediatric poisonings reported to poison control centers, 72.5% are usually managed by the family at home.[1] The remainder are usually referred to an emergency department for further treatment. Of all available poisons, the most common products children ingest include cosmetics and personal care products, cleaning substances, analgesics, plants, cough and cold preparations, foreign bodies, and topical products.[1] Interestingly, fewer than 20 types of drugs are involved in 90% of all toxic ingestions.[7]

NURSING CARE OF THE CHILD WITH A TOXICOLOGIC EXPOSURE

Assessment

Refer to Chapter 4, "Initial Assessment and Triage," for a review of the comprehensive initial assessment. Additional or specific assessment data related to a toxicologic exposure are listed in the following sections.

ADDITIONAL HISTORY

- When obtaining a history of toxic exposure, include the following questions specific to the exposure or substance using the "5 Ws":
  - Who?
    - Other family members exposed.
    - Other children exposed.
  - What?
    - Route of exposure.
    - Open bottles or containers found near the child.
    - Evidence of exposure, pill fragments in mouth, product spilled on clothing, pieces of plants.
    - Estimated amount of exposure. Have the caregiver count or measure remaining pills or liquid.
    - Treatment administered prior to arrival in the emergency department, including use of an antidote and prehospital care.
    - Contact with regional poison center and their recommendations for a home remedy or decontamination method.
  - When?
    - Time of exposure.
    - Time exposure discovered.
    - Estimated duration of exposure.
  - Where?
    - Availability of other products in the general area where the exposure occurred.
    - Location child found (e.g., home, baby-sitters, inside or outside house).
  - Why?
    - Intent of exposure: Self-harm, unintentional.
    - Circumstances of exposure: Error in medication administration, curiosity.

SIGNS AND SYMPTOMS

The symptoms, severity, and time of onset of symptoms will vary enormously, depending on the type and quantity of toxin involved. Signs and symptoms of each particular exposure are listed with each toxin.

DIAGNOSTIC PROCEDURES

A variety of radiographic and laboratory studies may be indicated based on the suspected etiology of the child's toxicologic exposure. Definitive diagnostic testing is performed as the resuscitation is in progress or after the child is stabilized. Specific diagnostic procedures will be listed in the interventions of the selected toxicologic emergencies.

Monitors

- Cardiac monitor.

- Pulse oximeter.

- Capnography for intubated patients.

Radiographic Studies

- Chest film to evaluate for evidence of infiltrate from aspiration or the presence of a foreign body.

- Abdominal film to evaluate for evidence of pills or objects, *bezoar* formation.

Laboratory Studies

- Based on the suspected or known toxin, laboratory studies may be ordered. The following may be considered:

  - Comprehensive toxicology screen using blood or urine.

  - Components of a toxicology screen vary among laboratories and may not be inclusive for the patient's suspected exposure.

  - A negative toxicology screen does not indicate absence of exposure.

  - Specific quantitative drug levels.

  - Specific quantitative levels such as methemoglobin, methanol, iron, lead, ethylene glycol.

- Other laboratory tests may be ordered based on the potential actions of the toxin and signs and symptoms exhibited by the patient.

Nursing Diagnoses, Interventions, and Expected Outcomes

NURSING DIAGNOSIS	INTERVENTIONS	EXPECTED OUTCOMES
Airway clearance, ineffective, related to: • Airway obstruction from toxic ingestion, edema • Irritation of respiratory tract • Altered level of consciousness	• Monitor airway patency and breathing effectiveness • Maintain position of comfort, as appropriate • Open and clear the airway • Position supine	The child will maintain a patent airway, as evidenced by: • Regular rate, depth, and pattern of breathing • Symmetric chest expansion • Absence of signs and symptoms of airway obstruction: Stridor, dyspnea, and hoarse voice • Clear sputum of normal amount without abnormal color or odor • Absence of signs and symptoms of retained secretions: Fever, tachycardia, and tachypnea • Effective cough and gag reflex

Aspiration, risk of, related to:
• Altered level of consciousness
• Increased secretions
• Impaired cough or gag reflex
• Seizure activity
	• Monitor airway patency and breathing effectiveness
	• Position supine or most effective position
	• Suction as needed
	• Consider endotracheal intubation
	• Give nothing by mouth
		The child will not experience aspiration, as evidenced by:
		• A patent airway
		• Clear and equal breath sounds
		• Regular rate, depth, and pattern of breathing
		• ABG values within normal limits:
		  ■ PaO_2 80 to 100 mm Hg (10.0 to 13.3 KPa)
		  ■ SaO_2 >95%
		  ■ $PaCO_2$ 35 to 45 mm Hg (4.7 to 6.0 KPa)
		  ■ pH between 7.35 and 7.45
		• Chest radiograph without abnormality
		• Ability to handle secretions independently

Breathing pattern, ineffective, related to:
• Hypoxia
• Effects of toxicologic exposure
• Altered level of consciousness
	• Monitor airway patency and breathing effectiveness
	• Position appropriately
	• Administer oxygen
	• Assist ventilation, if needed
	• Consider endotracheal intubation
		The child will maintain an effective breathing pattern, as evidenced by:
		• Symmetric chest expansion
		• Clear and equal breath sounds
		• Regular rate, depth, and pattern of breathing
		• ABG values within normal limits:
		  ■ PaO_2 80 to 100 mm Hg (10.0 to 13.3 KPa)
		  ■ SaO_2 >95%
		  ■ $PaCO_2$ 35 to 45 mm Hg (4.7 to 6.0 KPa)
		  ■ pH between 7.35 and 7.45
		• Absence of use of accessory muscles or nasal flaring
		• Absence of stridor, dyspnea, and cyanosis
		• Trachea midline
		• Chest radiograph without abnormality

NURSING DIAGNOSIS	INTERVENTIONS	EXPECTED OUTCOMES

Gas exchange, impaired, related to:
• Aspiration
• Inhalation of toxic fumes or gases
• Ineffective airway clearance
• Ineffective breathing pattern
	• Monitor airway patency and breathing effectiveness
	• Administer oxygen
	• Monitor oxygen saturation
	• Prepare for and assist with endotracheal intubation, as indicated
		The child will maintain adequate gas exchange, as evidenced by:
		• Oxygen saturation >95% by pulse oximetry
		• ABG values within normal limits:
		  ■ PaO_2 80 to 100 mm Hg (10.0 to 13.3 KPa)
		  ■ SaO_2 >95%
		  ■ $PaCO_2$ 35 to 45 mm Hg (4.7 to 6.0 KPa)
		  ■ pH between 7.35 and 7.45
		• Symmetric chest expansion
		• Clear and equal breath sounds
		• Skin normal color, warm, and dry
		• Improved level of consciousness
		• Regular rate, depth, and pattern of breathing

Cardiac output, decreased, related to: • Dysrhythmia • Decreased venous return secondary to peripheral vasodilation or myocardial compromise	• Obtain vascular access • Administer intravenous fluids, as ordered • Consider intravenous fluid bolus • Monitor cardiac rhythm • Initiate cardiopulmonary resuscitation, as needed	The child will maintain adequate circulatory function, as evidenced by: • Strong, palpable peripheral and central pulses • Adequate blood pressure for age • Pulse rate appropriate for age • Absence of dysrhythmias • Skin normal color, warm, and dry • Improved level of consciousness • Urine output of 1 to 2 ml/kg/hour
Fluid volume deficit related to: • Decreased circulating volume • Alternation in capillary permeability	• Obtain vascular access • Initiate intravenous fluid therapy • Insert indwelling urinary catheter	The child will have an effective circulatory volume, as evidenced by: • Improved level of consciousness • Skin normal color, warm, and dry • Urine output of 1 to 2 ml/kg/hour • Urine specific gravity within normal limits • Hematocrit of 30 ml/dl or hemoglobin of 12 to 14 gm/dl or greater • Moist mucous membranes • Stable vital signs appropriate for age • Strong, palpable peripheral pulses
Knowledge deficit (caregiver) related to: • Caregiver's lack of understanding about toxicologic dangers • Caregiver's lack of knowledge related to effect of toxin	• Inform caregiver of treatment plan • Provide information about appropriate storage of toxic substances • Provide age-appropriate information on childproofing home • Encourage caregiver to install locks on cabinets and take other preventive measures	The caregiver will experience reduced knowledge deficit, as evidenced by: • Expression of intentions to use appropriate measures to protect against exposures • Expression of knowledge of environmental hazards • Verbalization of understanding of normal expectations for child's behaviors and knowledge of normal growth and development • Participation in age-appropriate activities • Ability to verbalize understanding of nursing and medical management

NURSING DIAGNOSIS	INTERVENTIONS	EXPECTED OUTCOMES
Injury, risk of, related to: • Lack of knowledge and developmental factors • Continued exposure or absorption of toxic substance through dermal, gastric, or other contact	• Initiate appropriate decontamination measures • Provide a safe emergency department environment • Provide information about developmental level • Provide age-appropriate and developmentally appropriate prevention information • Assess for possibility of exposure of other family members	The child will be free from injury, as evidenced by: • Completion of decontamination interventions • Caregiver's expression of understanding of child's developmental level • Caregiver's expression of intentions to use appropriate measures to protect against exposures • Caregiver's expression of express knowledge of environmental hazards
Family process altered, related to: • Guilt, blame, or chaotic social situation • Child with acute illness or injury	• Inform caregivers of treatment plan and options • Keep family aware of child's progress • Convey an attitude of concern; provide psychosocial support for child and caregiver • Refer caregiver to appropriate social services or community agencies for support or intervention	The family will exhibit behaviors that indicate an improved family process, as evidenced by: • Caregiver's demonstration of understanding of treatment plan and child's progress • Caregiver's positive interaction with child • Caregiver's seeking family and individual support as needed • Verbalization of concerns among others in the family unit

Triage or Acuity Decisions

EMERGENT   All pediatric patients, symptomatic or asymptomatic, with an actual or suspected exposure to a toxic substance.

URGENT   An asymptomatic pediatric patient who has been exposed to a nontoxic substance confirmed by a poison control center.

Planning and Implementation

Refer to Chapter 4, "Initial Assessment and Triage," for a description of the general nursing interventions for pediatric patients with alterations in airway, breathing, or circulation. After a patent airway, effective ventilation, and adequate circulation are assured, the following interventions are initiated, as appropriate, for the child's condition.

ADDITIONAL INTERVENTIONS

- Continuously monitor airway patency and breathing effectiveness. The child with a toxic ingestion of corrosive substances or inhalation of certain substances is at risk for the development of airway complications or alterations in breathing pattern. (Nursing diagnoses: Ineffective airway clearance; aspiration; ineffective breathing pattern; impaired gas exchange).

- Prepare the child and family for specific interventions related to the toxicologic emergency. (Nursing diagnosis: Knowledge deficit).

- Assess for the possibility that others may have also sustained exposure to the substance. (Nursing diagnosis: Injury).

- Initiate decontamination measures. The aim of decontamination is to prevent further absorption of the substance and promote excretion. (Nursing diagnosis: Injury):

  - Initiate external dermal decontamination for the child with exposure to toxic or hazardous materials.

  - Initiate appropriate hazardous material decontamination, as indicated by institution policies and the agent involved.

  - Prompt decontamination will lessen exposure for patient, health care providers, and treatment areas.

- Initiate gastric decontamination on a timely basis (see Table 32)[2,7-9] (Nursing diagnosis: Injury.) When appropriate, initiate other decontamination methods, such as hemodialysis, hemoperfusion, urinary alkalization, or whole-bowel irrigation.

Whole-Bowel Irrigation

An additional intervention that may be implemented to decontaminate a poisoned child is whole-bowel irrigation. Consult a poison control center before initiation of this intervention. This method increased in use during the early 1980s and is recommended today to decontaminate the bowel of patients who have ingested toxins that cannot effectively be absorbed by activated charcoal, such as metals and sustained-release preparations.[10]

Whole-bowel irrigation is accomplished by the administration, either orally or through a gastric tube, of polyethylene glycol electrolyte solution at a rate of 500 ml/hour until effluents are clear. This solution is designed to pass through the intestinal tract without being absorbed. Whole-bowel irrigation is contraindicated for ileus or a bowel obstruction.[2,10] As with any method of decontamination, aspiration is a potential complication.

Evaluation and Ongoing Assessment

Children who have been exposed to a toxic substance require meticulous and frequent reassessment of airway patency, breathing effectiveness, circulatory status, and mental status. Initial improvements may not be sustained, and additional interventions may be needed. Monitoring of drug levels may be needed to achieve the desired outcomes.

Table 32

	GASTRIC DECONTAMINATION		
	Syrup of Ipecac	**Activated Charcoal**	**Gastric Lavage**
General information	Naturally occurring emetic: Derived from the dried roots of a plant found in Central America.	Fine, black, tasteless powder produced from organic materials.	More effective intervention than syrup of ipecac-induced emesis if properly performed.
Action	Induces vomiting by: • Triggering the chemo-receptor zone in the brain, activating the vomiting center. • Causes focal irritation in the gastrointestinal tract.	Absorbs substances in the stomach and gastrointestinal tract.	Washes out stomach contents with saline gastric tube.

Dosage and administration	Administer within 1 to 2 hours after ingestion:
	• Administer 15 ml to children 1 to 12 years of age; 30 ml to children older than 12 years of age.
	• Follow with 4 to 8 oz of clear fluid.
	• Repeat in 30 minutes if no emesis.
	• Discontinue oral fluids once vomiting begins.
		• Preparation should contain a cathartic (e.g., sorbital, magnesium citrate) to enhance elimination.
		• Mix activated charcoal with water or a cathartic to form a slurry. It may be helpful to add flavoring such as strawberry mix. Place in a cup with lid to conceal color. Provide a straw with a large hole. Doses:
		  ▪ Infant: 1 gm/kg.
		  ▪ Children: 25 to 50 g total dose.
		  ▪ Adults: 50 to 100 g total dose.
		• Administer orally or through the gastric tube.
			• Insert a large-bore gastric tube.
			• Place the child in the side-lying left lateral decubitus position.
			• Instill normal saline until the return is clear.

Contraindications	• Children younger than 1 year of age. • Caustic or corrosive substances: Acids or alkalis. • Drugs known to cause rapid onset of seizures or decreased level of consciousness. • Hydrocarbons or petroleum distillates. • Foreign-body ingestion. • Absence of gag reflex. • Child has vomited.	• Caustic and corrosive substances. • Rapidly absorbed toxins such as alcohol. • Low molecular weight toxins such as iron, lithium, alcohols. • Elemental metals such as iron, lithium, lead, mercury, arsenic.	• Ingestion of sharp objects. • Caustic or corrosive substances. • Hydrocarbons.

GASTRIC DECONTAMINATION		
	Syrup of Ipecac	**Activated Charcoal**	**Gastric Lavage**
Complications	• Esophageal tears. • Pneumomediastinum. • Aspiration. • Diaphragmatic rupture. • Subarachnoid hemorrhage. • Protracted vomiting.	• Aspiration. • Constipation. • Paralytic ileus.	• Aspirations. • Esophageal rupture. • Endotracheal intubation. • Gastrointestinal perforation. • Hypothermia. • Electrolyte imbalances.
Special considerations	• Most children will vomit three to four times in the first hour after administration; effect may last for hours. • Do not give if activated charcoal may be administered.	• Administration of a cathartic in infants should be done with caution. • Multiple doses of sorbitol may cause repeated episodes of diarrhea, predisposing the child to dehydration.	• Monitor the child closely for gastric distention which may interfere with ventilation. • May not be useful for all ingestions; consult poison control center.

SELECTED TOXICOLOGIC EMERGENCIES

The following selected emergencies are common pediatric exposures. However, frequency and type of toxicologic emergencies may vary by region. Consultation with regional poison experts to identify appropriate current treatment modalities is an essential component of emergency care, planning, and interventions. Additional history, signs and symptoms, and additional interventions specific to the selected toxicologic emergencies are listed. Standard assessment data and interventions outlined in Chapter 4, "Initial Assessment and Triage," and previously in this chapter are not repeated with each selected emergency but must also be applied.

Unknown Poison or Overdose

On occasion, a child who is unconscious or nonverbal will be seen in the emergency department for an exposure to an unknown poison. In these cases, the child's clinical presentation may provide clues toward identifying the poisoning agent. **For all exposures, treat the child and not the suspected poison.**

ADDITIONAL HISTORY

- Abnormal behavior for age.

- Exhibiting symptoms of an unknown etiology.

SIGNS AND SYMPTOMS

Table 33 provides an overview of signs and symptoms associated with some specific poison exposures. Consult a poison control center or toxicology expert to assist in identifying specific toxins.

Table 33

POISONS	
Signs and Symptoms	**Possible Poison**

● Odor:
    ■ Alcohol
    ■ Garlic
    ■ Oil of wintergreen
    ■ Bitter almond
	Ethanol, methanol, organophosphates, arsenic, menthyl salicylate, cyanide, and hydrocarbon.

● Decreased respirations	Alcohol, barbiturates, narcotics, sedatives, and hypnotics.
● Tachypnea	Carbon monoxide, cyanide, salicylate, amphetamines, and anticholinergic.
● Bradycardia	Narcotics, digitalis, beta-blockers, sedatives, and hypnotics.
● Tachycardia	Amphetamines, alcohols, sympathomimetic, salicylate, theophylline, cocaine, and tricyclic antidepressants.
● Dysrhythmia	Anticholinergics, tricyclic antidepressants, organophosphates, phenothiazines, digoxin, cyanide, and carbon monoxide.
● Hypothermia	Ethanol, carbon monoxide, tricyclic antidepressants, phenothiazines, and barbiturates.
● Methemoglobinemia	Nitrates, nitrites, and benzocaine.
● Coma, altered level of consciousness	Carbon monoxide, cyanide, and anticholinergics.
● Excessive salivation and lacrimation	Organophosphates and carbamates.
● Hypotension	Arsenic, calcium-channel-blockers, tricyclic antidepressants, digoxin, barbiturates, opioids, envenomation, beta-blockers.
● Seizures	Cocaine, camphor, carbon monoxide, salicylate, aminophylline, tricyclic antidepressants, organophosphates, and nicotine.

Adapted from Haddad L, Shannon M, Winchester J. *Clinical Management of Poisoning and Drug Overdose*. Philadelphia, Pa: WB Saunders; 1998. Used with permission.

Over-the-Counter Medications

ACETAMINOPHEN/*PARACETAMOL*

Acetaminophen/paracetamol is an analgesic and antipyretic commonly found in many over-the-counter and prescription preparations. Acetaminophen/paracetamol is one of the five most common drugs ingested by children, and one of the 10 most common drugs used by adolescents and adults in intentional self-poisonings.[1] There are several commercially available concentrations of products containing acetaminophen. Risk of improper dosing is increased by the variety of concentrations and packaging (e.g., infants drops, pediatric elixir, pediatric suspension, children's chewable, junior tablets).

Ingestion of acetaminophen/paracetamol may lead to hepatic failure and death. Toxicity can occur with a single large exposure or multiple exposures over hours or days. The onset of symptoms is generally dependent on the total amount of acetaminophen/paracetamol ingested per kg of body weight. However, each case must be considered individually and the poison control center consulted to assist with the analysis of toxicity and determination of total dose.

Acetaminophen/paracetamol levels can assist in assessing the severity and treatment needs of a child with acetaminophen/paracetamol toxicity. For children who have a single acute ingestion, a level drawn 4 hours after the ingestion must be plotted on the Rumack-Matthew nomogram. The nomogram is used to determine the risk of hepatic involvement and the need for antidote administration of *N*-acetylcysteine 20%, better known as Mucomyst.

Signs and Symptoms of Toxicity

Symptoms progress at a variable rate, depending on the dose and time of ingestion. Signs and symptoms of toxicity include:

- Anorexia, nausea, and vomiting.
- Increased liver enzymes.
- Renal function deterioration.
- Hepatic failure.

Diagnostic Procedures

Laboratory Studies

- Acetaminophen/paracetamol level.
- Liver enzymes.

Additional Interventions

- Anticipate and prepare for administration of antidote, depending on the severity of the ingestion:
  - *N*-acetylcysteine.
  - Administration is based on serum acetaminophen levels, patient assessment, and poison control center recommendations.
  - Follow poison center recommendations on method and route of administration.
  - When administering orally, the unpleasant taste and "rotten egg" smell may be masked somewhat if diluted in juice, poured over ice, placed in a covered cup, and sipped through a straw.
- Anticipate and prepare for the infusion of Parvolex IVI infusion which is the antidote for paracetamol. Administer as a slow intravenous infusion, as per hospital policy, within 24 hours of ingestion.

IRON

In 1996, more than 45,000 children ingested a toxic amount of vitamins.[1] Many attractively shaped, candy flavored, over-the-counter chewable multiple vitamins contain iron. Prenatal vitamins, which contain large amounts of iron, may be life-threatening even if the child ingests only a few.

Prediction of toxicity can be determined if the number of ingested tablets is known. The severity of iron poisoning is directly related to the amount of elemental iron ingested. A serum iron concentration greater than 300 mcg/dL has been associated with vomiting. A serum iron concentration of greater than 500 mcg/dL has been associated with coma.[2]

Symptoms of toxicity can occur as early as 30 minutes after ingestion. Decontamination using gastric lavage with a large-bore gastric tube must be initiated immediately to avoid further absorption.

Signs and Symptoms

Symptomatology of iron toxicity is divided into four stages:

Stage 1: Approximately 30 minutes to 6 hours after ingestion, gastrointestinal symptoms occur. These include vomiting, diarrhea, hematemesis, and abdominal pain.

Stage 2: Six to 12 hours after ingestion, the child may experience temporary alleviation of symptoms. This stage does not always occur.

Stage 3: More than 12 hours after ingestion, metabolic acidosis, circulatory failure, central nervous system depression leading to coma, and hepatic failure occur.

Stage 4: One to 2 months after ingestion, gastric scarring and strictures develop.

Note: There is often a rapid progression from stage 1 to stage 3.

Diagnostic Procedures

Laboratory Studies

- Serum iron levels are extremely important in the management of the child. However, interpretations of the levels may be difficult. Consultation with a poison control center is recommended.

- Coagulation studies.

- Electrolytes, complete blood count, serum glucose test.

- Stool for occult blood.

- Type and crossmatch.

Radiographic Studies

- Abdominal film:
    - Often used to determine the efficacy of gastric decontamination because iron is radiopaque.
    - A bezoar or iron concretion may be detected.

Additional Interventions (in addition to those previously described in this chapter):

- Anticipate possible whole-bowel irrigation if positive radiographic findings.

- Prepare for administration of deferoxamine mesylate which is an iron chelation agent for acute iron intoxication. Following administration of deferoxamine mesylate, the child's urine will turn a pink, salmon, or vin rose color. This indicates that the iron is binding with the deferoxamine mesylate.

Prescription Medications

TRICYCLIC ANTIDEPRESSANTS

The ingestion of tricyclic antidepressants can be potentially lethal to children.[7] Amitriptyline hydrochloride, amoxapine, desipramine hydrochloride, and doxepin hydrochloride are commonly ingested tricyclic antidepressant drugs. The amount of tricyclic antidepressants in the serum and its toxicity is not precise.[2,10] For some children, ingestion of as little as one tablet may cause symptoms.

Toxicity is manifested in a variety of neurologic and cardiovascular presentations. The signs and symptoms of a tricyclic antidepressant poisoning are related to the anticholinergic activity and quinidine-like effects. Significant complications occur within 1 to 4 hours after the ingestion of a toxic amount.[1,2] However, the patient may develop wide-complex dysrhythmias, hypotension, and seizures shortly after a toxic ingestion.

Because of the complex pharmacology of tricyclic antidepressant overdose, a number of medications routinely used for therapeutic intervention must be avoided. The lethal cardiac effects of tricyclic antidepressant overdose are not related to the anticholinergic properties of the drug.[2,11] Rather, the quinidine-like effects are responsible for intraventricular conduction delay, ventricular dysrhythmia, decreased cardiac output, and hypotension.[12] Physostigmine sulfate is contraindicated in the treatment of tricyclic antidepressant overdose because of its effect on ventricular conduction, the risk of increasing cardiac toxicity, and the lowering of the seizure threshold.[11,12] Asystole has been reported following the administration of physostigmine in these patients. The administration of other medications must be carefully evaluated prior to administration. Other medications that must be avoided include quinidine sulfate, procainamide hydrochloride, flumazenil, propranolol hydrochloride, and verapamil hydrochloride.[11,12]

Signs and Symptoms

- Altered level of consciousness: Drowsiness or sedation, confusion, agitation, hallucinations, coma.

- Seizures.

- Decreased respirations.

- Cardiovascular effects:

  - Dysrhythmias and widened QRS, sinus tachycardia.

  - Hypotension.

- Peripheral anticholinergic-related symptoms:
  - Flushing, dry mouth, and dilated pupils.
  - Tachycardia.
  - Hypertension.
  - Urine retention.
  - Decreased bowel sounds.
  - Hyperpyrexia.

Additional Interventions

- Perform 12-lead electrocardiogram.
- Administer medications, as indicated:
  - Sodium bicarbonate is used to treat the dysrhythmia. Consult a poison control center or a toxicology expert.
  - Hypotension may be treated with dopamine hydrochloride or norepinephrine bitartrate if the child remains hypotensive after fluid administration.[2]
- Initiate gastric decontamination once the airway is secured.
- Monitor electrolytes.

CARDIAC MEDICATIONS

Pediatric patients are not routinely prescribed cardiac medications. However, when these drugs are left within reach, children may ingest these potentially lethal medications. Three cardiac medication poisonings commonly seen in the emergency department are from beta-blockers, calcium-channel-blockers, and digitalis.[13] Even though beta-blockers and calcium-channel-blockers act on different receptors in the cardiovascular system, the signs and symptoms of toxic ingestion have a similar presentation.

Digoxin, a cardiac inotrope, is prescribed for young infants with congenital cardiac anomalies and for patients with congestive heart failure. Digoxin toxicity may be either acute or chronic.

Signs and Symptoms

- Cardiovascular (see Table 34).
- Neurologic (see Table 34).
- Hypoglycemia with beta-blockers.
- Hypercalcemia and metabolic acidosis with calcium-channel-blockers.
- Bronchospasm with beta-blockers.
- Hyperkalemia.
- Nausea.
- Vomiting.

Table 34

SIGNS AND SYMPTOMS OF CARDIAC MEDICATION OVERDOSE	
Cardiovascular Signs and Symptoms of Toxicity	
Beta-Blockers and Calcium-Channel-Blockers	**Digitalis**
Marked bradycardia Hypotension Atrioventricular block Accelerated junctional tachycardia	First-degree, second-degree, and third-degree blocks Bradycardia Ventricular dysrhythmias
Neurologic Signs and Symptoms of Toxicity	
Beta-Blockers and Calcium-Channel-Blockers	**Digitalis**
Seizures Coma	Lethargy Visual disturbances

Diagnostic Procedures

Monitors

- Cardiac monitor.

- 12-lead electrocardiogram.

Laboratory Studies

- Drug screen to determine the type of medication ingested.

- Digoxin level if appropriate.

- Serum electrolytes, especially K^+ and Ca^{++}.

- Serum or whole blood glucose test.

Additional Interventions

- Anticipate the need for whole-bowel irrigation if the child has ingested a sustained-release beta-blocker or calcium-channel-blocker.

- Anticipate need for administration of specific antidotes or pharmacologic agents, such as:

  - Calcium infusion for calcium-channel-blocker toxicity.[13,14]

  - Glucagon hydrochloride for both calcium-channel-blocker and beta-blocker toxicity.[13]

  - Digoxin-specific antibody fragments for digitalis toxicity.[13]

- Prepare for and assist with external cardiac pacing or placement of transvenous pacemaker to maintain cardiac output during initial resuscitation, as indicated.

Household Products

HYDROCARBONS AND PETROLEUM DISTILLATES

Most hydrocarbons are derived from petroleum, although others are derived from pine oil and plant wood. They can vary in toxicity and can be lethal exposures. Typically, the products most commonly involved in hydrocarbon poisonings include:

- Lamp oil.
- Solvents and thinners.
- Gasoline.
- Lighter fluid.
- Kerosene.
- Waxes containing mineral oil.
- Liquid polishes.

Additional History

- Coughing and choking with initial ingestion.
- Gradual increase in work of breathing.
- Odor of hydrocarbon on breath.

Signs and Symptoms

Hydrocarbon toxicity varies, depending on the type of agent and the risk for aspiration. Some agents can cause serious systemic effects, such as hepatic failure or central nervous system depression. Additional signs and symptoms include:

- Nausea and vomiting.
- Dry, persistent cough.
- Crackles, wheezes, and diminished breath sounds.
- Tachypnea.
- Altered mental status.
- Dysrhythmias, though less common in children.
- Dizziness.
- Signs of respiratory distress.

Additional Interventions

- Decontaminate skin by washing with soap and water. With prolonged contact, hydrocarbons may defat the skin and result in surface burns or continued exposure.

- Provide gastric decontamination as recommended by the poison control center:

  - Gastric decontamination methods are controversial and depend on the type of product ingested.

  - Vomiting should be avoided to lessen the risk of aspiration. Therefore, syrup of ipecac is contraindicated. Avoid the administration of activated charcoal.

- Trend respiratory assessment. Initially, the asymptomatic patient may develop respiratory symptoms that progress to distress within hours after ingestion. Anticipate the need for intubation with worsening respiratory symptoms.

HOUSEHOLD CLEANING AGENTS

Most caustic injuries are caused by exposure to an acid or alkali. Methods of treatment and initial presentation are similar, regardless of the pH of the substance. Commonly ingested products are toilet bowl cleaners, drain openers, pool cleaners, and floor wax strippers. Others include oven and grill cleaners, dishwasher detergents, and household bleach. Exposure may be the result of topical ingestion or the inhalation or absorption through mucous membranes.

Regardless of the mechanisms of each specific caustic agent, unless decontamination is completed, the end result may be direct tissue injury and possibly cellular death. When caustics are ingested, it is extremely difficult to determine if esophageal or stomach burns are present based on the presence or absence of oral burns. Therefore, recommendations from the poison control center are extremely helpful.

Additional History

- Unusual odor or stain on skin or clothing.
- Open container of household products.

Signs and Symptoms

- Drooling or dysphagia.
- Burns in or around the mouth.
- Vomiting.
- Stridor.
- Soft tissue swelling.

Additional Interventions

- Initiate immediate dilution and irrigation using water or available liquid. Do not give oral fluids after initial dilution until a further assessment is completed.

- If exposure to the skin or eyes has occurred, flush with copious amounts of water or saline until neutralized.

- Prevent gastric evacuation:
  - Syrup of ipecac and activated charcoal are contraindicated.
  - To avoid emesis, keep the child calm and do not administer anything by mouth after the initial dilution.

ALCOHOLS

For a child, alcohol ingestion can be a serious, life-threatening emergency. Depending on the type of alcohol, toxicity can occur with an ingestion of less than 1 tsp. Table 35 presents alcohol types and examples.

Table 35

TYPES AND EXAMPLES OF ALCOHOL	
Type	**Examples of Products**
Ethanol	Alcoholic beverages, perfumes, and mouthwash
Isopropyl	Rubbing alcohol and solvents
Ethylene glycol	Radiator antifreeze and deicers
Methanol	Windshield washer fluid, solvents and antifreeze, and gasoline

Signs and Symptoms

- Altered level of consciousness.
- Hyperthermia.
- Nausea and vomiting.
- Staggered gait.
- Slurred speech.
- Seizures.
- Respiratory depression.
- Muscle incoordination.

Diagnostic Procedures

Laboratory Studies

- Serum or whole blood glucose test.
- Specific alcohol (ethanol, methanol) level.
- Electrolytes.
- Blood gas.

Additional Interventions

- Treatment varies and ranges from simple oral dilution measures to infusion of an ethanol drip (i.e., for methanol poisoning). Consult a poison control center for treatment recommendations.

- Administer glucose, as indicated, if documented hypoglycemia is present. Children have low glycogen stores, placing them at higher risk for hypoglycemia when intoxicated. Therefore, monitor serum glucose levels closely. Consider administration of intravenous fluids with glucose for continuous or maintenance infusion.

- Anticipate and prepare for correction of acidosis.

- Prepare for hemodialysis in severe ethylene glycol and methanol ingestion.

LEAD

One of the most common preventable pediatric health problems in the United States is lead poisoning. Although lead poisoning is widespread among rural and urban youth, most children go undiagnosed and untreated because they have no obvious symptoms. However, lead encephalopathy and death are possible in children with high levels of lead. Symptomatic lead poisoning is a medical emergency. The blood level considered to indicate lead toxicity has progressively decreased. Appendix AA provides blood lead levels and treatment modalities.

Lead-based paint and lead-contaminated dust and soils remain the primary sources and pathways of lead exposure for children. Children are also exposed through caregivers' occupations and hobbies, air, water, and food. Although costly, lead paint abatement of housing is a critical measure in the prevention of lead poisoning.

Additional History

- Exposure to lead paint:
    - Living in a home painted before 1978, when lead content was not limited in residential paint.
    - Playground equipment painted with lead paint.
    - Nursery equipment painted with lead paint.
    - Recent renovation of an older home.
- Caregiver with hobby (e.g., pottery glaze, lead fishing sinkers, exposure to caregivers' clothing after using indoor firing ranges).
- Exposed to food from lead-soldered cans.
- Use of "traditional" medicine containing lead.
- Exposure to drinking water with high levels of lead (e.g., cisterns with lead liners, water systems with lead-soldered joints, water systems standing on lead surfaces).
- Eating from improperly fired pottery.

Signs and Symptoms

- Acute lead encephalopathy may include:

  - Coma.

  - Seizures.

  - Bizarre behavior.

  - Ataxia.

  - Apathy.

  - Incoordination.

  - Vomiting.

  - Loss of recently acquired skills.

  - Altered level of consciousness.

- Symptomatic lead poisoning without encephalopathy may include:

  - Lethargy.

  - Anorexia.

  - Sporadic vomiting.

  - Intermittent abdominal pain and constipation.

  - Decrease in play activity.

Diagnostic Procedures

Laboratory Studies

- Venous lead level.

- Serum iron and iron-binding capacity because iron deficiency can enhance lead absorption and toxicity.

- Ferritin.

Radiographic Studies

- Abdomen radiograph or flat plate, which may show radiopaque foreign materials ingested during the preceding 24 to 36 hours.

Additional Interventions

- Anticipate the need for chelation therapy in symptomatic children with toxic lead levels. Prepare for transport to pediatric center to provide chelation and supportive interventions.

- Refer to appropriate agencies for followup and environmental evaluation.

Bites and Stings

Each year, thousands of children are treated in the emergency department for various types of bites and stings. For example, dog bites account for 80% of bite injuries, and the majority of those bitten are children.[1,15] Although most of the creatures that inhabit the world around us are not harmful to humans, some can cause significant illness, injury, or death. Approximately 50 to 100 people die each year as a result of insect stings.[1] Venomous reptiles, arthropods, and marine animals are found throughout the world. It is important for emergency nurses to be familiar with the local environment and aware of local inhabitants that may cause envenomation.

Although venomous snakes are found in many areas of the United States, Australia is widely populated with many species of venomous snakes. More than 1,000 bites requiring treatment occur annually throughout Australia, of which 0.2% are fatal. Envenomation of children from snake bites carries a high morbidity or mortality rate if left untreated because of the higher metabolic rate and body surface area-to-weight ratio. Bite or fang marks may not be present with some types of Australian venomous snakes called elapids. These snakes have rather small, nonretractable fangs that tend to scratch the skin and leave no puncture marks.

If the insect, mammal, or reptile is poisonous, children are at a greater risk of developing systemic symptoms from the venom because of their smaller size and weight. Reactions to envenomation are based on[15-18]:

- Child's age and weight; younger children with higher metabolic rate are at greater risk.
- Health of the child.
- Amount of exertion after the envenomation:
  - Venom is transported through the lymphatic system, not the bloodstream.
  - Physical exertion will assist in the rapid spread of venom throughout the child's body.
- Type of bite or venom:
  - The amount of venom injected is not always proportional to the systemic effect.
  - Small amounts of venom from some creatures can result in serious anaphylactic and/or systemic reactions.
  - Bite injuries are frequently associated with crush injuries to the extremity.
  - Bite wounds can be contaminated with multiple organisms (see Table 36).
- Time elapsed from incident to definitive care.
- Prehospital care.

Table 36

ORGANISMS THAT MAY CONTAMINATE A BITE WOUND		
Aerobic Bacteria	**Anaerobic Bacteria**	**Other Pathogens**
• *Staphylococcus aureus* • *Streptococcus* • *Eikenella corrodens*	• *Bacteroides* • *Enterobacter cloacae* • *Proteus mirabilis*	• Hepatitis virus • *Clostridium tetani* • Herpes virus • Rabies virus

ADDITIONAL HISTORY

- Type of animal, insect, or reptile.
- Known allergies to insect bites.
- Asthma.
- Previous administration of antivenin.

SIGNS AND SYMPTOMS

Signs and symptoms will vary with the animal, reptile, arthropod, or insect involved. Symptoms may include:

- Edema of the airway.
- Respiratory distress:
  - Tachypnea.
  - Wheezes.
- Altered mental status.
- Abnormal skin color.
- Altered skin integrity:
  - Fang marks.
  - Bite marks.
  - Vesicles.
  - Edema, which may be progressive beyond the bite or sting.
  - Ulcerations.
  - Urticaria.
  - Wounds.
  - Tissue necrosis.
- Pain, which may be severe.
- *Myolysis.*
- Ptosis.
- Coagulopathy.
- Systemic symptoms due to envenomation from reptiles, marine animals, or arthropods include[19]:
  - Symptoms vary depending on the type and severity of the envenomation.
  - Gastrointestinal, cardiovascular, pulmonary, neurologic, and musculoskeletal symptoms.

- Systemic symptoms may include:
  - Fever.
  - Chills.
  - Malaise.
  - Nausea or vomiting.
  - Diarrhea.
  - Cardiac dysrhythmias.
  - Hypertension or hypotension.
  - Tachycardia.
  - Pulmonary edema.
  - Mulscle cramps.
  - Seizures.
  - Paresthesias.
  - Paralysis.
  - Weakness.
  - Syncope.
  - Confusion.

DIAGNOSTIC PROCEDURES

Laboratory Studies

- Creatinine phosphokinase.
- Complete blood count.
- Platelet count.
- Prothrombin time.
- Partial prothromboplastin time.
- Fibrinogen.
- Fibrin split products.
- Electrolytes.
- Blood urea nitrogen.
- Urinalysis.

Monitors

- 12-lead electrocardiogram.

ADDITIONAL INTERVENTIONS

- Immobilize the affected limb.

- Keep the child calm and still.

- Initiate treatment for anaphylaxis (see Figure 46).

- Remove any constricting clothing or jewelry around the bite or sting area.

- Consult a poison control center for assistance in the identification of venomous animals, reptiles, or arthropods, and for specific management information.

Figure 46

CARE OF THE CHILD WITH ANAPHYLAXIS

Establish a patent airway

↓

Obtain vascular access with two large-bore intravenous lines

↓

Administer medications, as indicated:
- Epinephrine hydrochloride, subcutaneous, intramuscular or intravenous
- Diphenhydramine hydrochloride, 25 to 50 mg, intramuscular or intravenous
- Corticosteroids
- H$_2$ blockers
- Dopamine hydrochloride if child remains hypotensive despite epinephrine hydrochloride and fluids

↓

Provide continuous assessment of the child's airway, breathing, and circulatory status

↓

Provide appropriate wound care

- Provide wound care (see Figure 47).

- Administer tetanus prophylaxis.

- Provide discharge teaching regarding wound care and prevention of reoccurrence.

Figure 47

WOUND CARE

Inspect the wound for the presence of foreign bodies
such as stingers, teeth, tentacles, pincers, barbs, or spines

Use appropriate technique to gently remove any remaining pieces of the foreign matter

Cleanse the wound with mild soap and water, if not contraindicated*

Copiously irrigate potentially contaminated wounds with normal saline

Apply cool compresses for comfort, if not contraindicated

Administer pain medication, as indicated

Administer tetanus prophylaxis, as indicated

Administer antibiotics, as indicated

In preparation for discharge:

● Instruct the child and caregivers regarding signs and symptoms of infection and other wound complications that may occur

● Instruct the child and caregivers regarding proper wound care at home

● Instruct the child and caregiver regarding follow-up recommendations and signs and symptoms that indicate a need to return to the emergency department or contact their physician

*Some wounds caused by venomous species may require other techniques initially. Consult a poison control center for these recommendations.

● Provide additional interventions for venomous snake bites by immobilizing the affected limb and compressing the superficial lymphatics to stop the systemic spread of venom:

■ Apply a pressure bandage, starting at the bite site, and progressing distally to the end of the fingers or toes and then proximally toward the shoulder or groin.

■ The bandage must be firm enough to slow venous return but must not impede arterial flow.

- Do not remove the bandage until antivenom is administered.

- Apply direct, continuous pressure to bites to the torso or head until definitive treatment is started.

- Determine the need for and administer specific antivenom, as indicated and directed by the poison control center or protocol. Antivenom may be prescribed for some spider bites (neurotoxic spider) as well as venomous snake bites. See Appendix BB for information on administration of antivenom for venomous snake bites.

- Administer prophylactic antibiotics (snake bites are often complicated by staphylococcal infection).

- Grade the amount of envenomation (see Table 37).

Table 37

AN EXAMPLE OF GRADING OF ENVENOMATION FOR SNAKE BITES	
Severity	**Findings**
None	• Fang marks only. • No local or systemic signs or symptoms.
Minimal	• Fang marks with slowly progressive local swelling. • No systemic symptoms.
Moderate	• History of single or multiple bites or provoked bites from a large venomous snake or highly toxic species. • Fang marks with rapid development of edema that extends beyond the bite area. • Systemic symptoms of nausea and vomiting. • Metallic taste. • Paresthesia.
Severe	• History of bite from a toxic snake. • Prolonged embedding of fangs. • Multiple bites. • Rapid, progressive swelling. • Subcutaneous hemorrhage. • Severe systemic signs and symptoms, including muscle fasciculations. • Shock.

Adapted from Hodge D, Trecklenberg F. Bites and stings. In: Fleisher GR, Ludwig S, eds. *Synopsis of Pediatric Emergency Medicine.* Baltimore, Md: Williams & Wilkins; 1996:463-476. Used with permission.

- Additional interventions for selected marine envenomation:

- Immerse affected area in hot water (up to 45°C [113°F]).

- Use detoxicant of 3 to 5% acetic acid to inactivate venom.

HEALTH PROMOTION

Prevention must focus on interventions that are directed at lessening toxic exposures. The following safety measures and family education must be stressed:

- Encourage safe storage of poisons and medications:
  - Store poisons in appropriately marked containers, well out of reach, and locked in a cabinet.
  - Store medications out of reach and in a locked cabinet.
  - Discard old medications.
- Provide the telephone number of a poison control center. In the event of an unintentional poisoning, caregivers must bring bottles or containers to the emergency department.
- Encourage caregivers to:
  - Install special locks for cabinets.
  - Teach their child safety habits.
- Refer the family to appropriate resources for information and prevention concerning:
  - Childproofing the home.
  - Appropriate storage of household products and cleaning chemicals.
  - Initial treatment of a toxic ingestion.
- Educate caregivers about reducing blood lead levels. Poison control centers can provide resources for prevention literature and additional prevention measures:
  - Instruct caregivers to make sure that the child does not have access to peeling paint or chewable surfaces painted with lead.
  - Instruct caregivers to wash the child's hands and face before they eat.
  - Instruct caregivers to wash toys and pacifiers frequently.
- Encourage measures to prevent bites and stings. Encourage caregivers to:
  - Become familiar with the insects, spiders, and snakes that populate the local environment.
  - Become familiar with the insects, spiders, and snakes that populate the local environment when a hike or trip is planned.
  - Cover exposed areas with light, tight-fitting clothes when working, walking, or hiking in an environment that may contain insects.
  - Always shake out clothing, sleeping bags, and boots before putting them on when camping or hiking.
  - Use an insect repellent or natural repellent to keep insects away. Be sure it is safe for the individual's age.

SUMMARY

A child who has been exposed to a toxic substance may be at risk for great harm. The pieces of the puzzle that fit together to decrease this risk include use of the poison control center as a source of information about the management of the ill child, use of public service agencies to educate families and communities about prevention, and becoming active as an advocate to assure that drugs are packaged safely and all caregivers receive age-appropriate education for their children.

REFERENCES

1. Litovitz T, Smilkstein M, Felberg L, Klein-Schwartz W, Berlin R, Morgan J. 1996 Annual report of the American Association of Poison Control Centers Toxic Exposure Surveillance System. *Am J Emerg Med.* 1997;15:447-455.

2. Haddad L, Shannon M, Winchester J. *Clinical Management of Poisoning and Drug Overdose.* Philadelphia, Pa: WB Saunders; 1998.

3. Centers for Disease Control and Injury Prevention. *Ten Leading Causes of Death by Age Group.* Hyattsville, Md: National Center for Health Statistics; 1995.

4. Weisman RS, Howlan MA, Reynolds JR, Smith C. Pharmacokinetic and toxicokinetic principles. In: Goldfrank LR, Flomenbaum NE, Lewin NA, Weiseman RS, Howland MA, Hoffman RS, eds. *Toxicologic Emergencies.* 5th ed. Norwalk, Conn: Appleton & Lange; 1994:85-98.

5. Fine JS. Reproductive and perinatal principles. In: Goldfrank LR, Flomenbaum NE, Lewin NA, Weiseman RS, Howland MA, Hoffman RS, eds. *Toxicologic Emergencies.* 5th ed. Norwalk, Conn: Appleton & Lange; 1994:421-437.

6. Bruckner JM. Pediatric pharmacology and intravenous therapy. In: Bruckner JM, Wallin KD, eds. *Manual of Pediatric Nursing.* Boston, Mass: Little, Brown, & Co; 1996:33-44.

7. Dean B. Ingestion and poisoning. In: Kelly SJ, ed. *Pediatric Emergency Nursing.* 2nd ed. Norwalk, Conn: Appleton & Lange; 1994:365-375.

8. Gorelick M. Gastric emptying. In: Dieckmann RA, Fiser D, Selbst SM, eds. *Pediatric Emergency and Critical Care Procedures.* St. Louis, Mo: Mosby-Year Book; 1997:557-566.

9. Melini LV. Poisoning: An overview. In: Thomas DO, ed. *Quick Reference to Pediatric Nursing.* Gaithersburg, Md: Aspen Publishers; 1991:231.

10. Barone MA, ed. *The Harriet Lane Handbook.* 14th ed. St. Louis, Mo: Mosby-Year Book; 1996:24-53.

11. Henretig FM, Shannon M. Toxicologic emergencies. In: Fleisher GR, Ludwig S, eds. *Textbook of Pediatric Emergency Medicine.* 3rd ed. Baltimore, Md: Williams & Wilkins; 1993:745-801.

12. Weisman RS, Howland MA, Hoffman RS, Cohen H. Cyclic antidepressants. In: Goldfrank LR, Flomenbaum NE, Lewin NA, Weiseman RS, Howland MA, Hoffman RS, eds. *Toxicologic Emergencies.* 5th ed. Norwalk, Conn: Appleton & Lange; 1994:725-759.

13. Henretig FM, Shannon M. Toxicologic emergencies. In: Fleisher GR, Ludwig S, Silverman BK, eds. *Synopsis of Pediatric Emergency Medicine.* Baltimore, Md: Williams & Wilkins; 1996:405-446.

14. Haddad LM. Resuscitation after nifedipine overdose exclusively with intravenous calcium chloride. *Am J Emerg Med.* 1996;14:602-603.

15. Hodge D, Trecklenberg F. Bites and stings. In: Fleisher GR, Ludwig S, Silverman BK, eds. *Synopsis of Pediatric Emergency Medicine.* Baltimore, Md: Williams & Wilkins; 1996:463-476.

16. Minton S, Bechtel HB. Arthropod envenomation and parasitism. In: Auerbach P, ed. *Wilderness Medicine.* St. Louis, Mo: Mosby-Year Book; 1995:742-768.

17. Reeves JA, Allison EJ, Goodman PE. Black widow spider bite in a child. *Am J Emerg Med.* 1996;14:469-471.

18. Stewart C. *Environmental Emergencies.* Baltimore, Md: Williams & Wilkins; 1990.

19. Tully SB, Wingert WA. Venomous animal bites and stings. In: Barkin RM, ed. *Pediatric Emergency Medicine: Concepts and Clinical Practice.* 2nd ed. St. Louis, Mo: Mosby-Year Book; 1997:465-473.

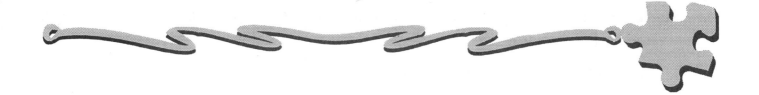

Crisis Intervention

OBJECTIVES

On completion of this lecture, the learner should be able to:

✦ Identify the nursing assessment of families in crisis.

✦ Plan appropriate interventions for families in crisis.

✦ Identify the key signs and symptoms of a family's crisis response.

✦ Identify two methods of stress reduction for the emergency care team.

INTRODUCTION

Perhaps no event is as traumatic as the serious illness, injury, or death of a child. *Stress* is defined as "a relationship between a person and the environment that is appraised by the person as taxing or exceeding his or her resources and endangering his or her well-being."[1] For some people, stress may facilitate the learning of new methods to cope with stress and the utilization of resources that have not previously been available. For others, stressful events can precipitate a crisis event.

A *crisis* is a state of disequilibrium that occurs when usual coping strategies are inadequate and immediate interventions are required.[2] Situations that may precipitate a crisis event vary among individuals and families. Depending on the concurrent individual or family stresses, a variety of situations may trigger a crisis event for that individual or family. The death of a child predictably initiates a crisis event for a family; however, less serious injuries or illness may also create additional stress and precipitate a crisis.

During a stressful event, habitual coping mechanisms may fail. The family's equilibrium may be suddenly threatened as a result of concern for their child's pain, injury, or death. Their usual coping mechanisms or methods of problem solving may be insufficient, leaving them without control of the situation. Tension and frustration increases as the event becomes more apparent, causing a loss of "mental energy." Finally, disequilibrium occurs, resulting in crisis.

The characteristics of the crisis event that will influence the family's response include[3]:

- Event onset: Was it gradual or sudden?

- Event predictability: Was it anticipated or unexpected?

- Previous experiences: Is the event similar to previous experiences, or it is unique?

- Confounding factors: Is the event an isolated event or did it occur in combination with other stressors?

- Rating of the event: Is the event the worst experience ever experienced, or is it less stressful than past experiences?

Understanding factors that influence the family's or individual's responses will increase the nurse's ability to assist children and their families in a crisis situation. The goals of crisis intervention for patients and their families are to assess intense emotional reactions rapidly, assist the family to cope with the initial stages of grieving, and reduce the long-term effects of the crisis.

NURSING CARE OF THE FAMILY IN CRISIS

Assessment

HISTORY

Consider all family members when assessing the impact of a crisis event associated with a critically ill or injured child. To avoid confusion and establish a trusting relationship, assign one or two members of the emergency care team to communicate with the family in crisis. The history must include:

- The family's perception of the event or situation. Do they share guilt feelings or place blame regarding the event? Are there other family problems that may contribute positively or negatively to the situation? Determine stressors or critical incidents that may have preceded the present situation or are currently present.[1]

- The availability of support systems for the child and the caregiver. Consider family, friends, clergy, or other spiritual leaders.

- Previous experience with illness or injury. Has anything like this ever happened before, and, if so, what happened? What coping mechanisms were used?

- Presence of any concurrent maturational crises within the family structure, such as divorce, separation, death, adolescence, marriage.

- The family's current level of functioning and usual coping mechanisms. Determine the problem-solving or coping strategies usually used and whether they were unsuccessful or successful in the past.[1]

FAMILY RESPONSES

Family members may react to stress or a crisis event in different ways. Reactions may be guided by culture and family rituals. Responses may include physiologic or behavioral changes.

Signs and Symptoms

Family members may exhibit any of the following signs and symptoms:

- Sympathetic nervous system response:
    - Tachycardia.
    - Sweaty palms.
    - Dry mouth.
    - Hyperventilation.
- Nausea.
- Headache.
- Chest pain.

Behaviors

- Withdrawal or isolation.
- Demanding behavior, restlessness, or pacing.
- Speaking loudly, quickly, or profanely.
- Poor eye contact.
- Loud crying, shouting, banging on walls or tables.
- Violent behavior or threats against members of the emergency care team and other survivors.
- Threats of, or actual, self-destructive behavior.
- Confronting or accusing one another.
- A stated feeling of helplessness, increased frustration, decreased coping and decision-making ability.
- Forgetfulness.
- Clumsiness.

Nursing Diagnoses, Interventions, and Expected Outcomes

NURSING DIAGNOSIS	INTERVENTIONS	EXPECTED OUTCOMES
Ineffective family coping, related to: • Situational crisis secondary to the child's illness or injury • Lack of support systems	• Encourage the family to participate in the care • Keep family informed • Facilitate family presence • Provide psychosocial support • Provide bereavement followup	The family members will demonstrate adaptation to situational crisis, as evidenced by: • Caregivers seeking family and individual support as needed. • Verbalization of concerns among others in the family unit • Caregiver's positive interaction with child
Anxiety and fear (child and caregiver) related to: • Unfamiliar environment • Situational crisis • Unpredictable nature and condition • Knowledge deficit • Invasive procedures • Actual or potential threat of loss • Separation	• Keep family informed • Facilitate family presence • Provide psychosocial support • Explain all procedures honestly and at a level the child and caregiver can understand • Let your concern and caring show • Avoid statements negating or minimizing feelings • Reassure siblings they are not to blame • Explain to siblings that people are sad due to the death	The family members will experience decreasing anxiety and fear, as evidenced by: • Orientation to surroundings • Ability to verbalize concerns and ask questions of the health care team • Use of effective coping skills • Ability to describe reasons for equipment and procedures used in treatment
Parental role conflict related to: • Effects of illness • Hospitalization of child	• Facilitate family presence • Encourage the family to participate in the care	The caregiver will continue caregiver role during child's hospitalization, as evidenced by: • Collaboration with health professionals • Relation of information regarding child's previous health status • Participation in child's care
Anticipatory grieving related to: • Anticipated, actual, or possible loss	• Provide psychosocial support • Provide privacy and time for family to say goodbye • Encourage family members to stay together • Facilitate family presence • Facilitate the baptism of the child • Use concrete words to inform family members the child has died • Let your concern and caring show • Provide opportunity to view, touch, and hold the child • Avoid statements negating or minimizing feelings • Provide support during requests for organ or tissue donation or autopsy • Offer mementos • Assist the family in making decisions • Provide written bereavement information • Provide follow-up telephone numbers • Avoid sedatives for family • Provide bereavement followup • Reassure siblings they are not to blame • Encourage caregivers not to protect siblings from pain • Provide explanations to caregivers to inform siblings of the death	Family members will begin to manifest grieving behavior, as evidenced by: • Verbalization of meaning of death and loss • Sharing of grief with significant others

Planning and Implementation

The emergency care team must be prepared to implement crisis intervention and stress reduction techniques to assist the family in regaining control, understanding the event, and using available support systems. Nursing interventions must be individualized to meet the spectrum of responses exhibited by the child and family.

- Provide psychosocial support. (Nursing diagnoses: Anxiety and fear; ineffective family coping):

    - Reassure the family that the health care team will do everything possible to reduce any pain the child may experience.

    - When appropriate, provide reassurance regarding the status of the child.

    - Call the child by name.

    - As appropriate, provide activities for the child (e.g., videos, books, drawing on paper).

    - Provide easy access to a telephone.

    - Offer to contact friends, family, or pastoral or spiritual support persons, as appropriate.

    - In cases of critical illness, injury, or resuscitation, provide a separate waiting area or quiet room for the family.

- Facilitate family presence. (Nursing diagnoses: Ineffective family coping; anxiety and fear; parental role conflict):

    - During emergency care situations, including resuscitation, provide the family members the option to be present in the treatment or resuscitation area. Ideally, this area is in a location where they can see and touch their child.

    - Reassess the needs of family members frequently. Encourage the caregivers to feel free to exit and re-enter the treatment area as needed.

    - If the caregivers choose not to remain with the child, support their choice.

    - Appoint one staff member to stay with the family, whether the family is inside or outside of the treatment area.

- Encourage the family to participate in the care of the child. (Nursing diagnoses: Ineffective family coping; parental role conflict).

- Keep the family informed of the status of the child. (Nursing diagnoses: Anxiety and fear; ineffective family coping):

    - Maintain a frequent dialogue with the family concerning the child's responses to treatment and the next steps of care when the family member is present in the room and when they are outside of the resuscitation or treatment area.

    - Some persons will benefit from detailed explanations, while others may want someone to sit quietly with them.

    - Assess for nonverbal cues to determine the family's needs. For example, a family member who reaches for a nurse's hand is requesting physical contact.

    - Validate the family's understanding of the child's condition; review information provided.

- Explain all procedures honestly and at the level the child and caregiver can understand. (Nursing diagnosis: Anxiety and fear):

  - Assign a nurse or physician to explain the treatment plan.

  - In all communications with the family, be consistent and honest.

  - Refer to the child by name or by "your baby or child." Ask the parent or family member the child's name if you have not been provided that information prior to your interaction with them.

  - Listen to the family; allow them to express feelings and concerns about the event. Silence must be accepted and honored.

  - Avoid telling the family members how they "should" feel or react, especially in the case of the critically ill or injured child.

  - Contact a social worker or chaplain to provide assistance in meeting the family's psychosocial and emotional needs.

CARE OF FAMILIES EXPERIENCING GRIEF RESULTING FROM THE DEATH OF A CHILD

It is unthinkable in our society that a child should die ahead of a caregiver or grandparent; however, thousands of children die annually from illness, injury, suicide, or murder. The family members' ability to successfully resolve grief is greatly affected by what occurs during the time immediately surrounding the death of a child. Sudden death eliminates the family members' opportunity to prepare for the grief that follows the death of a family member after a long illness or expected death.

Assessment

People who are grieving may exhibit a variety of reactions that help them to begin the grieving process.[1,5] Family reactions must be supported. Each cultural group has its own belief patterns regarding healing practices and death that affect their response to death. What may be acceptable grieving behaviors for one cultural group may be offensive to another. The nurse must have an awareness of varying rituals and beliefs to facilitate the establishment of a helping relationship with the family. "By recognizing the stages of emotional distress, the emergency nurse can intervene on a corresponding level, averting unnecessary hostility while providing the most therapeutic response to the family's emotional needs."[6]

Grief reactions include:

- Shock and disbelief.

- Numbness.

- Denial.

- Anger.

- Hostility.
- Physical complaints.
- Guilt.
- Shame.

Interventions for the Family When Death Has Occurred

- Facilitate family presence in the resuscitation area. (Nursing diagnosis: Anticipatory grieving).[7] Family members are often comforted, and the grief process is facilitated, when given the opportunity to say goodbye while a loved one is still alive.[8] A staff member must remain with the family, both inside and outside the resuscitation room. The family's needs include being kept informed of the patient's condition and the impending death in order to anticipate the loss.[4]

- Explain to the family what to expect, what they will see, and what they will hear when they are in the resuscitation room (Nursing diagnosis: Anxiety and fear).

- Facilitate the baptism of the child if the parents request it. (Nursing diagnosis: Anticipatory grieving). Parents may be unaware that baptism can be performed in the emergency department. Usually baptism is done prior to pronouncement of death.

- When informing the family that death has occurred, use concrete words such as "dead" or "has died." Usage of other terminology may cause confusion (e.g., "passed away," "expired," "left us"). (Nursing diagnosis: Anticipatory grieving).

- Let your concern and caring show. (Nursing diagnoses: Anxiety and fear; anticipatory grieving). Tell parents and family members you are sorry about their loss. Do not judge parents by their response or lack of response; everyone reacts differently to death.[4]

- Provide family members the opportunity to view, touch, and hold their child. (Nursing diagnosis: Anticipatory grieving). Some family members may not be comfortable with holding a dead child. Always offer, but do not assume that a family member wants to hold the child. Prepare family members before they see the child by telling them how the body looks and feels. Allow them to stay with the child as long as possible. Be available to answer any questions, but facilitate private time for family members to say goodbye.

- Avoid statements negating or minimizing their feelings and thoughts. (Nursing diagnoses: Anxiety and fear; anticipatory grieving). Do not use statements such as "it was really for the best," and "your little angel is in heaven." Instead of offering solutions, simply say you are sorry. Be gentle when talking to caregivers (e.g., terminology, mannerisms). Sit down if they are sitting and maintain eye contact.

- Provide support during requests for tissue or organ donation and requests for autopsy. (Nursing diagnosis: Anticipatory grieving). Most states have enacted required request laws that make this an obligatory action. Families often receive comfort knowing that some good has come from the child's death.

- Offer parents a lock of hair, a photograph, a footprint, or the hospital identification bracelet. (Nursing diagnosis: Anticipatory grieving).

- Provide information about delactation or offer the telephone numbers of breast-feeding support groups (e.g., LaLeche League) if the mother has been breast-feeding.

- Assist the family in making decisions. (Nursing diagnosis: Anticipatory grieving). Provide family with information concerning the disposition of the body, including the contact person and telephone number if they later have questions.[4]

- Provide written bereavement information for parents and family members. (Nursing diagnosis: Anticipatory grieving). Inform the family about community support groups that offer assistance to the bereaved. This must be part of a packet of information given to the caregiver while in the emergency department.[4] When giving verbal and written information, offer it to a supportive family member as well as the parents, who may not be processing the information at that time.

  Note to instructor: Discuss any bereavement information currently used in your institution.

- Provide as much time as the family needs to say goodbye. (Nursing diagnosis: Anticipatory grieving). Some families may need several hours, although this may not always be feasible in a busy emergency department with space limitations. Alternative sites within the hospital may need to be made available. Provide interventions to assist the family in reaching closure, therefore enabling them to leave the emergency department.

- Caregivers may have questions several days or weeks following their child's death. Before they leave the emergency department, provide follow-up telephone numbers and answer any questions that they may have. (Nursing diagnosis: Anticipatory grieving).

- Avoid the use of sedatives for grieving caregivers. (Nursing diagnosis: Anticipatory grieving). Caregivers who hide in a fog of sedatives will have more difficulty progressing through the grief process than those who experience the intensity of their emotions.

- Provide bereavement followup over the next few weeks or months. (Nursing diagnoses: Anticipatory grieving; ineffective family coping). Followup may include telephone calls or written communication. Families who have experienced a death resulting from homicide or suicide, or unexpected circumstances such as sudden infant death syndrome, may need additional information and resources to assist in resolving their grief.

CARE FOR SURVIVING SIBLINGS

Assessment

Although siblings may not fully understand the events at hand, their presence may be a source of comfort to the family. Arrangements must be made to allow their presence and to provide for their care when the family is involved in making necessary arrangements. Adjunctive personnel (e.g., chaplain, social worker, child life specialists) can be especially helpful in facilitating this process. Table 38 provides an overview of reactions that may be exhibited by siblings.

Table 38

REACTION OF SIBLINGS TO DEATH		
Age	**Concept**	**Reactions**
Birth to 2 years	• No real concept of death. • Has a sense of separation or abandonment; feels a sense of loss; senses that something is different. • For the small infant, it may be responses related to the disruption in routine.	• May express nonspecific forms of upset: Irritability, change in sleep or feeding patterns.
2 to 6 years	• Beginning to understand reality of death but is confused. • Realizes that being dead means not being alive; may see death as reversible. • May believe that the deceased person still physically exists. • May believe that he or she is responsible for death. • Fears punishment, fears death is a form of punishment. • Believes that death is contagious.	• May be curious, confused. • May ask body-oriented questions. • Response may be delayed until a time when the child may feel more safe. • Adults often miss the relationship between delayed responses to death.
6 to 12 years	• Learning to think logically and to solve problems. Death is concrete, with specific causes. • Understands biologic functioning. Death is considered a universal and irreversible event. • Beginning to deal with possibility of own mortality.	• Vacillates between emotions – may be angry or curious or may act as if nothing happened. • May still feel that somehow they were to blame. • May experience intense guilt about having wished their sibling were dead at some time in the past. • May overidentify and fear the future. • May become excessively demanding. • Feelings of isolation from family.
Over 12 years	• Thinks in abstract terms. Reality of own death surfaces. • Denial of own vulnerability.	• May exhibit exaggerated risk-taking behaviors. • May become embarrassed to talk about death. • May become isolated from peers and family.

Adapted from Emergency Nurses Association. Special patient population: pediatrics. In: *Emergency Nursing Orientation: Diversity in Practice.* Park Ridge, Ill: Author; 1999. Used with permission.

Interventions

Interventions for surviving siblings must be appropriate for their developmental level and facilitated by the presence of at least one family member:

- Use simple terms to tell preschool children what has occurred and how it might affect them. (Nursing diagnosis: Anticipatory grieving).

- Provide information as requested and answer all questions honestly. Children over 9 years of age may be provided with more detailed information. (Nursing diagnoses: Anxiety and fear; anticipatory grieving).

- Reassure siblings that they are not to blame. (Nursing diagnoses: Anxiety and fear; anticipatory grieving). Children's fantasies are often worse than reality and they interpret cause and effect in the more literal sense (e.g., "I was mean to Sally and now she is dead").

- Explain that people around them are sad because of the death and not because they are angry. (Nursing diagnosis: Anxiety and fear).

- Allow children the opportunity to view and touch their sibling. (Nursing diagnosis: Anticipatory grieving). Explain what they will see, feel, and smell. A family member, as well as hospital staff, must always be with the sibling.

- Encourage caregivers not to try to protect siblings from pain by excluding them from important family rituals or by hiding their own grief. (Nursing diagnosis: Anticipatory grieving). Remind caregivers to answer questions with simple, direct, and honest answers. Do not tell a child that a sibling has "gone to sleep."

- Provide the family with phrases to use in explaining death to siblings that are not present. (Nursing diagnosis: Anticipatory grieving). Explain that the child's response may not be the same as that of the adult. Young children will often continue with normal play, may not cry, and may not seem sad. They will also talk very openly about the deceased and the death.

CARE FOR THE EMERGENCY CARE TEAM

The death of patients and major devastating injuries among children are difficult events for any person involved in resuscitation efforts. Each new event may trigger sadness and a sense of failure for the team. Persons at risk for these feelings include team members involved at the bedside and others who have knowledge of the patient's presence in the emergency department, such as prehospital and security personnel, clerical staff, social workers, laboratory technicians, and pastoral care personnel.

Emergency departments must facilitate development of the following mechanisms to assist the emergency care team:

- Develop protocols and a checklist to guide staff members when assisting survivors. Clarify each team member's responsibilities.

- Allow "recovery time" for staff members involved in a stressful resuscitation. A brief discussion of 15 to 30 minutes in length, immediately after the event, may reduce associated stress.

- Provide a program to alert staff members to the signs of stress (e.g., altered job satisfaction, irritability, persistent lateness, frequent sick leave, sleep disturbance). Organize group sessions to discuss staff feelings regarding an unsuccessful resuscitation and provide support to one another.

- Determine one's own feelings about death. Feelings of anger, sadness, disappointment, failure, and fear when a child dies are normal. By acknowledging these feelings, staff members will find it easier to approach the child's survivors openly and supportively.

- Educate one's self about the grief process. Understanding the impact of death or injury on a family prepares the health care provider to be more effective in offering support. Awareness of the behavior and emotions that accompany grieving enables health care providers to reassure and assist caregivers in realizing that their reactions are normal.

- Encourage staff members to learn and accept their peers' reactions to stressful events.

A critical incident is any situation experienced by an emergency care provider that evokes unusually strong emotional reactions. These reactions have the potential to interfere with the ability to function. Examples of critical incidents that may trigger these reactions are[2]:

- Any event with significant emotional power that overwhelms usual coping mechanisms.

- Death of a child or a child who is injured by a malicious or careless adult.

- Victims who are children, relatives, or friends of the emergency care providers.

- Events that threaten the safety or life of staff.

Signs and Symptoms

Critical incidents may produce a characteristic set of physical, cognitive, emotional, and behavioral symptoms (see Table 39). Reactions to a critical incident may appear immediately, within a few hours, within days, several weeks, or even months later. Reactions may last for an indefinite period of time.

Interventions

Critical incident stress management is an organized program that provides intervention strategies designed to lessen stress. Critical incident stress management can assist emergency personnel in managing and recovering from significant stresses encountered in their work.[9] Education about stress reduction measures, risk factors for stress, and the provision of defusing and formal debriefings are all methods of critical incident stress management. After a critical incident, defusing and debriefing may expedite a quicker recovery from the stress-associated event.

Table 39

COMMON SIGNS AND SYMPTOMS OF STRESS	
Physical	**Cognitive**
• Fatigue • Tachypnea • Elevated blood pressure • Tachycardia • Thirst • Headaches • Dizziness • Gastrointestinal upset	• Confusion • Impaired decision-making ability • Loss of concentration • Memory lapses • Impaired problem-solving ability
Emotional	**Behavioral**
• Anxiety, apprehension, or fear • Guilt • Grief • Denial • Uncertainty • Loss of emotional control • Feeling of being overwhelmed • Depression • Intense anger • Irritability or agitation	• Withdrawal from others • Emotional outbursts • Suspiciousness • Changes in eating and drinking • Changes in resting and sleeping • Deceased personal hygiene • Changes in activity and speech

The debriefing is a peer-driven, clinician-guided discussion of a traumatic event with the goal of mitigating the psychological trauma and accelerating recovery from significant stress.[9] The discussion is guided by trained personnel who were not involved in the incident. Debriefings usually occur within 24 to 72 hours of the event. Using a seven-step process, the goals of a debriefing process are:

- Prevention of additional stress.

- Return of participants to a precrisis level of functioning.

- Organization and mobilization of resources.

- Clarification of the event.

The seven steps of debriefing include:

- Initial phase: The people in attendance are introduced and the rules of the debriefing are discussed. Only those involved in the event, including prehospital personnel, are allowed to attend. The issues discussed are considered confidential.

- Fact phase: Each individual discusses his or her role in the event and describes what was seen, done, heard, and smelled.

- Thought phase: Persons willing to speak are asked to share what they felt during the incident and how they personalized the experience.

- Reaction phase: Participants describe their reactions to the worst part of the incident. This allows a safe environment to discuss the psychological and physiologic effects of the incident.

- Symptom phase: The participants discuss any reactions to stress they have experienced since the incident. Mental health professionals determine the need for additional help for any group members.

- Teaching phase: Team members discuss stress management strategies and methods to support one another during the crisis.

- Re-entry phase: The group is given an opportunity to ask any additional questions. The events of the crisis are summarized, and referrals are made for additional help, if needed.

Defusings are shortened versions of the debriefing. Defusings always take place immediately after the critical incident and can last 20 to 40 minutes. They are led by trained persons and are designed to either eliminate the need to provide a formal debriefing or enhance the actual debriefing session.[9]

Debriefings and defusing are two methods of promoting wellness related to critical incident stress management. Overall, critical incident stress management accelerates the rate of "normal recovery, in normal people, who are having normal reactions to abnormal events."[9]

SUMMARY

Caring for the physiologic needs of an ill or injured child is the primary focus of the emergency care team. During this time, it is important to remember that the family is also in crisis. The emergency nurse can be instrumental in assisting family members to cope with the sudden tragic event by offering support and by providing information about available resources. Early intervention in the grief process may reduce the emotional and psychological consequences to survivors. To assist health care providers with their stress and grief, remember: "Being responsible for the life of a child is not the same as being responsible for their death."[10]

REFERENCES

1. Emergency Nurses Association. Psychological aspects of trauma care. In: *Trauma Nursing Core Course (Instructor) Manual.* 4th ed. Park Ridge, Ill: Author; 1995:325-345.

2. Mitchell J, Resnik H. *Emergency Response to Crisis.* Ellicott City, Md: Chevron Publishing; 1986.

3. Solursh DS. The family of the trauma victim. *Nurs Clin North Am.* 1990;25:155-162.

4. Emergency Nurses Association. *Presenting the Option for Family Presence.* Park Ridge, Ill: Author; 1995.

5. McFarland G, McFarlane E. *Nursing Diagnosis and Intervention; Planning Patient Care.* 2nd ed. St. Louis, Mo: Mosby-Year Book; 1993.

6 Sacchetti A, Lichenstein R, Carraccio C, Harris R. Family member presence during pediatric emergency department procedures. *Pediatr Emerg Care.* 1996;12:268-271.

7. Thomas DO. Crisis intervention and death. In: Soud TE, Rogers JS, eds. *Manual of Pediatric Emergency Nursing.* St. Louis, Mo: Mosby-Year Book; 1998:178-192.

8. Post H. Letting the family in during a code. *Nursing.* 1989;3:43-46.

9. Mitchell J, Everly G. *Critical Incident Stress Debriefing: CISD.* Ellicott City, Md: Chevron Publishing; 1993.

10. Thomas DO. Personal communication; 1993.

ADDITIONAL READINGS

1. Fraser S, Atkins J. Survivors' recollections of helpful and unhelpful emergency nurse activities surrounding sudden death of a loved one. *J Emerg Nurs.* 1990;4:13-16.

2. Lightner C, Hathaway N. *Giving Sorrow Words.* New York, NY: Warner; 1990.

3. Schlump-Urquhart SR. Families experiencing a traumatic accident: implications for nursing management. *AACN Clin Issues Crit Care Nurs.* 1990;1:522-534.

4. Neidig JR, Dalgas-Pelish P. Parental grieving and perceptions regarding health care professional's intervention. *Issues Compr Pediatr Nurs.* 1991;14:179-191.

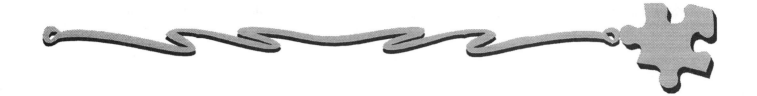

CHAPTER 14

Stabilization and Transport

OBJECTIVES

On completion of this lecture, the learner should be able to:

✦ Identify the indications for the transfer of the pediatric patient.

✦ Discuss the stabilization required prior to transfer.

✦ Compare and contrast ground and air transport of pediatric patients.

✦ Describe the personnel that are needed to safely transport the ill or injured child.

INTRODUCTION

Competent care of pediatric patients requires specialized skills, equipment, and personnel. If these components of care are unavailable, the child must be transferred to a facility specialized in the care of children. Indication for transport include[1]:

● Need for pediatric expertise.

● Need for a diagnostic procedure.

● Potential for deterioration because of a child's illness or injury.

● Requested transfer.

Transfer Requirements

If all the provisions regarding consent have been met, additional transfer requirements must be met. These include:

● A physician at the receiving facility must agree to accept the patient.

● The receiving facility must have adequate space and personnel to care for the individual.

- Medical records related to the emergency medical condition must accompany the patient to the receiving facility.

- The transfer must utilize qualified personnel and adequate equipment, as determined by the sending physician.

UNITED STATES
Consolidated Omnibus Budget Reconciliation Act (COBRA)

Prior to 1986, there were many accounts of emergency departments refusing to care for indigent patients.[2] In 1986, the Consolidated Omnibus Budget Reconciliation Act (COBRA), which addresses issues related to transfer and refusal for treatment, was passed.[3] Since then, there have been several additions and modifications to the COBRA provisions. General provisions include[2]:

- COBRA covers any individual who comes to an emergency department that participates in Medicaid for examination of a medical condition. The hospital is obligated to provide a screening examination. If the patient has an emergency medical condition, the hospital must provide one of the following:
  - Stabilization of a patient within the skill and capability of the hospital resources.
  - Transfer of the patient to another medical facility with additional care resources. The patient cannot be transferred unless the patient or his or her guardian requests the change. A physician must sign a certificate that the medical benefits of the transfer outweigh the risks to the transfer of the patient (must have evidence that the patient received and understood the risks and benefits associated with the transfer).
- In 1994, one section of the COBRA legislation, the Emergency Medical Treatment and Active Labor Act (EMTALA), was further clarified to state that there are two circumstances when the unstable patient may be transferred[4]:
  - The patient or their family requests a transfer.
  - The physician or referring personnel determine that the benefits of transfer outweigh the risks of not transferring the child.

COMPONENTS OF THE TRANSFER SYSTEM

Policies and Procedures

Each referring hospital must have written policies, procedures, and transfer guidelines that include:

- Which patients must be transferred.

- Procedures for initial stabilization prior to transport.

- Available modes of transport according to geographical area.

- Personnel and equipment to accompany the child.

Communication

The transfer process begins once the referring facility contacts the receiving hospital. It is important to confirm that the child has been accepted for admission to the receiving facility. The referring facility must provide the following information[5]:

- Chief complaint or problem as the diagnosis may not be available.
- Age.
- Indications for transfer.
- Vital signs.
- Treatment rendered.
- Location of the patient (e.g., emergency department, intensive care unit).
- Past medical history.
- Weight.
- Previous admission of the child to the receiving or referring facility.

Transport Resources

GENERAL TRANSPORT CONSIDERATIONS

Once the decision has been made to transfer the pediatric patient, the method of transport must be considered. Factors that influence this decision include:

- Geography; landing sites for helicopters or fixed-wing vehicles.
- Composition of the transport crew and competence and experience with pediatric patients.
- Condition of the child.
- Distance and transport time between the two facilities.
- Traffic and road conditions.
- Weather.
- Availability of appropriate equipment and supplies.
- Available modes of transport in a given area.

Table 40 provides potential advantages and disadvantages of ground and air transport.

Table 40

GROUND VERSUS AIR TRANSPORT: ADVANTAGES AND DISADVANTAGES	
Ground Transport	
Advantages	**Disadvantages**
• Availability • Space in the vehicle • Can travel in any weather • Ability to carry several prehospital personnel • Ability to carry more equipment • Family may accompany child in vehicle	• Transport can take up to three times longer by ground than by rotor wing • Traffic and road conditions can interfere with transport • Loss of vehicle to the community
Air Transport	
Advantages	**Disadvantages**
• Saves time • Improved communication ability • Heightened emergency response at receiving facility because of experience with helicopter transport patients • Continued availability of ground emergency medical services resources within the referral area	• Weather restrictions • Lack of availability • Cost • Physiologic impact • Noise • Vibrations • Temperature changes • Gas expansion with altitude • Fear of flying • Space and weight restrictions

Once the mode of transport has been chosen, an estimated time of arrival and instructions for patient preparation must be communicated to the receiving facility.

RISKS OF TRANSPORT

Regardless of the method of transport, certain risks are involved. These include[6,7]:

- Possibility of a transport vehicle crash (e.g., ambulance, helicopter, fixed wing aircraft).

- Potential for death or further injury related to inadequate equipment or an inexperienced crew during transport.

- Delay in arrival related to mechanical failure or environmental obstacles.

- Loss of radio communication related to system malfunction.

PERSONNEL CONSIDERATIONS

The composition of transport teams varies. Ideally, the team that transports pediatric patients is a dedicated pediatric team. However, in some areas of the country, pediatric transport personnel are not accessible. Members of the team involved in the transport of children must have pediatric training and the ability to deliver the appropriate level of care to patients of various ages with a wide array of illnesses and injuries. An emergency nurse involved in the transport of children must be trained to provide the necessary interventions during transport. It is recommended that the pediatric transport team consist of at least three members, with the primary member being a transport nurse.[5-8] Other members of the team may include a physician, paramedic, respiratory therapist, and the driver or pilot.

EQUIPMENT CONSIDERATIONS

Preparation of the pediatric patient for transport begins with anticipation. Transport equipment must meet the following criteria[5]:

- Accommodate a wide range of ages, sizes, and weights.
- Be useful in the transport setting.
- Be lightweight, durable, portable, and perhaps fulfill several functions, such as a monitor that has a built-in defibrillator and an external pacemaker.
- Be easily cleaned and maintained.
- Have a power source that will last the length of the transport.

Documentation

Copies of the child's records (e.g., nursing and medical record, laboratory results, x-rays) must accompany the child to the receiving hospital. Include a copy of the written permission for transfer. Many facilities have specific forms that are used during the transport of a patient.

STABILIZATION PRIOR TO TRANSFER

Stabilization of the pediatric patient prior to transfer involves meeting the immediate needs and anticipating any change of condition that may occur during transport. The priorities of stabilization are listed below.

Airway

- Maintain a patent airway.
- Maintain immobilization of the cervical spine if trauma is suspected.
- Continue the delivery of supplemental oxygen, as indicated.

- If the child is intubated, reconfirm tube placement each time the patient is moved and assure the following documentation is completed:

  - Time of intubation.

  - Endotracheal tube size and cuffed versus noncuffed tube.

  - Depth of endotracheal tube placement, location of tube at lip, teeth, or gum line.

  - Medications administered for intubation procedure and continued sedation.

- Insert a gastric tube to decompress the stomach if the child is intubated.

Breathing

- Reassess the child's respiratory status before transport (e.g., breath sounds, work of breathing, oxygen saturation).

- For patients being transported by air, anticipate and prepare for additional interventions based on air physiology (e.g., placement of chest tube for a small pneumothorax).

Circulation

- Secure intravenous lines in preparation for transport.

- Calculate intake and output; document total intravenous fluid and blood product administration.

Other

- Apply sterile dressings to all open soft tissue injuries.

- Splint all suspected fractures prior to transport.

- Conduct and document neurovascular assessment of all splinted or injured extremities.

INTRAHOSPITAL TRANSPORT OF THE PEDIATRIC PATIENT

Transport of children within the hospital environment also requires consideration. Members of the team involved in the transfer of pediatric patients to diagnostic departments and patient care units must have the ability to deliver the appropriate level of care during the intrahospital transport process. The emergency nurse must evaluate the patient's potential care needs during the transport process to determine the appropriate staff to accompany the patient. When the patient is transported to a diagnostic department for a procedure or study, the time required to complete the procedure and the number of department staff in attendance must also be weighed.

The composition of the team transporting the child varies. A combination of nurses, respiratory therapist, physicians, and assistant personnel are used. Continuous monitoring, assessment, and interventions are imperative for seriously and critically ill or injured children. Therefore, the team composition is determined by the patient's acuity level, current treatment, and complexity of care as well as potential needs during intrahospital transport. Suitable equipment, supplies, and medications must also be readily available to the transporting staff.

CARE OF FAMILY MEMBERS

To reduce the stress and uncertainty of the family, and depending on the transport system's policies and procedures regarding passengers, consider allowing a family member to accompany the child. When it is being determined if a caregiver may accompany their child during transport, the space available on the vehicle or space and weight limitations of the aircraft must be considered.

Use the following guidelines when discussing the child's transport with the family:

- Explain why the child needs to be transferred.
- Obtain consent as required, before transport.
- Provide an explanation if family members cannot accompany their child during transport.
- Strongly recommend that the family observe all traffic laws.
- Do not allow the family to leave the institution until the child leaves.
- Provide the family with maps and directions to the receiving facility.
- If the family member or caregiver is alone, assist with transportation arrangements as needed.
- Allow the family to see the child before transport.

SUMMARY

Transfer of the pediatric patient must be an organized procedure that includes prearranged agreements between referring and receiving facilities, transfer policies and protocols, standards of care for stabilization and transport, appropriate equipment, and consideration of the emotional needs of the child and family.

REFERENCES

1. American College of Emergency Physicians. Principles of appropriate transfer. *Ann Emerg Med.* 1990;19:337-338.

2. Trauma Nursing Coalition. *Resource Document for Nursing Care of the Trauma Patient.* 2nd ed. Park Ridge, Ill: Author; 1997.

3. Southard P. COBRA legislation: Complying with ED provisions. *J Emerg Nurs.* 1989;15:23-25.

4. Department of Health and Human Services. Health Care Financing Administration Interim Final Rule. *Federal Register.* 1994;59:32-86.

5. Boyd C, Hungerpillar J. Patient risk in prehospital transport: air versus ground. *Emerg Care Q.* 1990;5:48-55.

6. Jaimovich D, Vidyasagar D. *Handbook of Neonatal and Transport Medicine.* St. Louis, Mo: Mosby-Year Book; 1996.

7. McCloskey K, Orr R, eds. *Pediatric Transport Medicine.* St. Louis, Mo: Mosby-Year Book; 1995.

8. Emergency Nurses Association. *Interfacility Transport of the Critically Ill or Injured Patient.* Park Ridge, Ill: Author; 1997.

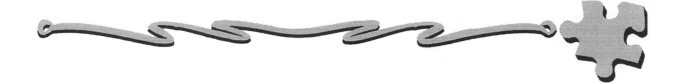

Emergency Nursing Pediatric Course

Pediatric Multiple Trauma Skill Station

EQUIPMENT FOR THE STATION

- Two tables (one for mannikin, one for supplies)
- Five chairs
- One child mannikin
- One pediatric nonrebreather mask
- One rigid tonsil suction
- One bag-valve-mask device (1,000-ml)
- Resuscitation masks (sizes appropriate for mannikins)
- One endotracheal tube (size appropriate for mannikin)
- One 4 × 4-inch gauze pad
- One chest tube (20-French)
- One blanket or similar type of warming device
- One penlight
- One stethoscope
- Intravenous catheters (20-gauge, 24-gauge)
- One blood-collecting tube
- One 500-ml lactated Ringer's solution or 0.9% normal saline, and intravenous tubing
- Three electrocardiogram electrodes
- One pulse oximeter probe
- One gastric tube (10-French or larger)
- One pediatric indwelling urinary catheter
- One clipboard (testing day)
- Personal protective equipment
- One backboard

- One rigid splint for femur
- Rigid cervical collars (infant, small)
- Lateral stabilization devices (rolled towels, blanket, foam blocks)
- Blankets for immobilization
- Adhesive tape (2-inch) or backboard straps

STATION PREPARATION

1. Assemble all equipment and ensure that it is in working order.

2. Arrange equipment and the mannikin on the tables.

3. Place chairs around the table with the mannikin.

4. Display the case scenarios and the A through I mnemonic on a chalkboard, flipchart, or poster.

	Moulage Instructions
Case A	Blood on face; deformity of left forearm; ecchymosis on left anterior chest; abrasion on left iliac crest; ecchymosis on left upper quadrant.
Case B	Contusion on right parietal area; ecchymosis on right lower chest; abrasions on face; contusion on right side of forehead; ecchymosis on right upper quadrant; abrasions on extremities.
Case C	Deformity of right upper leg; abrasions on left side of face; blood on left ear, abrasions on extremities.
Case D	Ecchymosis on left lateral and lower chest, down to left abdomen; 3-cm laceration on left lower leg; ecchymosis on left lateral back.

INTRODUCTION TO THE SKILL STATION

1. The instructor will discuss and/or demonstrate a primary and a secondary assessment or learners will view the station demonstration videotape.

2. The instructor will demonstrate or play the videotape demonstrating the sizing and application of a cervical collar and immobilization of a child on a backboard. Learners will practice this skill as a group. This demonstration and return demonstration should be completed before the case scenarios are practiced (see Chapter 6, "Pediatric Trauma," for an explanation of these procedures).

3. Each learner will be presented with a case scenario and will:

- Conduct the primary and secondary assessment of a multiply injured child. During the assessment, learners must describe appropriate inspection techniques and demonstrate appropriate palpation and auscultation techniques.

- Determine the management priorities for the injured child.

- Demonstrate the need for universal precautions when caring for the injured child.

4. Four multiple trauma scenarios are included for teaching. Each learner is provided with a different scenario to practice. Each scenario integrates abnormalities that require appropriate interventions in the primary and/or secondary assessment.

5. One student should be assigned as the team leader responsible for completing the assessment and directing the team. The other members of the group can assist by performing bag-valve-mask ventilation, manual stabilization of the cervical spine, etc. On evaluation day, each student is evaluated by himself or herself with no other group members in the room.

6. The instructor will provide responses to the learner's questions about the case scenarios. The instructor will also provide specific information related to the case progression as appropriate.

7. The instructor will inform learners:

- The sequence of the primary assessment is important.

- To be successful, the steps with double asterisks (**) must be performed in order. Once the learner begins the assessment of E through I, the instructor will assume that the learner has completed the primary assessment. It is acceptable for the learner to identify interventions such as placing the child on the cardiac monitor, initiating pulse oximetry, inserting an indwelling urinary catheter or gastric tube, or other diagnostic studies during the primary assessment. This does not constitute the learner "leaving" the primary assessment.

- Patency of intravenous access established by prehospital personnel must be assessed.

- Appropriate palpation and auscultation must be demonstrated during the assessment as indicated on the evaluation form.

- The effectiveness of interventions which are expected to have an immediate effect on the patient must be evaluated (e.g., auscultation of breath sounds after intubation, effectiveness of bag-valve-mask ventilation, effectiveness of a fluid bolus, effectiveness of suctioning the airway, assessment of breathing following chest tube insertion).

- For those scenarios that have the patient arriving by private auto, initiate manual spinal immobilization while simultaneously assessing the airway.

- If the patient is unconscious on arrival, the airway must be manually opened to assess airway patency.

- To assess circulation, obtain central **AND** peripheral pulse rate and quality, and skin color **AND** temperature during the primary assessment.

PRINCIPLES OF PEDIATRIC MULTIPLE TRAUMA ASSESSMENT AND INTERVENTIONS AND SPINAL IMMOBILIZATION

The care of the injured pediatric patient is based on performance of a systematic assessment and initiation of the appropriate interventions. The management priorities are based on the life-threatening injuries found in the primary assessment and other injuries found in the secondary assessment, as well as the child's age and the resources available for providing care.

The primary assessment is a brief assessment of airway, breathing, circulation, and disability. Life-threatening conditions are identified and treated before the assessment continues. The secondary assessment is a systematic approach to identifying additional problems and determining the priorities of care.

Simultaneous assessment, diagnosis, and intervention may be required for the child who is severely injured. The priorities for intervention will depend on the complexity of the child's injuries and the availability and qualifications of the emergency care providers. Those injuries that have the greatest potential to compromise the airway, breathing, circulation, and/or disability are given the highest priority.

The child must be re-evaluated after any interventions that have an immediate effect on him or her to determine their effectiveness. The evaluation and ongoing assessment begin at the completion of the secondary assessment. These include primary reassessment and a re-evaluation of vital signs.

The systematic assessment can be remembered as follows:

 A = Airway with simultaneous cervical spine stabilization

 B = Breathing

 C = Circulation

 D = Disability – brief neurologic assessment

 E = Exposure and environmental control

 F = Full set of vital signs and family presence

 G = Give comfort measures

 H = Head-to-toe assessment and history

 I = Inspect the posterior surfaces

Tables 41, 42, and 43 provide guidelines for conducting the primary and secondary assessments and identifying the appropriate interventions.

Table 41

PRIMARY ASSESSMENT	
Assessments	**Potential Interventions**
A = Airway and Cervical Spine Stabilization	
While maintaining spinal stabilization (see pages 167-170 for explanation of the technique for spinal stabilization and immobilization): • Vocalization • Tongue obstruction • Loose teeth or foreign objects • Vomitus or other secretions • Bleeding • Edema • Drooling • Dysphagia • Abnormal airway sounds (stridor or snoring)	• Position the patient • Open the airway with jaw thrust • Suction or remove foreign objects • Insert oropharyngeal/nasopharyngeal airway • Perform endotracheal intubation/rapid sequence induction • Prepare for needle or surgical cricothyroidotomy
B = Breathing	

• Level of consciousness
• Spontaneous respirations
• Rate and depth of respirations
• Symmetric chest rise and fall
• Presence and quality of bilateral breath sounds
• Work of breathing:
  ■ Nasal flaring
  ■ Retractions
  ■ Expiratory grunting
  ■ Accessory muscle use
• Jugular vein distention and position of trachea
• Paradoxical respirations
• Soft tissue and bony chest wall integrity
	• Provide supplemental oxygen
	• Provide bag-valve-mask ventilation
	• Perform endotracheal intubation/rapid sequence induction
	• Insert gastric tube to reduce abdominal distention
	• Perform needle thoracentesis
	• Insert chest tube
	• Apply nonporous dressing taped on three sides

C = Circulation	
• Rate and quality of central and peripheral pulses • Skin color, temperature • Capillary refill • External bleeding	• Apply direct pressure over uncontrolled bleeding sites • Insert two large-bore intravenous catheters with warmed lactated Ringer's solution • Administer 20-ml/kg fluid bolus of isotonic crystalloid solution • Obtain intraosseous access • Obtain blood sample for typing • Perform cardiopulmonary resuscitation and advanced life-support measures • Administer blood or blood products • Correct electrolyte and acid-base balance • Prepare for surgery
D = Disability	
• Level of consciousness (AVPU) • Pupils	• Perform further investigation during the secondary assessment • Immobilize spine • Administer pharmacologic therapy

Table 42

SECONDARY ASSESSMENT	
Assessment	**Potential Interventions**
E = Exposure and Environmental Control	
• Obvious underlying injuries • Additional signs of illness • Sources of heat loss	• Save clothes for forensic evidence • Apply warm blankets • Provide overhead warming lights • Provide radiant warmer or other approved warming device • Maintain warm ambient environment • Increase room temperature as needed • Administer warm intravenous fluids • Administer warm humidified oxygen
F = Full Set of Vital Signs	
• Rate and depth of respirations • Rate and quality of pulse • Blood pressure • Temperature • Weight	• Place on cardiorespiratory monitor • Trend vital signs • Estimate weight using length-based resuscitation tape
F = Family Presence	
• Needs of the family • Need for additional support and desire to be in resuscitation room • Identification of the family members and their relationship to the child	• Facilitate and support family involvement • Assign health care professional to provide explanations about procedures and to be with the family • Assign a staff member to provide family support
G = Give Comfort Measures	

• Presence and level of pain	• Facilitate family presence for support of the child
	• Initiate pain management measures:
	  ▪ Use age-appropriate nonpharmacologic methods to facilitate coping
	  ▪ Administer analgesics and other appropriate medications to manage procedural pain and pain from interventions
	  ▪ Initiate physical measures (splints, dressings, ice)

H = Head-to-Toe Assessment	
Head and face • Inspect for wounds, ecchymosis, deformities, drainage from nose and ears, and pupils • Palpate anterior and posterior fontanelles in infants for fullness, bulging, or depression, deformities, crepitus	
Neck • Inspect for jugular vein distention, wounds, ecchymosis, and deformities • Palpate for tracheal position, tenderness, or deformity	

SECONDARY ASSESSMENT

Assessment	Potential Interventions
Chest ● Inspect for breathing rate and depth, work of breathing, use of accessory muscles, abdominal muscles, and paradoxical respirations ● Auscultate breath and heart sounds ● Palpate for tenderness, subcutaneous emphysema, crepitus, and deformity	
Abdomen and flanks ● Inspect for wounds, distention, ecchymosis, and scars ● Auscultate bowel sounds ● Palpate all four quadrants for tenderness, rigidity, guarding, and masses	
Pelvis and perineum ● Inspect for wounds, deformities, ecchymosis, priapism, and blood at the urinary meatus or in the perineal area ● Palpate the pelvis, anal sphincter tone, and femoral pulses	
Extremities ● Inspect for ecchymosis, movement, wounds, deformities, circulatory status, and motor function ● Palpate pulses, skin temperature, sensation, tenderness, deformities, and bony crepitus	
H = History	
History ● MIVT ● CIAMPEDS	
I = Inspect Posterior Surfaces	
Posterior surfaces ● Maintain cervical spine stabilization and support injured extremities while the patient is logrolled. ● Inspect posterior surfaces for wounds, deformities, and ecchymosis ● Palpate posterior surfaces for tenderness and deformities ● Palpate anal sphincter tone (if not assessed previously)	

Table 43

PLANNING AND IMPLEMENTATION		
Area	**Diagnostic Studies**	**Interventions**
General		• Prepare for operative intervention • Arrange admission or transfer • Determine Pediatric Coma Scale score and Revised Trauma Score • Provide psychosocial support for patient and family • Administer pain medication, as prescribed
Head and face	Radiographic studies, laboratory studies	• Position patient • Administer medications, as prescribed • Monitor intracranial pressure
Neck	Radiographic studies, laboratory studies	• Immobilize vertebral column • Administer steroids, as prescribed
Chest	Radiographic studies, laboratory studies, electrocardiogram, central venous pressure monitoring	• Insert chest tube • Perform autotransfusion
Abdomen and flanks	Radiographic studies, laboratory studies, ultrasound, and diagnostic peritoneal lavage	• Insert urinary catheter • Insert gastric tube
Pelvis and perineum	Radiographic studies, laboratory studies	• Insert urinary catheter • External pelvic fixator
Extremities	Radiographic studies, laboratory studies	• Immobilize affected limb • Provide elevation, ice
Posterior surfaces	Radiographic studies, laboratory studies	• Immobilize spine
Surface trauma		• Irrigate wound • Provide wound care • Provide ice • Provide care for amputated parts • Administer tetanus prophylaxis and antibiotics

STEPS IN SKILL PERFORMANCE

The instructor will demonstrate or play the videotape demonstrating spinal immobilization of the pediatric patient. The learners will practice as a group, determining the correct size of a rigid cervical collar, applying the rigid cervical collar, and immobilizing the child on a backboard.

Once the learners have practiced spinal immobilization, each learner will be presented a case scenario depicting a child who is en route or has presented to the emergency department following a traumatic event. The script and steps in skill performance are listed on pages 370-389.

The instructor will tell the learner: "I will describe a case scenario of a multiply injured child. As you assess the child and evaluate interventions, I will give you additional information."

SUMMARY

During evaluation, the learner must demonstrate all critical steps designated with one (*) and two (**) asterisks, and 70% of the total number of points. Each learner will be evaluated using a new and different scenario. Therefore, concentrate on understanding the principles of the station and not memorizing the specific case scenarios. Learners will not be evaluated on the ability to perform spinal immobilization.

Certain critical steps must be demonstrated or described in order during the primary assessment. These are designated with ** on the evaluation form. The total number of critical steps (**) in any scenario is 6 to 8. Critical steps designated with ** may include:

- Assesses airway patency.

- Identifies one appropriate airway intervention.

- Assesses breathing effectiveness.

- Identifies one appropriate intervention for ineffective breathing.

- Assesses perfusion status.

- States one appropriate intervention for ineffective circulation.

- Assesses the level of consciousness (AVPU).

Additional critical steps that must be demonstrated or described during the remainder of the station are designated with an asterisk (*) on the evaluation form. All of these steps must also be performed to successfully complete the station.

- States one measure to prevent heat loss.

- Identifies appropriate diagnostic studies or interventions.

At the completion of the demonstration, the learner will be asked if there is anything he or she wants to add or revise. Learners may not add to or revise any of the ** steps.

MULTIPLE TRAUMA INTERVENTION

Teaching Case A

Parents present to the triage desk carrying a 6-year-old boy who is crying. The mom states that he fell two stories, struck the rail, and then landed on the deck. The boy's face is covered with dried blood. The parents state that he has not stopped crying since the fall. The Pediatric Assessment Triangle reveals that he is alert and crying, his respirations are unlabored, and his skin is pale. You notice a deformed left forearm. The patient is taken to the trauma room. A support person responds to the trauma room to provide family support. Please proceed with your primary and secondary assessments and appropriate interventions.

Instructor Responses	Skill Steps	Demonstrated		
		Yes		No
	1. Assesses airway patency AND initiates cervical spine stabilization (at least three of the following):	** _____		_____
Crying	• Vocalization			
No tongue obstruction	• Tongue obstruction			
Two front teeth missing; no foreign objects	• Loose teeth or foreign objects			
No vomitus or other secretions	• Vomitus or other secretions			
Dried blood on face from missing teeth	• Bleeding			
No edema	• Edema			
No drooling	• Drooling			
No dysphagia	• Dysphagia			
No abnormal airway sounds	• Abnormal airway sounds			
Instructor response: "The airway is patent and the cervical spine is manually stabilized."				

Instructor Responses	Skill Steps	Demonstrated		
		Yes		No
	2. Assesses breathing effectiveness (at least three of the following):	** _____		_____
Alert, crying	• Level of consciousness			
Spontaneous shallow respirations present	• Spontaneous breathing			
Respiratory rate of 36 breaths/minute and shallow	• Rate and depth of respirations			
Symmetric chest rise and fall	• Symmetric chest rise and fall			
Breath sounds diminished on left base and shallow	• Presence and quality of breath sounds			
	• Work of breathing (at least three of the following):			
No nasal flaring	■ Nasal flaring			
No retractions	■ Retractions			
No expiratory grunting	■ Expiratory grunting			
No accessory muscle use	■ Accessory muscle use			
No jugular vein distention; trachea midline	• Jugular vein distention and tracheal position			
No paradoxical respirations	• Paradoxical respirations			
Ecchymosis on lower left anterior chest wall	• Soft tissue and bony chest wall integrity			
	3. States need for oxygen via nonrebreather mask	** _____		_____
	4. Assesses perfusion status (at least two of the following):	** _____		_____
Central pulse strong, rate 130 beats/minute; peripheral pulses weak	• Central AND peripheral pulse rate and quality			
Skin pale and warm	• Skin color AND temperature			
Capillary refill 3 seconds	• Capillary refill			
Bleeding from mouth controlled. No other evidence of external bleeding.	5. Inspects for uncontrolled external bleeding	_____		_____
Intravenous access obtained	6. States need to obtain vascular access at two sites	** _____		_____
Fluid bolus administered	7. States need to administer a 20-ml/kg fluid bolus	_____		_____
	8. Obtains blood sample for typing	_____		_____
	9. Reassesses perfusion status (at least two of the following):	_____		_____
Central pulse 115 beats/minute; peripheral pulses stronger	• Central AND peripheral pulse rate and quality			
Skin pale and warm	• Skin color AND temperature			
Capillary refill 2 seconds	• Capillary refill			

Instructor Responses	Skill Steps	Demonstrated		
		Yes		No
Responds to verbal stimuli, intermittently crying	10. Assesses level of consciousness (AVPU)	** ___		___
Pupils equal and reactive	11. Assesses pupils	___		___
Secondary Assessment				
Ecchymosis on left anterior chest, abrasion on left iliac crest	12. Removes all clothing	___		___
	13. States one measure to prevent heat loss: ● Warm blankets ● Overhead warming lights or other warming device ● Warm ambient environment ● Warm intravenous fluids ● Warm humidified oxygen	* ___		___
BP = 96/58 mm Hg P = 115 beats/minute R = 28 breaths/minute T = 37°C (98.6°F) Weight = 25 kg, estimated by length-based resuscitation tape	14. States need to get a complete set of vital signs	___		___
Electrocardiogram = normal sinus rhythm	15. Places cardiac monitor leads on patient and evaluates rhythm	___		___
Oxygen saturation 96% on nonrebreather mask	16. Places pulse oximeter on patient	___		___
Complains of pain in his chest, left forearm, left shoulder, and mouth	17. States need to evaluate for presence of pain or discomfort	___		___

Demonstrates and describes the head-to-toe assessment by describing appropriate inspection techniques (e.g., lacerations, abrasions, contusions, ecchymosis), demonstrating appropriate palpation techniques, and demonstrating appropriate auscultation techniques.

Dried blood on face from missing teeth; abrasion on tip of nose; abrasion on chin; upper lip slightly swollen. Both upper central incisors disrupted.	18. Inspects AND palpates head AND face for injuries	___		___
"I'll maintain stabilization while you assess the neck" No abnormalities	19. Inspects AND palpates neck for injuries	___		___
Ecchymosis on left anterior lower chest. No crepitus.	20. Inspects AND palpates chest for injuries	___		___
Breath sounds diminished in left base. Heart sounds normal.	21. Auscultates breath AND heart sounds	___		___
Faint ecchymosis on left upper quadrant	22. Inspects the abdomen for injuries	___		___
Bowel sounds absent	23. Auscultates bowel sounds	___		___

Instructor Responses	Skill Steps	Demonstrated		
		Yes		No
Tenderness in left upper quadrant and pain in left shoulder with palpation, abdomen nondistended and soft	24. Palpates all four quadrants of the abdomen for injuries	_____		_____
Abrasion on left iliac crest. No tenderness to palpation.	25. Inspects AND palpates the pelvis for injuries	_____		_____
No abnormalities	26. Inspects the perineum for injuries	_____		_____
No abnormalities to lower extremities. Normal neurovascular status in lower extremities. Edema with mild deformity of left distal forearm. No other injuries to other extremities. Normal neurovascular status in all extremities.	27. Inspects AND palpates all four extremities for neurovascular status and injuries	_____		_____
	28. Describes method to maintain spinal stabilization when patient is logrolled	_____		_____
No abnormalities	29. Inspects AND palpates posterior surfaces for injuries	_____		_____
"The team is completing spinal immobilization. Proceed with your assessment."	30. States need to complete spinal immobilization	_____		_____
Fell two stories striking his chest on the railing and then falling to the deck. No past medical history; no allergies; immunizations current	31. States need to obtain a history using: ● MIVT ● CIAMPEDS	_____		_____

Instructor response: "You have identified certain injuries during the assessment. Now that you have completed the secondary assessment, list five additional diagnostic studies or interventions for this patient."

Note to instructor: If the learner has previously identified any of the appropriate diagnostic studies or interventions listed, include the diagnostic study or intervention in the total of five.

Instructor Responses	Skill Steps	Demonstrated		
		Yes		No
	32. Identifies appropriate diagnostic studies or interventions (at least five of the following):	*_____		_____
	• Forearm radiograph			
	• Calculate Pediatric Coma Scale score and Revised Trauma Score			
	• Cervical spine radiograph			
	• Chest radiograph			
	• Clean and dress abrasions			
	• Continue to provide psychosocial support to the family			
	• Computerized tomography scan of the chest and abdomen			
	• Computerized tomography scan of the chest			
	• Dental consultation			
	• Laboratory studies			
	• Pain control measures			
	• Prepare for admission or transfer			
	• Splint, elevate, and ice extremity			
Instructor response: "What is the evaluation and ongoing assessment for this patient?"				
	33. States need to re-evaluate primary assessment	_____		_____
	34. States need to re-evaluate vital signs	_____		_____

MULTIPLE TRAUMA INTERVENTION

Teaching Case B

Prehospital Radio Report:

An advanced life-support ambulance is en route with an 18-month-old toddler from a motor vehicle crash. The child was being held in the mother's arms and was thrown against the dashboard. Both parents are unconscious at the scene. The Pediatric Assessment Triangle reveals that she responds to verbal stimuli but appears sleepy, her respirations are unlabored, and her skin is pale. She moves all extremities. Her blood pressure is 78/54 mm Hg, her pulse is 190 beats/minute, and her respiratory rate is 44 breaths/minute. A contusion is noted in the right parietal area. The child is immobilized on a half backboard with a rigid cervical collar. Oxygen is being administered via nonrebreather mask. The patient has just arrived in the emergency department. Please proceed with your primary and secondary assessments and appropriate interventions.

Instructor Responses	Skill Steps	Demonstrated		
		Yes		**No**
	1. **Assesses airway patency while maintaining spinal immobilization (at least three of the following):**	** _____		_____
Crying and gurgling	• **Vocalization**			
No tongue obstruction; vomitus noted in mouth	• **Tongue obstruction**			
No loose teeth; vomitus noted	• **Loose teeth or foreign objects**			
Vomitus noted	• **Vomitus or other secretions**			
No bleeding; vomitus noted	• **Bleeding**			
No edema	• **Edema**			
No drooling; vomitus noted	• **Drooling**			
No dysphagia	• **Dysphagia**			
Mild snoring	• **Abnormal airway sounds**			
	2. **Demonstrates suctioning the airway**	** _____		_____
Instructor response: "The airway is now patent."				

Instructor Responses	Skill Steps	Demonstrated		
		Yes		No
	3. Assesses breathing effectiveness (at least three of the following):	** ____		____
Opens eyes to verbal stimuli	● **Level of consciousness**			
Present	● **Spontaneous breathing**			
Respiratory rate 44 breaths/minute and shallow	● **Rate and depth of respirations**			
Symmetric chest rise and fall	● **Symmetric chest rise and fall**			
Equal and clear bilaterally	● **Presence and quality of breath sounds**			
	● **Work of breathing (at least three of the following):**			
No nasal flaring	■ **Nasal flaring**			
No intercostal retractions	■ **Retractions**			
No expiratory grunting	■ **Expiratory grunting**			
No accessory muscle use	■ **Accessory muscle use**			
No jugular vein distention; trachea midline	● **Jugular vein distention and tracheal position**			
No paradoxical respirations	● **Paradoxical respirations**			
Ecchymosis on right lower chest; bony chest wall integrity intact	● **Soft tissue and bony chest wall integrity**			
	4. **States need to continue oxygen via nonrebreather mask**	** ____		____
	5. **Assesses perfusion status (at least two of the following):**	** ____		____
Central pulses present at 190 beats/minute; peripheral pulses difficult to palpate	● **Central AND peripheral pulse rate and quality**			
Skin pale and cool	● **Skin color AND temperature**			
Capillary refill 4 seconds	● **Capillary refill**			
No uncontrolled bleeding	6. **Inspects for uncontrolled external bleeding**	____		____
Intravenous access obtained	7. **States need to obtain vascular access at two sites**	** ____		____
Fluid bolus administered	8. **States need to administer a 20-ml/kg fluid bolus**	____		____
	9. **Obtains blood sample for typing**	____		____
	10. **Reassesses perfusion status (at least two of the following):**	____		____
Central pulse 188 beats/minute; peripheral pulses remain absent	● **Central AND peripheral pulse rate and quality**			
Skin pale and cool	● **Skin color AND temperature**			
Capillary refill 4 seconds	● **Capillary refill**			
Fluid bolus administered	11. **States need to administer a repeat 20-ml/kg fluid bolus**	____		____

Instructor Responses	Skill Steps	Demonstrated		
		Yes		No
Central pulse 170 beats/minute; peripheral pulses palpable Skin pale but warmer Capillary refill 3 seconds	12. Reassesses perfusion status (at least two of the following): ● **Central AND peripheral pulse rate and quality** ● **Skin color AND temperature** ● **Capillary refill**	_____		_____
Instructor response if the learner has administered the second fluid bolus: "The patient is demonstrating improvement. Continue with your assessment."				
Responds to verbal stimuli	13. **Assesses level of consciousness (AVPU)**	******____		_____
Pupils equal and reactive	14. **Assesses pupils**	_____		_____
Secondary Assessment				
Multiple abrasions	15. **Removes all clothing**	_____		_____
	16. **States one measure to prevent heat loss:** ● **Warm blankets** ● **Overhead warming lights or other warming device** ● **Warm ambient environment** ● **Warm intravenous fluids** ● **Warm humidified oxygen**	*_____		_____
BP = 74/50 mm Hg P = 160 beats/minute R = 40 breaths/minute Rectal T = 36.6°C (97.8°F) Weight = 14 kg, estimated by length-based resuscitation tape	17. **States need to get a complete set of vital signs**	_____		_____
Electrocardiogram = normal sinus rhythm	18. **Places cardiac monitor leads on patient and evaluates rhythm**	_____		_____
Oxygen saturation 95% on a nonrebreather mask	19. **Places pulse oximeter on patient**	_____		_____
Crying at intervals, difficult to assess	20. **States need to evaluate for presence of pain or discomfort**	_____		_____
Demonstrates and describes the head-to-toe assessment by describing appropriate inspection techniques (e.g., lacerations, abrasions, contusions, ecchymosis), demonstrating appropriate palpation techniques, and demonstrating appropriate auscultation techniques.				
Instructor response: "Based on the patient's current perfusion status and vital signs, the trauma surgeon has decided to administer packed red blood cells for transfusion. The team is administering the fluid. Continue with your head-to-toe assessment."				
Hematoma palpated on occiput. Contusion to right forehead; pieces of glass noted in hair. Multiple abrasions on face.	21. **Inspects AND palpates head AND face for injuries**	_____		_____

Instructor Responses	Skill Steps	Demonstrated		
		Yes		No
"I'll maintain stabilization while you assess the neck" No abnormalities *"I'll replace the collar"*	22. Inspects AND palpates neck for injuries	————		————
Ecchymosis on right lower chest. No crepitus.	23. Inspects AND palpates chest for injuries	————		————
Breath sounds clear and equal bilaterally. Heart sounds normal.	24. Auscultates breath AND heart sounds	————		————
Ecchymosis on right upper quadrant	25. Inspects the abdomen for injuries	————		————
Bowel sounds absent	26. Auscultates bowel sounds	————		————
Abdomen flat and firm. Cries during palpation of right upper quadrant.	27. Palpates all four quadrants of the abdomen for injuries	————		————
No abnormalities	28. Inspects AND palpates the pelvis for injuries	————		————
No abnormalities	29. Inspects the perineum for injuries	————		————
Scattered abrasions. Moving legs, normal pulses; capillary refill 3 seconds in lower extremities. Moving upper extremities; capillary refill 3 seconds in upper extremities.	30. Inspects AND palpates all four extremities for neurovascular status and injuries	————		————
	31. Describes method to maintain spinal stabilization when patient is logrolled	————		————
No abnormalities	32. Inspects AND palpates posterior surfaces for injuries	————		————
Paramedics state she was sitting in the right front passenger seat being held by mother. Windshield spidered. Moderate damage to front end of car. No family available. Moving upper extremities, capillary refill 3 seconds in upper extremities.	33. States need to obtain a history using: ● MIVT ● CIAMPEDS	————		————
	34. States need to consider insertion of gastric tube	————		————
Urinary catheter inserted	35. States need to insert urinary catheter	————		————

Instructor response: "140 ml of packed red cells are being infused. Capillary refill is now 2 seconds. Pulse is 140 beats/minute; blood pressure is 86/56 mm Hg. Skin is pale and warm. You have identified certain injuries during the assessment. Now that you have completed the secondary assessment, list five additional diagnostic studies or interventions for this patient."

Note to instructor: If the learner has previously identified any of the appropriate diagnostic studies or interventions listed, include the diagnostic study or intervention in the total of five.

Instructor Responses	Skill Steps	Demonstrated		
		Yes		No
	36. **Identifies appropriate diagnostic studies or interventions (at least five of the following):**	*_____		_____
	● **Calculate Pediatric Coma Scale score and Revised Trauma Score**			
	● **Cervical spine radiograph**			
	● **Chest radiograph**			
	● **Clean and dress abrasions**			
	● **Consider the need for operative intervention**			
	● **Computerized tomography scan of the abdomen**			
	● **Computerized tomography scan of the head**			
	● **Laboratory studies**			
	● **Pain management and sedation measures**			
	● **Pelvis radiograph**			
	● **Prepare for admission or transfer**			
Instructor response: "What is the evaluation and ongoing assessment for this patient?"				
	37. States need to re-evaluate primary assessment	_____		_____
	38. States need to re-evaluate vital signs	_____		_____

MULTIPLE TRAUMA INTERVENTION

Teaching Case C

Prehospital Radio Report:

An advanced life-support ambulance is en route with a 6-year-old child who was riding a bike and was struck by a van. The child is unresponsive. His right upper leg is swollen and deformed, but pedal pulses are good. The child's color is pale, with capillary refill of 3 seconds. His blood pressure is 110/70 mm Hg, his pulse is 120 beats/minute, and his respirations are 20 breaths/minute. He is immobilized on a backboard with a rigid cervical collar. Oxygen is being administered via nonrebreather mask at 15 liters/minute. Intravenous access is obtained, and 500 ml lactated Ringer's solution is infused. The right femur is splinted.

He has just arrived in the emergency department. The Pediatric Assessment Triangle reveals that he is unresponsive, exhibits snoring respirations, and is pale. A support person responds to the trauma room to provide support to the family. Please proceed with your primary and secondary assessments and appropriate interventions.

Instructor Responses	Skill Steps	Demonstrated		
		Yes		No
	1. Demonstrates manually opening the airway	_____		_____
	2. Assesses airway patency while maintaining spinal immobilization (at least three of the following):	** _____		_____
Not vocalizing; gurgling noted	• Vocalization			
Snoring respirations resolved with jaw thrust; vomitus noted	• Tongue obstruction			
No loose teeth or foreign objects; vomitus noted	• Loose teeth or foreign objects			
Vomitus noted in mouth	• Vomitus or other secretions			
No bleeding; vomitus noted	• Bleeding			
No edema; vomitus noted	• Edema			
No drooling; vomitus noted	• Drooling			
No dysphagia	• Dysphagia			
Snoring respirations resolved; gurgling noted	• Abnormal airway sounds			
	3. Demonstrates suctioning the airway	** _____		_____
Instructor response: "The airway is patent and spinal immobilization is being maintained."				

Instructor Responses	Skill Steps	Demonstrated		
		Yes		No
	4. Assesses breathing effectiveness (at least three of the following):	** _____		_____
Unresponsive	● **Level of consciousness**			
Present but slow and shallow	● **Spontaneous breathing**			
Respirations slowing to 14 breaths/minute and shallow	● **Rate and depth of respirations**			
Symmetric chest rise and fall, but shallow	● **Symmetric chest rise and fall**			
Equal but diminished bilaterally	● **Presence and quality of breath sounds**			
	● **Work of breathing (at least three of the following):**			
No nasal flaring	■ **Nasal flaring**			
No intercostal retractions	■ **Retractions**			
No expiratory grunting	■ **Expiratory grunting**			
No accessory muscle use	■ **Accessory muscle use**			
No jugular vein distention; trachea midline	● **Jugular vein distention and tracheal position**			
No paradoxical respirations but shallow	● **Paradoxical respirations**			
No soft tissue injury; bony chest wall intact	● **Soft tissue and bony chest wall integrity**			
	5. Demonstrates bag-valve-mask ventilation with 100% oxygen	**		_____
	6. Assesses effectiveness of assisted ventilations:	_____		_____
Bilateral chest rise and fall	● **Chest rise and fall**			
Breath sounds present	● **Presence of breath sounds**			
	7. States need for intubation	_____		_____

Instructor response: "The team is preparing the equipment and medications for rapid sequence induction for intubation. Please continue your assessment."

Instructor Responses	Skill Steps	Demonstrated		
	8. Assesses perfusion status (at least two of the following):	** _____		_____
Central pulses present at 110 beats/minute; peripheral pulses strong	● **Central AND peripheral pulse rate and quality**			
Skin pale and warm	● **Skin color AND temperature**			
Capillary refill 2 seconds	● **Capillary refill**			
No uncontrolled bleeding	**9. Inspects for uncontrolled external bleeding**	_____		_____
Prehospital intravenous access patent	**10. Assesses patency of prehospital intravenous access**	_____		_____
Intravenous access obtained	**11. States need to obtain a second vascular access**	** _____		_____

Instructor Responses	Skill Steps	Demonstrated		
		Yes		No
	12. Infuses fluid at a maintenance rate	_____		_____
	13. Obtains blood sample for typing	_____		_____
Instructor response: "The child is now intubated. Demonstrate and describe your immediate evaluation of endotracheal tube placement."				
Symmetric chest rise and fall Bilateral equal breath sounds; epigastric sounds absent End-tidal CO_2 device placed; reading indicates positive placement	14. Demonstrates and describes endotracheal tube placement (at least two of the following): ● Observes chest rise and fall ● Listens for breath sounds in the axillary areas and over epigastric area ● Assesses end-tidal CO_2 via monitor or device (if available)	_____		_____
Unresponsive	15. Assesses level of consciousness (AVPU)	**_____		_____
Pupils midposition and sluggish	16. Assesses pupils	_____		_____
Secondary Assessment				
Multiple abrasions to upper and lower extremities; deformity on right femur	17. Removes all clothing	_____		_____
	18. States one measure to prevent heat loss: ● Warm blankets ● Overhead warming lights or other warming device ● Warm ambient environment ● Warm intravenous fluids ● Warm humidified oxygen	*_____		_____
BP = 110/70 mm Hg P = 100 beats/minute R = ventilations assisted at 24 breaths/minute Rectal T = 37.4°C (99.3°F) Weight = 23 kg, estimated by length-based resuscitation tape	19. States need to get a complete set of vital signs	_____		_____
Electrocardiogram = normal sinus rhythm	20. Places cardiac monitor leads on patient and evaluates rhythm	_____		_____
Oxygen saturation 100% with assisted ventilations	21. Places pulse oximeter on patient	_____		_____
Rapid sequence induction included the administration of an analgesic, sedative, and paralytic; adequately sedated at this time	22. States need to evaluate for presence of pain or discomfort	_____		_____

Demonstrates and describes the head-to-toe assessment by describing appropriate inspection techniques (e.g., lacerations, abrasions, contusions, ecchymosis), demonstrating appropriate palpation techniques, and demonstrating appropriate auscultation techniques.

Instructor Responses	Skill Steps	Demonstrated		
		Yes		No
Boggy area with palpable step-off in left parietal area; bleeding from left ear; multiple abrasions on left side of face	23. Inspects AND palpates head AND face for injuries	_____		_____
"I'll maintain stabilization while you assess the neck" No abnormalities *"I'll replace the collar"*	24. Inspects AND palpates neck for injuries	_____		_____
No abnormalities. No crepitus.	25. Inspects AND palpates chest for injuries	_____		_____
Breath sounds clear and equal bilaterally with assisted ventilations. Heart sounds normal.	26. Auscultates breath AND heart sounds	_____		_____
No abnormalities noted	27. Inspects the abdomen for injuries	_____		_____
Bowel sounds present in all quadrants	28. Auscultates bowel sounds	_____		_____
Abdomen soft and nondistended	29. Palpates all four quadrants of the abdomen for injuries	_____		_____
No abnormalities noted	30. Inspects AND palpates the pelvis for injuries	_____		_____
No abnormalities	31. Inspects the perineum for injuries	_____		_____
Scattered abrasions. Deformity on right thigh. Normal pulse and brisk capillary refill in lower extremities. Right leg splinted. Normal pulses and brisk capillary refill in upper extremities.	32. Inspects AND palpates all four extremities for neurovascular status and injuries	_____		_____
	33. Describes method to maintain spinal stabilization when patient is logrolled	_____		_____
No abnormalities	34. Inspects AND palpates posterior surfaces for injuries	_____		_____
Paramedics report that child crossed in front of the van, which was traveling at approximately 25 mph. Patient struck by left front bumper. Was witnessed to be thrown approximately 10 feet, striking his head on the curb. He was not wearing a helmet. No allergies or medications; no medical history. Immunizations current. Last food consumed 2 hours prior to crash.	35. States need to obtain a history using: ● **MIVT** ● **CIAMPEDS**	_____		_____

Instructor Responses	Skill Steps	Demonstrated		
		Yes		No
Gastric tube inserted	36. **States need to insert gastric tube**	_____		_____
Urinary catheter inserted	37. **States need to insert urinary catheter**	_____		_____
Instructor response: "You have identified certain injuries during the assessment. Now that you have completed the secondary assessment, list five additional diagnostic studies or interventions for this patient." Note to instructor: If the learner has previously identified any of the appropriate diagnostic studies or interventions listed, include the diagnostic study or intervention in the total of five.				
	38. **Identifies appropriate diagnostic studies or interventions (at least five of the following):** • **Arterial blood gas** • **Calculate Pediatric Coma Scale score and Revised Trauma Score** • **Cervical spine radiograph** • **Chest radiograph** • **Clean and dress abrasions** • **Continue to provide psychosocial support to the family** • **Computerized tomography scan of the head; consider computerized tomography scan of the abdomen** • **End-tidal CO_2 monitoring** • **Femur radiograph** • **Laboratory studies** • **Pain management and sedation measures** • **Pelvis radiograph** • **Prepare for admission or transfer** • **Prepare for possible operative intervention**	*_____		_____
Instructor response: "What is the evaluation and ongoing assessment for this patient?"				
	39. **States need to re-evaluate primary assessment**	_____		_____
	40. **States need to re-evaluate vital signs**	_____		_____

MULTIPLE TRAUMA INTERVENTION

Teaching Case D

Parents bring in a 12-year-old adolescent who was driving a small motorized minibike and was thrown from the bike. The parents bring him in to triage in a wheelchair. The Pediatric Assessment Triangle reveals that he is alert, his respirations are rapid and shallow, and his skin is pale. He is complaining of pain in the left flank. He is immediately placed in the trauma room. A support person responds to the trauma room to provide family support. Please proceed with your primary and secondary assessments and appropriate interventions.

Note to instructor: The case was developed to reflect an adolescent scenario; do not change the age in the scenario. An adult mannikin may be used.

Instructor Responses	Skill Steps	Demonstrated		
		Yes		No
	1. **Assesses airway patency AND initiates cervical spine stabilization (at least three of the following):**	** ____		____
Answering questions	● **Vocalization**			
No tongue obstruction	● **Tongue obstruction**			
No loose teeth	● **Loose teeth or foreign objects**			
No vomitus or other secretions	● **Vomitus or other secretions**			
No bleeding	● **Bleeding**			
No edema	● **Edema**			
No drooling	● **Drooling**			
No dysphagia	● **Dysphagia**			
No abnormal sounds	● **Abnormal airway sounds**			
Instructor response: "The airway is patent. The cervical spine is being manually stabilized."				

Instructor Responses	Skill Steps	Demonstrated		
		Yes		No
	2. Assesses breathing effectiveness (at least three of the following):	** _____		_____
Alert	● **Level of consciousness**			
Present	● **Spontaneous breathing**			
Respiratory rate 28 breaths/minute and shallow	● **Rate and depth of respirations**			
Asymmetric chest rise and fall on left	● **Symmetric chest rise and fall**			
Breath sounds diminished on left	● **Presence and quality of breath sounds**			
	● **Work of breathing (at least three of the following):**			
Mild nasal flaring	■ **Nasal flaring**			
Intercostal retractions	■ **Retractions**			
No expiratory grunting	■ **Expiratory grunting**			
Accessory muscle use	■ **Accessory muscle use**			
No jugular vein distention; trachea midline	● **Jugular vein distention and tracheal position**			
No paradoxical respirations	● **Paradoxical respirations**			
Ecchymosis on left, lateral lower chest	● **Soft tissue and bony chest wall integrity**			
	3. States need for oxygen via nonrebreather mask	** _____		_____
	4. States need to prepare for chest tube insertion	_____		_____
	5. Assesses perfusion status (at least two of the following):	** _____		_____
Central pulse present at 126 beats/minute; peripheral pulses present	● **Central AND peripheral pulse rate and quality**			
Skin pale and warm	● **Skin color AND temperature**			
Capillary refill 2 seconds	● **Capillary refill**			
No uncontrolled bleeding	**6. Inspects for uncontrolled external bleeding**	_____		_____
Intravenous access obtained	**7. States need to obtain vascular access at two sites**	** _____		_____
Fluid bolus administered	**8. States need to administer a 20-ml/kg fluid bolus**	_____		_____
	9. Obtains blood sample for typing	_____		_____
	10. Reassesses perfusion status (at least two of the following):	_____		_____
Central pulse 110 beats/minute; peripheral pulses present	● **Central AND peripheral pulse rate and quality**			
Skin pale and warm	● **Skin color AND temperature**			
Capillary refill 2 seconds	● **Capillary refill**			

Instructor Responses	Skill Steps	Demonstrated		
		Yes		No
Alert	11. Assesses level of consciousness (AVPU)	**_____		_____
Pupils equal and reactive	12. Assesses pupils	_____		_____
Instructor response: "A chest tube is inserted and an immediate rush of air is obtained. Minimal bleeding is noted from the chest tube. The chest tube is connected to a drainage unit. Describe the appropriate reassessment of the patient following placement of a chest tube."				
	13. Reassesses breathing effectiveness (at least three of the following):	_____		_____
Awake	● Level of consciousness			
Present	● Spontaneous breathing			
Rate 20 breaths/minute	● Rate and depth of respirations			
Symmetric chest rise and fall	● Symmetric chest rise and fall			
Equal breath sounds	● Presence and quality of breath sounds			
	● Work of breathing (at least three of the following):			
No nasal flaring	■ Nasal flaring			
No retractions	■ Retractions			
No expiratory grunting	■ Expiratory grunting			
No accessory muscle use	■ Accessory muscle use			
No jugular vein distention; trachea midline	● Jugular vein distention and tracheal position			
No paradoxical movement	● Paradoxical movement			
Secondary Assessment				
Multiple abrasions	14. Removes all clothing	_____		_____
	15. States one measure to prevent heat loss:	*_____		_____
	● Warm blankets			
	● Overhead warming lights or other warming device			
	● Warm ambient environment			
	● Warm intravenous fluids			
	● Warm humidified oxygen			
BP = 110/70 mm Hg P = 100 beats/minute R = 20 breaths/minute Oral T = 37°C (98.6°F) Weight = 58 kg	16. States need to get a complete set of vital signs	_____		_____
Electrocardiogram = normal sinus rhythm	17. Places cardiac monitor leads on patient and evaluates rhythm	_____		_____
Oxygen saturation 98% on a nonrebreather mask	18. Places pulse oximeter on patient	_____		_____

Instructor Responses	Skill Steps	Demonstrated		
		Yes		No
Rates pain at chest tube site at 8 on a scale of 1 to 10; an analgesic is ordered	19. States need to evaluate for presence of pain or discomfort	————		————
Demonstrates and describes the head-to-toe assessment by describing appropriate inspection techniques (e.g., lacerations, abrasions, contusions, ecchymosis), demonstrating appropriate palpation techniques, and demonstrating appropriate auscultation techniques.				
No abnormalities; he was wearing a helmet	20. Inspects AND palpates head AND face for injuries	————		————
"I'll maintain stabilization while you assess the neck" No abnormalities	21. Inspects AND palpates neck for injuries	————		————
Ecchymosis on left, lower lateral chest. Mild crepitus and subcutaneous emphysema over ecchymotic area.	22. Inspects AND palpates chest for injuries	————		————
Breath sounds clear and equal bilaterally. Heart sounds normal.	23. Auscultates breath AND heart sounds	————		————
Abrasion extending down left lateral aspect of abdomen	24. Inspects the abdomen for injuries	————		————
Bowel sounds present	25. Auscultates bowel sounds	————		————
Abdomen flat; tender to palpation in left upper quadrant	26. Palpates all four quadrants of the abdomen for injuries	————		————
No abnormalities	27. Inspects AND palpates the pelvis for injuries	————		————
No abnormalities	28. Inspects the perineum for injuries	————		————
3-cm laceration to left lower leg. Normal neurovascular status in lower extremities. Normal neurovascular status in upper extremities.	29. Inspects AND palpates all four extremities for neurovascular status and injuries	————		————
	30. Describes method to maintain spinal stabilization when patient is logrolled	————		————
Ecchymosis on left lateral back. CVA tenderness present with palpation.	31. Inspects AND palpates posterior surfaces for injuries	————		————
"The team is completing spinal immobilization"	32. States need to complete spinal immobilization	————		————
	33. States need to obtain a history using:	————		————
Patient states he struck a rock and lost control of the bike, propelling him forward over the handlebars. He was wearing a helmet.	• MIVT			
History of asthma; last ate 4 hours ago. Medications – inhalers; allergies – environmental. Current on immunizations.	• CIAMPEDS			

Instructor Responses	Skill Steps	Demonstrated		
		Yes		No
	34. States need to consider insertion of urinary catheter	_____		_____

Instructor response: "You have identified certain injuries during the assessment. Now that you have completed the secondary assessment, list five additional diagnostic studies or interventions for this patient."

Note to instructor: If the learner has previously identified any of the appropriate diagnostic studies or interventions listed, include the diagnostic study or intervention in the total of five.

	Skill Steps	Yes		No
	35. Identifies appropriate diagnostic studies or interventions (at least five of the following):	*_____		_____
	• Calculates Pediatric Coma Scale score and Revised Trauma Score			
	• Cervical spine radiograph			
	• Chest radiograph			
	• Clean and suture laceration			
	• Continue psychosocial support for the family			
	• Computerized tomography scan of the abdomen			
	• Laboratory studies; urinalysis			
	• Pain management and sedation measures			
	• Pelvis radiograph			
	• Prepare for admission or transfer			

Instructor response: "What is the evaluation and ongoing assessment for this patient?"

	Skill Steps	Yes		No
	36. States need to re-evaluate primary assessment	_____		_____
	37. States need to re-evaluate vital signs	_____		_____

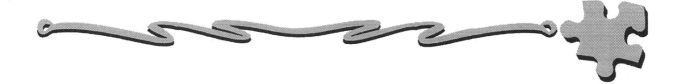

Emergency Nursing Pediatric Course

Triage Skill Station

EQUIPMENT FOR THE STATION

- One table
- Five to seven chairs
- Pictures that correspond to the case scenarios

STATION PREPARATION

1. Place chairs around the table.

2. Display scenario pictures on table.

3. Display A through I and CIAMPEDS mnemonics on a chalkboard, flipchart, or poster.

INTRODUCTION TO THE SKILL STATION

1. The instructor will discuss:

   - The assessment using the Pediatric Assessment Triangle
   - The triage physical assessment
   - The triage history
   - The triage decision

2. Learners will work in pairs during the teaching station to complete the triage assessment. However, each learner will be evaluated separately.

3. Given three assessments using the Pediatric Assessment Triangle, learners (working in groups of two or three) will complete a triage assessment. Only one patient will be discussed at any given time. Show the learners the photograph of each patient that corresponds to the assessment triangle.

4. The instructor will respond to the learners' questions about the patients. As the learners ask a question, the instructor will provide specific information. If the information is not available, the instructor will assume there are no significant findings.

5. Learners may use the CIAMPEDS mnemonic to obtain the history or any other method they choose.

6. The instructor will inform the learners that the ability to recognize the sick child, based on the Pediatric Assessment Triangle, is not being tested. The learners may begin by selecting any of the three scenarios.

7. The instructor will inform the learners that, for the purposes of this station, pulse oximetry is not available in the triage area. However, the area is secluded to allow a limited physical assessment (e.g., lifting the shirt to assess the chest and abdomen). Discussions regarding the learner's triage settings, personnel, training, or equipment requirements at their institution should be avoided.

8. The instructor will inform the learners that, once they have asked all of their questions and have begun assessment of another patient, they may not return to the previous patient.

9. The instructor will inform the learners that, once they have finished the assessment of all three patients, the learners will determine the priority of treatment. If the learners state, "I would take them all back," or something similar, the instructor will respond with, "You can do that, however, what is your order of priority for care?"

10. The instructor will inform the learners that they do not need to determine a medical diagnosis. Instead, determining the triage priority is the goal of the station.

11. The instructor will inform the learners to record the information as it is obtained in the appropriate area on the flow sheet. A sample completed flow sheet can be found at the end of this skill station.

    - There is a column for history and physical assessment for each patient.

    - It may be helpful to tell learners to abbreviate the information that they are recording (e.g., entering "normal" in the appropriate area on the flow sheet rather than the comprehensive information).

    - The chief complaint and scenario are printed at the top of the flow sheet. There are two blank flow sheets in the Provider manual (one for each teaching set). A flow sheet with the responses is also included as a study tool for learners.

PRINCIPLES OF TRIAGE AND INITIAL ASSESSMENT

1. Observation of the child's status should occur before the child is touched. This is referred to as the Pediatric Assessment Triangle ("across-the-room assessment") and includes:

    - General appearance – What is the general impression the triage nurse perceives when initially looking at the child? Does the child look well or look ill, or is the triage nurse not sure?

    - Airway status – What is the position of comfort to facilitate air entry? Are there audible upper airway sounds, such as stridor or snoring? If stridor is present, what is the potential for a foreign body to be the cause? If the child is coughing, what does the cough sound like? Is it productive, is it dry, or does it have a barking quality?

- Breathing status – Is the respiratory rate within normal limits for this child's age, or is the rate too slow or too fast? Are the respirations shallow or deep? Are signs of accessory muscle use evident (with clothing on)? Is the child's skin color normal, pale, or dusky?

- Circulatory status – Is the child flushed, normal color, mottled, or dusky? Is there any obvious bleeding?

- Disability (brief neurologic assessment) – Is the child running, walking, requiring assistance to ambulate, or being held? Is the child alert, irritable, or sleepy? Is the muscle tone good or are the extremities flaccid?

2. The triage assessment starts with a rapid evaluation of the primary assessment. If the child has life-threatening alterations, the child is immediately taken to a resuscitation area. Tables 44 and 45 describe the A through I assessment and the initial physical assessment in triage.

3. The history is obtained from the caregiver of the infant or young child or from both the caregiver and older child or adolescent. The CIAMPEDS mnemonic (see Table 46) organizes the components of the basic pediatric history.

4. The following findings are emergent or urgent findings:

- Signs of airway obstruction

- Signs of moderate or severe respiratory distress

- Pallor or mottled skin color with delayed capillary refill

- Lethargy; decreased response to environment; decreased response to pain

- "Paradoxical irritability" (inability to comfort child)

- Bulging or sunken anterior fontanelle in infants

- Fever higher than 38°C (100.4°F) in any infant younger than 2 to 3 months of age

- Hypothermia in the neonate

- History inconsistent with illness or injury

- History of existing illness such as sickle cell disease, cystic fibrosis, or congenital heart defect

Table 44

PRIMARY ASSESSMENT

A = Airway

Assess:
- Vocalization
- Tongue obstruction
- Loose teeth or foreign objects
- Vomitus or other secretions
- Preferred posture
- Bleeding
- Edema
- Drooling
- Dysphagia
- Abnormal airway sounds (stridor or snoring)

B = Breathing

Assess:
- Level of consciousness
- Spontaneous breathing
- Rate and depth of respirations
- Symmetric chest rise and fall
- Presence and quality of breath sounds
- Work of breathing:
  - Nasal flaring
  - Retractions
  - Head bobbing
  - Expiratory grunting
  - Accessory muscle use
- Jugular vein distention and tracheal position
- Paradoxical respirations
- Soft tissue and bony chest wall integrity

C = Circulation

Assess:
- Central and peripheral pulse rate and quality
- Skin color and temperature
- Capillary refill
- Uncontrolled external hemorrhage

D = Disability

Assess:
- Level of consciousness (AVPU)
- Pupils

Table 45

SECONDARY ASSESSMENT
In some circumstances, modification of the secondary assessment may be necessary in the triage area because of space, privacy, or time limitations. Any components of the secondary assessment not completed during the triage process may be completed when the patient is placed in the treatment area.
E = Exposure and Environmental Control
Observe for: ● Obvious underlying injuries. ● Additional signs of illness. ● Heat loss. Initiate measure to maintain normothermia.
F = Full Set of Vital Signs
Measure complete set of vital signs: Respiratory rate, heart rate, temperature, blood pressure, and weight.
F = Family Presence
● Identify the family members and their relationship to the child. ● Assess the needs of the family, the need for additional support, and the desire to remain with the child.
G = Give Comfort Measures
Evaluate the presence and level of pain and discomfort (physical and psychological); initiate measures to relieve pain.
H = Head-to-Toe Assessment
Perform a focused head-to-toe assessment. At triage, the head-to-toe assessment is guided by the chief complaint, history, and assessment findings of the primary assessment.
H = History
Obtain the history using the CIAMPEDS format.
I = Inspect Posterior Surface
Inspect for rashes, petechia, edema; palpate for tenderness.

Table 46

TRIAGE HISTORY	
Format	**Questions**
(C) Chief Complaint	Why was the child brought to the emergency department? What is the primary problem or concern and duration of complaint?
(I) Immunizations	Are they up to date? When were they last given?
Isolation	Has the child recently been exposed to any communicable diseases?
(A) Allergies	Does the child have any known allergies? Is the child allergic to any medications? What was the child's reaction to the medication?
(M) Medications	Is the child taking any prescription drugs or over-the-counter drugs (e.g., acetaminophen)? When was the last dose administered and how much was given? Is the child on immunosuppressive medications?
(P) Past Medical History	Does the child have a history of any significant illness, injury, or hospitalization? Does the child have a known chronic illness?
Parents Impression of Child's Condition	What is different about the child's condition that concerns the caregiver?
(E) Events Surrounding the Illness or Injury	How long has the child been ill? Was the onset rapid or slow? Has anyone else in the family been ill? If the emergency visit is for an injury, when did the injury occur, was it witnessed, and what happened?
(D) Diet	How much has the child been eating and drinking? When was the last time the child ate or drank?
Diapers	When was the child's last void? How much was it? When was the child's last bowel movement? What did it look like and how large was the stool?
(S) Symptoms Associated with the Illness or Injury	What other symptoms are present? When did the symptoms begin? Has the condition gotten better or worse?

STEPS IN THE SKILL PERFORMANCE

The instructor will tell the learners: "I am going to provide you with the findings of the Pediatric Assessment Triangle of three children. Please proceed through a systematic assessment of each child. As you ask questions, I will provide additional information. I will only provide the information that you request. When you have finished asking all of the questions related to one case scenario, you may proceed to the next patient. You will not be allowed to return to a previous patient. Once you have assessed all three children, you will be asked to prioritize their order of treatment. Here is the first set of case scenarios."

Triage Teaching Case Scenarios – Set #1

Case A: A 5-year-old boy is sitting in his father's lap while his mother waits in the triage line. He is pale, does not appear to be in respiratory distress, and has a dressing on the side of his head with a small amount of bloody drainage.

Case B: A mother is carrying a 3-year-old girl toward the triage desk. She is alert, her skin color is normal, and she is observing ED activities.

Case C: A male adolescent is standing with his mother in the triage line. His skin color is normal and he is coughing intermittently.

Triage Teaching Case Scenarios – Set #2

Case A: A woman is waiting in the triage line. She is holding a 3-week-old infant bundled in a blanket. The infant's skin color is normal.

Case B: A hysterical mother rushes toward the triage desk carrying a 19-month-old toddler. You notice a bandage over the eye. The child's skin color is normal.

Case C: You see a 12-year-old female adolescent sitting slumped in a chair. She appears tired, and her face is flushed. Her respirations are rapid and deep.

SUMMARY

1. During evaluation, learners are evaluated individually, not as a group as they were in the teaching station.

2. During evaluation, pencil or pen and paper will be provided for the learner to record his or her findings.

3. Each learner will be evaluated for his or her ability to correctly prioritize the order of treatment for the three patients. Therefore, learners should concentrate on understanding the principles of the station and not memorizing the specific case scenarios.

4. Learners may ask as few or as many questions as needed to determine the appropriate priority.

5. The learners should be reminded that, once they have asked all of their questions and have begun assessment of another patient, they may not return to the previous patient.

6. The learners should be informed that there are a variety of scenarios used during the evaluation station.

Triage Teaching Case Scenarios – Set #1

A 5-year-old boy is sitting in his father's lap while his mother waits in the triage line. He is pale, does not appear to be in respiratory distress, and has a dressing on the side of his head with a small amount of bloody drainage.

CASE A			
Chief Complaint: "He fell and hurt his head 1 hour ago."			
Physical		**History**	
A		I	
B		A	
C		M	
D		P	
E		E	
F		D	
G - I		S	

Triage Teaching Case Scenarios – Set #1

A mother is carrying a 3-year-old girl toward the triage desk. She is alert, her skin color is normal, and she is observing ED activities.

CASE B			
Chief Complaint: "He had a seizure just a little bit ago."			
Physical		**History**	
A		I	
B		A	
C		M	
D		P	
E		E	
F		D	
G - I		S	

Triage Teaching Case Scenarios – Set #1

A male adolescent is standing with his mother in the triage line. His skin color is normal and he is coughing intermittently.

CASE C			
Chief Complaint: "He has been wheezing since this morning."			
Physical		**History**	
A		I	
B		A	
C		M	
D		P	
E		E	
F		D	
G - I		S	

Triage Teaching Case Scenarios – Set #2

A woman is waiting in the triage line. She is holding a 3-week-old infant bundled in a blanket. The infant's skin color is normal.

CASE A			
Chief Complaints: "She has been fussy for 3 days, not eating and sleeping well."			
Physical		**History**	
A		I	
B		A	
C		M	
D		P	
E		E	
F		D	
G - I		S	

Triage Teaching Case Scenarios – Set #2

A hysterical mother rushes toward the triage desk carrying a 19-month-old toddler. You notice a bandage over the eye. The child's skin color is normal.

CASE B			
Chief Complaint: "My baby hit her head and it's bleeding."			
Physical		**History**	
A		I	
B		A	
C		M	
D		P	
E		E	
F		D	
G - I		S	

Triage Teaching Case Scenarios – Set #2

You see a 12-year-old female adolescent sitting slumped in a chair. She appears tired, and her face is flushed. Her respirations are rapid and deep.

CASE C			
Chief Complaint: "My daughter is just not feeling well. She has been too tired lately."			
Physical		**History**	
A		I	
B		A	
C		M	
D		P	
E		E	
F		D	
G - I		S	

Triage Teaching Case Scenarios – Set #1

A 5-year-old boy is sitting in his father's lap while his mother waits in the triage line. He is pale, does not appear to be in respiratory distress, and has a dressing on the side of his head with a small amount of bloody drainage.

CASE A			
Chief Complaint: "He fell and hurt his head 1 hour ago."			
Physical		**History**	
A	Clear.	I	Has completed the recommended vaccine series for age. No exposure to communicable diseases.
B	Respiratory rate of 24 breaths/minute, not labored; breath sounds clear to auscultation.	A	None.
C	Skin color pale, cool, and moist; capillary refill 2 seconds. Pulses regular with rate 110 beats/minute and strong. Heart sounds normal.	M	None.
D	Pupils equal and reactive. Unable to sit up – leans on dad or against back of chair; opens eyes when name is called but is not answering questions. Able to move all extremities.	P	Previously healthy with no underlying illness. Mom is concerned because he is not as active as usual.
E	Scalp laceration is 4 cm long and begins to ooze blood when the dressing is removed. No other noticeable injuries.	E	About 1 hour ago he tripped at school and hit his head against a metal fence. According to his mother, there is a laceration under the dressing.
F	Pulse – 110 beats/minute. Respiratory rate – 24 breaths/minute. Blood pressure – 100/60 mm Hg. Temperature – 37.1°C (98.8°F). Weight – 18 kg.	D	Ate a large lunch about 4 hours ago. Last void was several hours ago at school.
G - I	*(G)* Unable to assess presence of pain. *(H, I)* There are no additional findings on focused secondary assessment.	S	No loss of consciousness. Has vomited twice since he hit his head. Mom says that he is now acting sleepy and is just not himself. She states that he seemed confused at home.

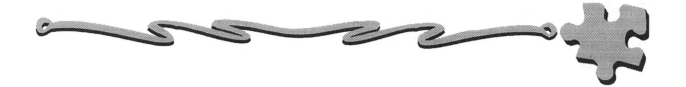

Emergency Nursing Pediatric Course

Pediatric Considerations Skill Station

EQUIPMENT FOR THE STATION

- One table
- Five to seven chairs
- One infant and one child mannikin
- One infant intubation mannikin
- One pillowcase
- One short backboard or pediatric immobilization board and three straps
- One lateral cervical immobilization device
- One rigid cervical collar (smallest size)
- One child restraint seat
- Three towels
- Three bath blankets
- One roll of adhesive tape
- Burn dressing or sheet
- One intraosseous needle
- One regular-drip intravenous tubing or blood tubing
- One 3-way stopcock
- One large syringe (20-ml or 35-ml)
- Intravenous catheters (24-gauge, 22-gauge, 20-gauge)
- One clear, occlusive intravenous dressing
- One 4 × 4-inch gauze pad
- One syringe (3-ml)
- One-inch needle (22-gauge)
- One-and-a-half-inch needle (19-gauge)

- Topical anesthetic agent and/or iontophoresis electrode (optional)

- One pulse oximeter probe

- Three electrocardiogram electrodes

- One end-tidal CO_2 detector (optional)

- One stethoscope

- One length-based resuscitation tape

- One oropharyngeal airway (variety of pediatric sizes)

- One tongue blade

- One simple oxygen mask (pediatric)

- One nonrebreather oxygen mask (pediatric)

- One suction catheter

- One rigid tonsil suction

- One bag-valve-mask device (1,000-ml)

- Resuscitation mask (sizes appropriate for scenario)

- Uncuffed endotracheal tubes (3.0-mm and 5.5-mm)

- One cuffed endotracheal tube (6.5-mm)

- One nebulizer with mask

- Metered-dose inhaler with spacer (optional)

- Distraction supplies: Bottle of bubbles, glitter wand, child's storybook (optional)
- Personal protective equipment

- One child or small adult blood pressure cuff (optional)

STATION PREPARATION

1. Assemble all equipment and ensure that it is in working order.

2. Arrange equipment and mannikins on the table.

3. Arrange chairs to separate learners into two teams.

    - If the group has six learners, two teams of three or three teams of two may be organized.

    - If the group has fewer than four learners, the learners may function as one team.

4. Place the table and equipment in a location that is conducive for the team to demonstrate selected skills. Arrange in a manner that allows all learners to observe the skill being demonstrated.

5. The case scenarios and questions are on pages 409-415 of this manual.

INTRODUCTION TO THE SKILL STATION

1. The instructor will inform the learners that this is a teaching station.

2. The instructor will read the case scenarios and corresponding questions to the learners. The learners will demonstrate the skill specified in the scenario. The following strategies may be used to select the order of the scenarios and questions presented:

    *   The instructor may randomly present questions from each category, alternating among categories and between the learner teams. The first case scenario for each category must be completed during the station.

    *   The instructor may ask the learners to select the category for the next scenario.

    *   The instructor may post the categories on cards and allow the learners to select from these cards. Cards with the scenarios or a number that identifies the scenario for the instructor may also be placed under the corresponding category. The learners would then select the category and the scenario. The questions can be arranged by heading, assigned a point value, and arranged using a format based on the "Jeopardy" game.

3. The learners will be presented with case scenarios that require interventions related to:

    *   Positioning and immobilization techniques

    *   Vascular access

    *   Pain management and medication administration

    *   Respiratory interventions

4. The learners will demonstrate or observe the following skills:

    *   Removal of a child from a car seat while maintaining cervical spine immobilization

    *   Sizing and insertion of an oral airway

    *   Oxygen delivery

    *   Endotracheal tube management

    *   Site selection for intramuscular injection, intravenous access, and intraosseous insertion

    *   Positioning for comfort techniques

    *   Positioning an infant for a lumbar puncture

    *   Nonpharmacologic pain management techniques

5. The instructor will provide specific information related to the case scenarios and ensure that the learners demonstrate appropriate techniques. The instructor will ensure that all interventions for the scenario have been demonstrated or discussed.

6. A minimum of eight scenarios, with at least two from each category, will be presented to the learners. As time allows, additional scenarios may be presented. Total time for this station is 60 minutes.

7. All content related to the case scenario interventions is provided in the Pediatric Considerations following Chapters 3, 5, 6, 7, and 11.

PRINCIPLES OF PEDIATRIC INTERVENTIONS

A variety of interventions are performed during the care of children in the emergency department and in other emergency care settings or situations. An essential aspect of providing these interventions is the availability of equipment in the appropriate sizes for all age groups, newborns through adolescents. Determining the correct equipment size for a specific patient can be a challenge. Formulas and charts have been developed to assist in this process. Products such as the Broselow™ tape and color-coded equipment storage systems are valuable tools in assisting with rapid selection of the appropriate-sized equipment.

The priorities of intervention depend on the complexity and acuity of the child's illness or injury. The approach to these interventions is governed by the child's development and psychosocial needs as well as the physiologic status. Integrating the priorities of intervention with a developmentally appropriate approach is essential in planning and implementing care that meets the needs of children and their families. Although emergency interventions include an array of procedures, many pediatric interventions include one or more of the following components: positioning or immobilization techniques, vascular access, pain management and medication administration, and respiratory interventions.

SUMMARY

Pediatric Considerations is a teaching station in which the learner has an opportunity to integrate the principles of growth and development with priorities of intervention. The case scenarios provide the learner an opportunity to incorporate multiple components of care into the planning and implementation of specific interventions.

Case 1: Positioning and Immobilization Techniques

Sara is an 8-month-old infant involved in a motor vehicle crash. She was alert and stable at the scene and was transported by ambulance to your emergency department for evaluation. Sara is alert and interactive and immobilized in her car seat. You need to remove her from the car seat.

- Demonstrate removing the infant from a car seat while maintaining spinal immobilization, and immobilizing her on a backboard.

- Describe techniques to keep the infant calm during this procedure.

Note to instructor: The learners work as a team to remove the infant mannikin from the car seat, to maintain cervical spine immobilization, and to immobilize the mannikin on a backboard. If learners are unfamiliar with this procedure, provide verbal instructions as they perform the steps.

Content outlining the procedure is found in Pediatric Considerations: Cervical and Spinal Immobilization at the end of Chapter 6. Content on comfort measures and distraction is found in Chapter 3, "The Pediatric Patient," and the Pediatric Considerations: Pain Management and Medication Administration at the end of Chapter 3.

Case 2: Positioning and Immobilization Techniques

David is a 4-week-old infant with fever who is brought to the emergency department by his parents. As part of his workup for possible sepsis, a lumbar puncture will be performed. Universal and isolation precautions have been initiated.

- Demonstrate, with the infant mannikin, how to position and hold the infant for the procedure.

- Describe the appropriate assessment during the procedure.

Note to instructor: The learner may choose to position the mannikin in the lateral decubitus position or the upright position. Ensure that the learner uses an appropriate positioning technique. **Discuss with the group the alternative position for a lumbar puncture and the risks associated with hyperflexion and vigorous holding. The learner should observe the infant's color, respiratory pattern, and muscle tone during the procedure.**

Content outlining positioning lumbar puncture is located in Pediatric Considerations: Positioning for Medical Procedures at the end of Chapter 11.

Case 3: Positioning and Immobilization Techniques

Meredith is a 3-year-old child who fell about 10 feet from the deck in her back yard, landing on the grass. She is transported to your emergency department by family car. On her arrival, you initiate cervical spine immobilization. Her vital signs are within normal limits for her age, and she is very active. She is immobilized on a full-sized backboard and twice has pulled her legs out from under the strap positioned above her knees.

- Describe and demonstrate two interventions you may use to assist in maintaining her immobilization.

Note to instructor: The learner should identify the need to place blanket or towel rolls along her lower body to restrict movement. Demonstrate the technique for learners as needed. Distraction techniques should also be initiated and used until the child is cleared for removal from the backboard.

Information on cervical and spinal immobilization is located in Pediatric Considerations: Cervical and Spinal Immobilization at the end of Chapter 6. Information on distraction techniques is located in Pediatric Considerations: Pain Management and Medication Administration at the end of Chapter 3.

Case 4: Positioning and Immobilization Techniques

Jimmie is a 5-year-old child who presents to the emergency department with a 4-cm laceration to the forehead, requiring sutures for subcutaneous and skin closure. The procedure for the laceration repair has been explained to him.

- Demonstrate a method to restrict his movement during the laceration repair.

- In addition to preparation for the procedure, what other strategies may you use to gain cooperation?

Note to instructor: The learner should identify that the least restrictive methods should be used in conjunction with age-appropriate distraction and pain management. The use of a restraint board may be considered, but it should be the last alternative. A less restrictive approach, supplemented by distraction and an appropriate topical or local anesthetic, should be the first consideration. The use of medications for sedation may also be considered, as appropriate for the patient situation and per hospital protocol.

Information on distraction, physically restrictive devices, and anesthetics is located in Pediatric Considerations: Pain Management and Medication Administration at the end of Chapter 3.

Case 1: Vascular Access

Mary is an 8-week-old infant who arrives by ambulance in full cardiopulmonary arrest. She is orally intubated and cardiac compressions are in progress. An intraosseous needle was placed in the left tibia by the paramedic.

- What are the indications for intraosseous insertion?

- Name two preferred sites for intraosseous insertion in the infant.

- Locate landmarks and sites for intraosseous insertion in the tibia and the femur.

- Describe how to evaluate patency of the intraosseous access and the signs of intraosseous infusion site infiltrate or extravasation.

- If the intraosseous access is not functional, can another intraosseous needle be placed in the same bone?

Note to instructor: Discussion for each question is listed below. Preferred alternative sites for this infant would include the right tibia and both distal femurs. Show the intraosseous needle to the learners.

Information on intraosseous insertion and management is located in Pediatric Considerations: Vascular Access at the end of Chapter 7.

Case 2: Vascular Access

Mackenzie is a 4-year-old child who presents following the development of a fever and rash. Her vital signs are pulse 190 beats/minute; respirations 36 breaths/minute; blood pressure 90/48 mm Hg; and temperature 38.6°C (101.4°F). Capillary refill is 3 seconds; her skin is cool and pale. A petechial rash is noted on her chest, abdomen, and extremities. Appropriate isolation precautions have been initiated. An intravenous line is established in the left hand with a 22-gauge catheter. A rapid bolus of 0.9% normal saline is ordered. The patient's weight is 18 kg.

- How many ml/kg should be administered for the fluid bolus?

- What is the total volume of fluid to be administered?

- Describe and demonstrate the use of a stopcock to rapidly infuse the intravenous fluid.

- What are other methods to rapidly infuse fluids?

Note to instructor: The patient should be given 20 ml/kg of 0.9% normal saline (total volume = 360 ml). The learner is to assemble the equipment needed, demonstrating the technique described below.

Information on rapid fluid administration is located in Pediatric Considerations: Pain Management and Medication Administration at the end of Chapter 3.

Case 3: Vascular Access

Andy is a 6-month-old infant who presents to the emergency department with a 3-day history of vomiting and diarrhea and decreased intake. He is clinically dehydrated but stable. Andy requires intravenous fluids for rehydration.

- What intravenous sites would be most appropriate for an infant this age?

- What catheter size would you anticipate using?

- Describe how you would secure the catheter and protect it from accidental dislodgment.

Note to instructor: Discussion for each question is listed below. Information on peripheral intravenous insertion and management is located in Pediatric Considerations: Vascular Access at the end of Chapter 7.

Case 1: Pain Management and Medication Administration

Steven is a 14-year-old adolescent who is referred by his primary care provider for a headache, fever, vomiting, and photophobia. He appears ill but is alert and oriented. His vital signs are within normal limits for his age. Respirations are unlabored, his color is pale but warm, and capillary refill is less than 2 seconds. A lumbar puncture is going to be performed. He is very anxious. Appropriate universal and isolation precautions have been initiated.

- Describe what strategies you can use to prepare the adolescent for this procedure.

- Discuss potential strategies for nonpharmacologic pain management.

- What pharmacologic interventions may facilitate this procedure?

Note to instructor: The learner should discuss issues related to preparing children or adolescents for procedures and coping skills as listed below. Pharmacologic interventions should focus on local or dermal anesthetics as described below.

Information on preparation for procedures, coping and distraction strategies and pharmacologic interventions is located in Pediatric Considerations: Pain Management and Medication Administration at the end of Chapter 3.

Case 2: Pain Management and Medication Administration

Joshua is a 1-year-old infant brought in by his mother for a high fever. His workup is completed and he will be discharged home following an intramuscular injection of ceftriaxone sodium.

- On the mannikin, locate the preferred injection site.

- What volume can be injected into a single site for a child this age?

- What may be done to reduce the pain of the injection?

- Describe and demonstrate how you would position the patient for the injection.

Note to instructor: The learner should locate the vastus lateralis muscle on the mannikin. A discussion for each question is provided below. Review with the learners positioning for comfort techniques. The caregiver could hold the child on his or her lap in a chest-to-chest position for the injection.

Information on intramuscular injections and positioning is located in Pediatric Considerations: Pain Management and Medication Administration at the end of Chapter 3.

Case 3: Pain Management and Medication Administration

Elizabeth is a 12-year-old female adolescent who is brought in by her parents after she fell from a trampoline. She is holding her right arm against her body and grimaces with every step. She states that she flipped off the trampoline, landing on her right arm, palm down, on the grass. She is alert, oriented, and cooperative. The Glasgow Coma Scale score is 15. She rates her pain as 8 on a scale of 0 to 10. Her examination is normal, other than the obvious angulated deformity to her right forearm. The neurovascular status is intact distal to the injury. She has no other injuries. Her radiographs are completed. She has a distal fracture of the radius and ulna. Her fracture will be reduced after administration of sedation and analgesia (conscious sedation).

- Name three interventions that may be initiated to assist in reducing the pain associated with the injury.

- Describe the personnel and equipment required at the bedside when sedatives and analgesics are used for procedural pain management.

Note to instructor:

- The learner should name at least three interventions, as discussed below. The learner should also consider the administration of an intravenous narcotic analgesic (morphine sulfate), per practitioner's order, before the radiographs are obtained.

- Equipment and personnel required during sedation are listed below. Review the important points after the second question is answered.

Information on basic care measures and sedation and analgesia for painful procedures is located in Pediatric Considerations: Pain Management and Medication Administration at the end of Chapter 3.

Case 4: Pain Management and Medication Administration

Stephanie is a 2-year-old toddler who presents with partial-thickness burns. Her caregiver reports that Stephanie pulled a cup of hot coffee from the table. She is alert and crying continuously. You note partial-thickness burns to the neck, chest, upper abdomen, and left arm.

- Describe pain management measures appropriate for this patient.

Note to instructor: The learner should identify that the burn wound should be covered with a sterile dressing as quickly as possible to decrease air flow across the wound. Air flow across a burn wound increases pain. Because of the extent and depth of the burn injury, the administration of an intravenous narcotic is also indicated. Morphine sulfate is an appropriate selection. The learner should encourage the caregiver's participation in comforting Stephanie and using some distraction techniques.

Information on pain management and distraction is located in Pediatric Considerations: Pain Management and Medication Administration at the end of Chapter 3. Information on care of the pediatric burn patient is located in Chapter 8, "Burns."

Case 1: Respiratory Interventions

Daniel is a 5-year-old child who presents by family car following an ingestion of an unknown medication. Daniel is unresponsive to painful stimuli, has a patent airway with manual positioning (jaw thrust), and spontaneous respirations of adequate rate and depth. Manual positioning of his airway is required to maintain patency.

- Describe indications for use of an oropharyngeal airway.

- Describe and demonstrate the sizing and insertion of an airway adjunct to assist in maintaining a patent airway until intubation is performed.

- Describe two methods to determine endotracheal tube size and depth for this patient.

Note to instructor: The learner should identify the use of an oropharyngeal airway as an initial adjunct. The points related to sizing and insertion are discussed below.

Information on oropharyngeal airways is located in located in Pediatric Considerations: Respiratory Interventions and Diagnostic Procedures at the end of Chapter 5.

Case 2: Respiratory Interventions

Jennifer is a 2-year-old toddler who presents with difficulty breathing and wheezing. Her mother reports one previous wheezing episode about 6 months previously. Jennifer is alert and interactive. She is tachypneic, with labored respirations, nasal flaring, and subcostal and intercostal retractions. Her color is slightly pale; capillary refill is 2 seconds. Her pulse is 132 beats/minute, her respirations are 48 breaths/minute, her blood pressure is 90/60 mm Hg, and her axillary temperature is 36.6°C (97.8°F).

- What strategies may assist in gaining the child's cooperation for administration of oxygen or inhaled medications?

- Describe your initial interventions for this patient.

Note to instructor: The learner should identify that the child should remain in a position of comfort. Additional interventions would include obtaining a pulse oximeter reading, administering oxygen, and administering albuterol by nebulizer or metered-dose inhaler with a spacer. Points on gaining cooperation and administration techniques are discussed below.

Information on respiratory interventions and pulse oximetry is located in Pediatric Considerations: Respiratory Intervention and Diagnostic Procedures at the end of Chapter 5.

Case 3: Respiratory Interventions

Jack is a 4-year-old child transported by ambulance following a generalized tonic-clonic seizure. Just prior to arrival at the emergency department, his respirations become shallow and slow. Bag-valve-mask ventilation was initiated. An intravenous line was established by the paramedic prior to arrival. The primary and secondary assessment has been completed and the nurse practitioner is preparing to intubate the patient. The appropriate equipment is at the bedside.

- Describe the patient assessment and nursing interventions during intubation.

- Describe two methods to confirm endotracheal tube placement once intubation is completed.

- Demonstrate a method to tape the endotracheal tube in place.

Note to instructor: Inform the learner there are four steps for this scenario; the learner will be asked to provide information in response to each of the four questions or steps. The points related to each question or request are discussed below.

Information on endotracheal intubation procedure is located in Pediatric Considerations: Respiratory Interventions and Diagnostic Procedures at the end of Chapter 5.

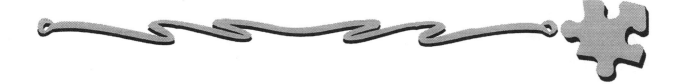

Emergency Nursing Pediatric Course

Pediatric Resuscitation Skill Station

EQUIPMENT FOR THE STATION

- Two tables (one for mannikin, one for supplies)
- Five to seven chairs
- One child mannikin
- One infant mannikin
- One pediatric nonrebreather mask
- One infant partial rebreather mask
- One rigid tonsil suction
- One uncuffed endotracheal tube (sizes appropriate for mannikins)
- One roll of adhesive tape
- One pediatric bag-valve-mask device (500-ml for infant scenarios, 1,000-ml for child scenarios)
- Resuscitation masks (sizes appropriate for mannikins)
- One blanket or similar type of warming device
- One penlight
- One stethoscope
- One each intravenous catheters (20-gauge, 24-gauge)
- One blood-collecting tube (any color)
- One 0.9% normal saline intravenous solution
- Three electrocardiogram electrodes
- One pulse oximeter probe
- One gastric tube (10-French or larger)
- One pediatric indwelling urinary-catheter
- Cardiac rhythm strips appropriate for scenarios
- One clipboard (testing day)

- Personal protective equipment
- One length-based resuscitation tape (optional)
- One end-tidal CO_2 detector (optional)

STATION PREPARATION

1. Assemble all equipment and ensure it is in working order.

2. Arrange equipment and mannikin on the tables.

3. Place chairs around the table with the mannikin.

4. Display the case scenarios and the A through I mnemonic on a chalkboard, flipchart, or poster.

INTRODUCTION TO THE SKILL STATION

1. The instructor will discuss and/or demonstrate a primary and a secondary assessment, or learners will view the station demonstration videotape.

2. Each learner will be presented with a case scenario and will:
   - Conduct the primary and secondary assessment of the child in respiratory distress, failure, shock, or cardiopulmonary arrest. During the secondary assessment, learners must state the need for a head-to-toe assessment. The ability to describe appropriate inspection techniques and demonstrate appropriate palpation and auscultation techniques are evaluated in the Pediatric Multiple Trauma station.
   - Determine the management priorities for the child in respiratory distress, failure, shock, or cardiopulmonary arrest.
   - Discuss the need for universal precautions when caring for the pediatric patient requiring resuscitation.

3. One student should be assigned as the team leader responsible for completing the assessment and directing the team. The other members of the group can assist by performing bag-valve-mask ventilation, cardiac compressions, etc. On evaluation day, each student is evaluated alone with no other group members in the room.

4. Six teaching scenarios are included in the Provider manual. The first four scenarios must always be used. Scenarios 5 and 6 can be used if there is a 1:6 ratio in the psychomotor skill station.

5. The instructor will inform learners:

- The sequence of the primary assessment is important.

- To be successful, the steps with double asterisks (**) must be performed in order. Once the learner begins the assessment of E through I, the instructor will assume that the learner has completed the primary assessment. It is acceptable for the learner to identify interventions such as placing the child on the cardiac monitor or pulse oximeter, inserting an indwelling urinary catheter or gastric tube, or other diagnostic studies during the primary assessment. This does not constitute the learner "leaving" the primary assessment.

- The instructor will provide responses to the learner's questions about the case scenarios. The instructor will also provide specific information related to the case progression as appropriate.

- Appropriate palpation and auscultation during the assessment as indicated on the evaluation form must be demonstrated.

- The effectiveness of interventions which are expected to have an immediate effect on the patient must be evaluated (e.g., auscultation of breath sounds after intubation, effectiveness of bag-valve-mask ventilation, effectiveness of a fluid bolus, effectiveness of suctioning the airway).

- To assess airway patency in the unresponsive child, first position the child and then demonstrate manually opening the airway.

- To assess circulation, obtain central AND peripheral pulse rate and quality, and skin color AND temperature during the primary assessment.

PRINCIPLES OF PEDIATRIC RESUSCITATION

The care of the critically ill pediatric patient is based on performance of a systematic assessment and initiation of the appropriate interventions. The management priorities are based on the life-threatening conditions found in the primary assessment and other problems found in the secondary assessment, as well as the child's age and the resources available for providing care.

The primary assessment is a brief assessment of airway, breathing, circulation, and disability. Life-threatening conditions are identified and treated before the assessment continues. The secondary assessment is a systematic approach to identifying additional problems and determining the priorities of care.

Simultaneous assessment, diagnosis, and intervention may be required for the child who is critically ill. The priorities for intervention will depend on the complexity of the child's illness and the availability and qualifications of the emergency care providers. Those conditions that have the greatest potential to compromise the airway, breathing, circulation, and/or disability are given the highest priority.

The child must be re-evaluated after any interventions are performed in the primary assessment to determine the effectiveness. The evaluation and ongoing assessment begin at the completion of the secondary assessment. These include a primary reassessment and re-evaluation of the vital signs.

The systematic assessment can be remembered as follows:

A = Airway

B = Breathing

C = Circulation

D = Disability – brief neurologic assessment

E = Exposure and environmental control

F = Full set of vital signs and family presence

G = Give comfort measures

H = Head-to-toe assessment and history

I = Inspect the posterior surfaces

Tables 47 and 48 provide guidelines for conducting the primary and secondary assessments and identifying the appropriate interventions.

STEPS IN SKILL PERFORMANCE

Each learner will be presented with a case scenario depicting a critically ill child who is en route or has presented to the emergency department. The script and steps in skill performance are listed on pages 424-445.

Tell the learner: "I will describe a case scenario of a child who is critically ill. As you assess the child and evaluate interventions, I will give you additional information."

Table 47

PRIMARY ASSESSMENT	
Assessments	**Potential Interventions**
A = Airway	
<ul><li>Vocalization</li><li>Tongue obstruction</li><li>Loose teeth or foreign objects</li><li>Vomitus or other secretions</li><li>Edema</li><li>Preferred posture</li><li>Drooling</li><li>Dysphagia</li><li>Abnormal airway sounds (stridor or snoring)</li></ul>	<ul><li>Position the patient</li><li>Open the airway with jaw thrust or chin lift</li><li>Suction or remove foreign objects</li><li>Insert an oropharyngeal/nasopharyngeal airway</li><li>Perform endotracheal intubation/rapid sequence induction</li><li>Prepare for needle or surgical cricothyroidotomy</li></ul>
B = Breathing	
<ul><li>Level of consciousness</li><li>Spontaneous respirations</li><li>Rate and depth of respirations</li><li>Symmetric chest rise and fall</li><li>Presence and quality of breath sounds</li><li>Work of breathing:<ul><li>Nasal flaring</li><li>Retractions</li><li>Head bobbing</li><li>Expiratory grunting</li></ul></li><li>Accessory muscle use</li><li>Jugular vein distention and tracheal position</li></ul>	<ul><li>Maintain position of comfort</li><li>Provide supplemental oxygen</li><li>Provide bag-valve-mask ventilation</li><li>Perform endotracheal intubation/rapid sequence induction</li><li>Insert gastric tube to reduce abdominal distention</li><li>Prepare for needle thoracentesis</li></ul>
C = Circulation	
<ul><li>Rate and quality of central and peripheral pulse</li><li>Skin color and temperature</li><li>Capillary refill</li></ul>	<ul><li>Perform cardiopulmonary resuscitation and advanced life-support measures</li><li>Control any obvious bleeding</li><li>Prepare for defibrillation/synchronized cardioversion</li><li>Obtain intravenous or intraosseous access</li><li>Administer 20-ml/kg fluid bolus of isotonic crystalloid solution</li><li>Administer medications</li><li>Administer blood or blood products</li><li>Correct electrolyte and acid-base imbalance</li></ul>
D = Disability	
<ul><li>Level of consciousness (AVPU)</li><li>Pupils</li></ul>	<ul><li>Perform further investigation during secondary assessment</li><li>Administer pharmacologic therapy</li></ul>

Table 48

SECONDARY ASSESSMENT	
Assessments	**Potential Interventions**
E = Exposure and Environmental Control	
• Obvious underlying injuries • Additional symptoms of illness • Sources of heat loss	• Apply warm blankets • Provide overhead warming light • Provide radiant warmer or approved warming device • Maintain warm ambient environment • Increase room temperature as needed • Administer warm intravenous fluids • Administer warm humidified oxygen
F = Full Set of Vital Signs	
• Rate and depth of respirations • Rate and quality of pulse • Blood pressure • Temperature • Weight	• Place on cardiorespiratory monitors • Trend vital signs • Estimate weight using length-based resuscitation tape (e.g., Broselow™ tape)
F = Family Presence	
• Identification of family members and their relationship to the child • Needs of the family • Need for additional support and desire to be in resuscitation room	• Facilitate and support family involvement • Assign health care professional to liaison with family and provide explanation of procedures, plan of treatment • Assign a staff member to provide family support
G = Give Comfort Measures	

• Presence and level of pain	• Facilitate family presence for support of the child
	• Initiate pain management measures:
	  ■ Use age-appropriate nonpharmacologic methods to facilitate coping
	  ■ Administer analgesics and other appropriate medications
	  ■ Initiate physical measures (splints, dressing, ice)

H = Head-to-Toe Assessment	
• Head-to-toe assessment using inspection, palpation, and auscultation techniques • Reassessment of airway, breathing, and circulation status once head-to-toe assessment is completed	• Initiate appropriate interventions based on findings
H = History	
• Complete history (CIAMPEDS) • Specialized history • Social history • Family history	• Initiate social service consult as needed
I = Inspect Posterior Surfaces	
• Rashes, lesions, petechia, edema, ecchymosis • Tenderness	• Logroll patient to maintain airway patency and spinal alignment

SUMMARY

During evaluation, the learner must demonstrate all critical steps designated with one (*) and two (**) asterisks, and 70% of the total number of points. Each learner will be evaluated using a new and different scenario. Therefore, the learner should concentrate on understanding the principles of the station and not on memorizing the specific case scenarios.

Certain critical steps must be demonstrated or described in order during the primary assessment. These are designated with ** on the evaluation form. The total number of critical steps (**) in any scenario is 6 to 8. Critical steps designated with ** may include:

- Assesses airway patency

- Identifies one appropriate airway intervention

- Assesses breathing effectiveness

- Identifies one appropriate intervention for ineffective breathing

- Assesses perfusion status

- States one appropriate intervention for ineffective circulation

- Assesses the level of consciousness (AVPU)

Additional critical steps that must be demonstrated or described during the remainder of the station are designated with an asterisk (*) on the evaluation form. All of these steps must also be performed to successfully complete the station.

- States one measure to prevent heat loss

- Identifies appropriate diagnostic studies or interventions

At the completion of the demonstration, the learner will be asked if there is anything he or she wants to add or revise. Learners may not add to or revise any of the ** steps.

SKILL: PEDIATRIC RESUSCITATION

Teaching Case A

A 3-month-old infant is brought to the emergency department by her mother. The mother states that the child has been vomiting, is not eating well, and is breathing very fast. She has had a runny nose, cough, and a fever. The Pediatric Assessment Triangle reveals that the child is pale, her respirations are difficult to assess, and she is lethargic. The infant's weight is 6 kg. A support person responds to the resuscitation room to provide support to the mother. Please proceed with your primary and secondary assessments and appropriate interventions.

Instructor Responses	Skill Steps	Demonstrated		
		Yes		No
	1. Assesses airway patency (at least three of the following):	****** _____		_____
Weak cry	• **Vocalization**			
No visible obstruction	• **Tongue obstruction**			
No loose teeth or foreign objects	• **Loose teeth or foreign objects**			
Some nasal secretions	• **Vomitus or other secretions**			
No edema	• **Edema**			
Lying in mother's arms	• **Preferred posture**			
No drooling	• **Drooling**			
No dysphagia	• **Dysphagia**			
No abnormal airway sounds	• **Abnormal airway sounds**			
	2. Assesses breathing effectiveness (at least three of the following):	****** _____		_____
Lethargic	• **Level of consciousness**			
Present but shallow	• **Spontaneous respirations**			
Respiratory rate 80 breaths/minute and shallow	• **Rate and depth of respirations**			
Symmetric chest rise and fall	• **Symmetric chest rise and fall**			
Expiratory wheezes; breath sounds equal	• **Presence and quality of breath sounds**			
	• **Work of breathing (at least three of the following):**			
Nasal flaring present	▪ **Nasal flaring**			
Severe substernal and intercostal retractions	▪ **Retractions**			
No head bobbing	▪ **Head bobbing**			
No grunting	▪ **Expiratory grunting**			
Using accessory muscles	▪ **Accessory muscle use**			
No jugular vein distention; trachea midline	• **Jugular vein distention or tracheal deviation**			

Instructor Responses	Skill Steps	Demonstrated		
		Yes		No
Infant tolerates mask	3. Applies oxygen via highest concentration	**_____		_____
Central and peripheral pulses rapid and strong. Heart rate is 160 beats/minute.	4. Assesses perfusion status (at least two of the following): • Central AND peripheral pulse rate and quality	**_____		_____
Skin pale and slightly cool	• Skin color AND temperature			
Capillary refill 2 seconds	• Capillary refill			
Intravenous access is achieved	5. States need to obtain vascular access	**_____		_____

Instructor response: "There has been a change in the child's color. The patient has extreme pallor, mucous membranes are pale, nailbeds are dusky."

Note to instructor: If the learner does not realize the need to reassess the airway and breathing, stop the learner and discuss the change in patient condition and the importance of identifying the cause for the change.

Instructor Responses	Skill Steps	Demonstrated		
	6. Reassesses airway patency (at least three of the following):	_____		_____
No longer crying	• Vocalization			
No visible obstruction	• Tongue obstruction			
No loose teeth or foreign objects	• Loose teeth or foreign objects			
No vomitus or other secretions	• Vomitus or other secretions			
No edema	• Edema			
No drooling or dysphagia	• Drooling or dysphagia			
No abnormal airway sounds	• Abnormal airway sounds			
	7. Reassesses breathing effectiveness (at least three of the following):	_____		_____
Unresponsive	• Level of consciousness			
Spontaneous respirations present with periods of apnea	• Spontaneous respirations			
Respiratory rate 40 breaths/minute; periods of apnea	• Rate and depth of respirations			
Chest rise symmetric but shallow	• Symmetric chest rise and fall			
Wheezes and crackles with poor air entry	• Presence and quality of breath sounds			
	• Work of breathing (at least three of the following):			
Nasal flaring continues	■ Nasal flaring			
Retractions present but not as severe	■ Retractions			
No head bobbing	■ Head bobbing			
Expiratory grunting noted	■ Expiratory grunting			
Using accessory muscles	■ Accessory muscle use			
No jugular vein distention; trachea midline	• Jugular vein distention and tracheal position			

Instructor Responses	Skill Steps	Demonstrated		
		Yes		No
	8. States need to assist ventilations	_____		_____
	9. Demonstrates bag-valve-mask ventilation with 100% oxygen	** _____		_____
	10. Assesses effectiveness of assisted ventilations:	** _____		
Symmetric and adequate chest rise with assisted ventilations	• Chest rise and fall			
Bilateral breath sounds present	• Presence of breath sounds			
	11. States need for intubation	_____		_____
Instructor response: "The child is now intubated using rapid sequence induction. Demonstrate and describe your immediate evaluation of endotracheal tube placement."				
	12. Demonstrates and describes assessment of endotracheal tube placement (at least two of the following):	_____		_____
Good chest rise and fall	• Observes chest rise and fall			
Equal breath sounds and absent epigastric sounds	• Listens for breath sounds in the axillary areas AND over epigastric area			
End-tidal CO_2 device is placed; reading indicates positive placement	• Assesses end-tidal CO_2 monitor or device (if available)			
Instructor response: "Endotracheal tube is in place and is secured."				
	13. Inserts gastric tube			
	14. Reassesses perfusion status (at least two of the following):	_____		_____
Peripheral pulses strong; rate 140 beats/minute	• Central AND peripheral pulse rate and quality			
Skin color improved; skin temperature warmer	• Skin color AND temperature			
Capillary refill <2 seconds	• Capillary refill			
Unresponsive	15. Assesses level of consciousness (AVPU)	** _____		_____
Pupils equal and reactive	16. Assesses pupils	_____		_____
Secondary Assessment				
No additional signs of illness	17. Removes all clothing	_____		_____
	18. States one measure to prevent heat loss:	* _____		_____
	• Warm blankets			
	• Overhead warming lights or other warming device			
	• Warm ambient environment			
	• Warm intravenous fluids			
	• Warm humidified oxygen			

Instructor Responses	Skill Steps	Demonstrated		
		Yes		No
BP = 92/50 mm Hg T = 37.8°C (100°F) P = 150 beats/minute R = assisted ventilations at 32 breaths/minute Weight = 6 kg	19. States need to get a complete set of vital signs	_____		_____
Electrocardiogram = sinus tachycardia without ectopy	20. Places cardiac monitor leads on patient	_____		_____
Oxygen saturation = 100% with 100% oxygen	21. Places pulse oximeter on patient	_____		_____
Patient has received a sedative agent, paralytic, and analgesic for intubation. No obvious pain or discomfort.	22. States need to evaluate for presence of pain or discomfort	_____		_____

Instructor response: "Normally, you would now conduct a head-to-toe assessment. It has been done. There are no significant findings."

Mother states child has had a cold with fever and runny nose. Poor feeding over the past couple of days. No allergies or medications. Immunizations current. Previously healthy.	23. States need to obtain a history using CIAMPEDS	_____		_____

Instructor response: "What additional diagnostic studies or interventions may be completed?"

Note to instructor: If the learner has previously identified any of the appropriate diagnostic studies or interventions listed, include the diagnostic study or intervention in the total of five.

	24. Identifies appropriate diagnostic studies or interventions (at least five of the following): ● Arterial blood gas ● Bedside glucose test ● Chest radiograph ● Consider nasal washing for respiratory syncytial virus antigen test ● Continue psychosocial support for the family ● End-tidal CO_2 monitor ● Laboratory studies ● Medications ● Place child in contact isolation ● Prepare for admission or transfer ● Urinary catheter	*_____		_____

Instructor response: "What is the evaluation and ongoing assessment of this patient?"

	25. States need to re-evaluate primary assessment	_____		_____
	26. States need to re-evaluate vital signs	_____		_____

SKILL: PEDIATRIC RESUSCITATION

Teaching Case B

A 2-year-old boy is brought to the emergency department by his father after being found floating face down in the bathtub. The father states "I just grabbed him and ran." The child is wrapped in a bath towel and his hair is wet. The Pediatric Assessment Triangle reveals that he is unresponsive, limp, apneic, and dusky. The child's weight is 15 kg. A support person responds to the resuscitation room to provide support. Please proceed with your primary and secondary assessments and appropriate interventions.

Instructor Responses	Skill Steps	Demonstrated		
		Yes		No
	1. Positions the patient AND demonstrates manually opening the airway	_____		_____
	2. Assesses airway patency (at least three of the following):	** _____		_____
No vocalization	• Vocalization			
No tongue obstruction visible; vomitus noted	• Tongue obstruction			
No loose teeth or foreign objects; vomitus noted	• Loose teeth or foreign objects			
Vomitus and water noted in mouth	• Vomitus or other secretions			
No edema; vomitus noted	• Edema			
Limp, supine on stretcher	• Preferred posture			
No drooling; vomitus noted	• Drooling			
None	• Dysphagia			
None	• Abnormal airway sounds			
Airway clear	3. Suctions the airway	** _____		_____

Instructor Responses	Skill Steps	Demonstrated		
		Yes		No
Note to instructor: If the learners identify that there are no respirations, they can move to the intervention without obtaining information about three indicators of breathing effectiveness.	4. **Assesses breathing effectiveness (at least three of the following):**	_____		_____
Unresponsive	● **Level of consciousness**			
Apneic	● **Spontaneous respirations**			
Apneic	● **Rate and depth of respirations**			
None	● **Symmetric chest rise and fall**			
No spontaneous respirations	● **Presence and quality of breath sounds**			
Apneic	● **Work of breathing (at least three of the following):**			
	■ **Nasal flaring**			
	■ **Retractions**			
	■ **Head bobbing**			
	■ **Expiratory grunting**			
No accessory muscle use	■ **Accessory muscle use**			
No jugular vein distention; trachea midline	● **Jugular vein distention and tracheal position**			
	5. **Demonstrates effective bag-valve-mask ventilation with 100% oxygen**	******_____		_____
	6. **Assesses effectiveness of assisted ventilations:**	******_____		_____
Symmetric and adequate chest rise with assisted ventilations	● **Chest rise and fall**			
Bilateral breath sounds present	● **Presence of breath sounds**			
	7. **States need for endotracheal intubation**	_____		_____
Instructor response: "The team is preparing the equipment for intubation. Proceed with your assessment."				
Note to instructor: If the learners identify that there is no central pulse, they do not need to assess peripheral pulses.	8. **Assesses perfusion status (at least two of the following):**	******_____		_____
Central pulse absent	● **Central AND peripheral pulse rate and quality**			
Skin dusky and cold	● **Skin color AND temperature**			
Capillary refill >5 seconds	● **Capillary refill**			
	9. **States need to initiate chest compressions**	******_____		_____
Electrocardiogram = asystole	10. **Places cardiac monitor leads on patient**	_____		_____
	11. **States need to obtain vascular access**	_____		_____
Instructor response: "The team is attempting peripheral access. The patient is intubated. Demonstrate and describe your immediate evaluation of endotracheal tube placement."				

Instructor Responses	Skill Steps	Demonstrated		
		Yes		No
Symmetric chest rise and fall Bilateral breath sounds present; epigastric sounds absent End-tidal CO_2 device placed; reading indicates positive placement	**12. Demonstrates and describes assessment of endotracheal tube placement (at least two of the following):** ● **Observes chest rise and fall** ● **Listens for breath sounds in the axillary areas AND over epigastric area** ● **Assesses end-tidal CO_2 via monitor or device (if available)**	**_____		_____
Instructor response: "The endotracheal tube is secured. Cardiac compressions are continued. Intravenous access is not yet established. Cardiac rhythm remains asystole. A gastric tube is inserted."				
Epinephrine administered	**13. States need to administer epinephrine via endotracheal tube**	_____		_____
Instructor response: "Intraosseous access is established in the right tibia. The patient remains in asystole. No palpable pulses."				
Epinephrine administered	**14. States need to administer epinephrine via the intraosseous access**	_____		_____
Central pulse present at 140 beats/minute; peripheral pulses not palpable Skin pale and cold Capillary refill 4 seconds	**15. Stops compressions and reassesses perfusion status (at least two of the following):** ● **Central AND peripheral pulse rate and quality** ● **Skin color AND temperature** ● **Capillary refill**	_____		_____
Instructor response: "Monitor indicates sinus rhythm."				
	16. States need to administer a 20-ml/kg fluid bolus	_____		_____
Instructor response: "Monitor indicates sinus rhythm."				
Central pulse 120 beats/minute; strong peripheral pulses present Skin cool and pale Capillary refill 3 seconds	**17. Reassesses perfusion status (at least two of the following):** ● **Central AND peripheral pulse rate and quality** ● **Skin color AND temperature** ● **Capillary refill**	_____		_____
Note to instructor: If a learner chooses to give a second fluid bolus, explain that the cool, pale skin and delayed capillary refill may be due to the drowning event, hypothermia, and continued exposure. Therefore, a second fluid bolus may not be indicated. The learner should obtain additional assessment information before making the decision about administering additional fluid. Refer to Chapter 6 for further information.				
Unresponsive	**18. Assesses level of consciousness (AVPU)**	**_____		_____
Pupils fixed and dilated	**19. Assesses pupils**	_____		_____
Secondary Assessment				
Patient arrived wrapped in a towel. Towel removed at the onset of resuscitation. No additional signs of illness or injury.	**20. Removes all clothing**	_____		_____

Instructor Responses	Skill Steps	Demonstrated		
		Yes		No
	21. States one measure to prevent heat loss: • **Warm blankets** • **Overhead warming lights or other warming device** • **Warm ambient environment** • **Warm intravenous fluids** • **Warm humidified oxygen**	*_____		_____
BP = 88/56 mm Hg P = 120 beats/minute R = respirations assisted at 24 breaths/minute Rectal T = 35.8°C (96.4°F) Weight = 15 kg	22. States need to get a complete set of vital signs	_____		_____
Oxygen saturation = 98% with assisted ventilations	23. Places pulse oximeter on patient	_____		_____
Unresponsive; no evidence of pain or discomfort	24. States need to evaluate for presence of pain or discomfort	_____		_____
Instructor response: "Normally, you would now conduct a head-to-toe assessment. It has been done. There are no significant findings."				
The father states that he left the child alone in the bathtub for a minute to answer the telephone. When he returned he found him face down in the bathtub. When he took him out of the tub he was limp. No allergies or medications. Immunizations current. No past medical history.	25. States need to obtain a history using **CIAMPEDS**	_____		_____
Instructor response: "What additional diagnostic studies or interventions may be completed?" Note to instructor: If the learner has previously identified any of the appropriate diagnostic studies or interventions listed, include the diagnostic study or intervention in the total of five.				
	26. Identifies appropriate diagnostic studies or interventions (at least five of the following): • **Arterial blood gas** • **Bedside glucose test** • **Chest radiograph** • **Continue psychosocial support** • **End-tidal CO_2 monitor** • **Laboratory studies** • **Pain management and sedation measures** • **Prepare for admission or transfer**	*_____		_____
Instructor response: "What is the evaluation and ongoing assessment for this patient?"				
	27. States need to re-evaluate primary assessment	_____		_____
	28. States need to re-evaluate vital signs	_____		_____

SKILL: PEDIATRIC RESUSCITATION

Teaching Case C

An unresponsive 3-year-old child is brought to the emergency department by a basic life-support ambulance. The child was found in an abandoned refrigerator. Patient arrives with cardiopulmonary resuscitation in progress. The child is transferred from the ambulance stretcher to the emergency stretcher; you note vomitus at the corner of the child's mouth and poor chest rise with assisted ventilation. The Pediatric Assessment Triangle reveals that he is unresponsive, apneic, and pale. Cardiac compressions are resumed. The child is placed on the cardiac monitor. A support person responds to the resuscitation room to provide support. Please proceed with your primary and secondary assessments and appropriate interventions.

Instructor Responses	Skill Steps	Demonstrated		
		Yes		No
	1. Positions the child AND demonstrates manually opening the airway	_____		_____
	2. Assesses airway patency (at least three of the following):	**_____		_____
No vocalization	• Vocalization			
Tongue continues to block the airway	• Tongue obstruction			
No loose teeth or foreign objects; vomitus present	• Loose teeth or foreign objects			
Mouth full of vomitus	• Vomitus or other secretions			
No edema; vomitus present	• Edema			
In cardiopulmonary arrest	• Preferred posture			
No drooling; vomitus noted at corners of mouth	• Drooling			
In cardiopulmonary arrest	• Dysphagia			
No airway sounds because of apnea	• Abnormal airway sounds			
	3. Describes and demonstrates the required interventions to clear the airway obstruction (must verbalize all three interventions): • Suctions the mouth • Repositions head to neutral position • Opens the airway	**_____		_____

Instructor response: "The airway is now patent."

Note to instructor: If the learner does not identify airway obstruction resulting from tongue and vomitus, cue them to identify the second obstruction.

Instructor Responses	Skill Steps	Demonstrated		
		Yes		No
Note to instructor: If the learners identify that there are no respirations, they can move to the intervention without obtaining information about three indicators of breathing effectiveness.	4. Assesses for breathing effectiveness (at least three of the following):	** _____		_____
Unresponsive	• Level of consciousness			
No spontaneous respirations	• Spontaneous respirations			
No respirations	• Rate and depth of respirations			
No chest rise and fall	• Symmetric chest rise and fall			
No breath sounds	• Presence and quality of breath sounds			
No work of breathing	• Work of breathing (at least three of the following):			
	▪ Nasal flaring			
	▪ Retractions			
	▪ Head bobbing			
	▪ Expiratory grunting			
Apneic	▪ Accessory muscle use			
No jugular vein distention; trachea midline	• Jugular vein distention and tracheal position			
Assisted ventilations resumed	5. States need to resume assisted ventilation with bag-valve-mask and 100% oxygen	_____		_____
	6. Demonstrates effective bag-valve-mask ventilation with 100% oxygen	** _____		_____
	7. Assesses effectiveness of assisted ventilations:	** _____		_____
Symmetric and adequate chest rise with assisted ventilations	• Chest rise and fall			
Bilateral breath sounds present	• Presence of breath sounds			
The team is preparing the equipment for intubation. Bag-valve-mask ventilation is continued.	8. States need to intubate the patient	_____		_____
Note to instructor: If the learners identify that the pulse is absent without chest compressions, they do not need to assess skin color, temperature, or capillary refill.	9. Assesses perfusion status (at least two of the following):	** _____		_____
Central pulses absent without compressions	• Central AND peripheral pulse rate and quality			
Skin pale and cold	• Skin color AND temperature			
Capillary refill > 5 seconds	• Capillary refill			
Electrocardiogram = asystole	10. States need to evaluate cardiac rhythm	_____		_____
Pulses palpable with chest compressions	11. States need to resume chest compressions and obtain vascular access	** _____		_____

Instructor Responses	Skill Steps	Demonstrated		
		Yes		No
Instructor response: "An intraosseous needle has been placed in the left tibia. Proceed with your assessment and interventions."				
Epinephrine administered	**12. States the need to administer epinephrine via the intraosseous needle**	_____		_____
Note to instructor: If the learners identify that the pulse is absent without chest compressions, they do not need to assess skin color, temperature, or capillary refill.	**13. Reassesses perfusion status (at least two of the following):**	_____		_____
Pulses remain absent without compressions	● **Central AND peripheral pulse rate and quality**			
Skin pale and cold	● **Skin color AND temperature**			
Capillary refill remains >5 seconds	● **Capillary refill**			
Asystole on monitor; cardiac compressions resumed	**14. Reassesses cardiac rhythm**	_____		_____
Epinephrine administered	**15. States need to administer a second dose of epinephrine**	_____		_____
Instructor response: "The patient has been orally intubated. Demonstrate and describe your immediate evaluation of endotracheal tube placement."				
Note to instructor: If the learners identify that the pulse is absent without chest compressions, they do not need to assess skin color, temperature, or capillary refill.	**16. Demonstrates and describes assessment of endotracheal tube placement (at least two of the following):**	_____		_____
Good chest rise and fall	● **Observes chest rise and fall**			
Equal breath sounds and absent epigastric sounds	● **Listens for breath sounds in the axillary areas AND over epigastric area**			
End-tidal CO$_2$ device is placed; reading indicates positive placement	● **Assesses end-tidal CO$_2$ via monitor or device (if available)**			
Gastric tube placed	**17. States need to insert a gastric tube**	_____		_____
Instructor response: "The endotracheal tube is in place and is secured. It has been 2 minutes since the last dose of epinephrine. Cardiac compressions continue."				
	18. Stops compressions and reassesses perfusion status (at least two of the following):	_____		_____
Pulses remain absent without compressions	● **Central AND peripheral pulse rate and quality**			
Skin pale and cold	● **Skin color AND temperature**			
Capillary refill remains >5 seconds	● **Capillary refill**			
Asystole on monitor, cardiac compressions resumed	**19. Reassesses cardiac rhythm**	_____		_____
Instructor response: "The child is being ventilated and compressions are being done. Please continue your assessment."				

Instructor Responses	Skill Steps	Demonstrated		
		Yes		No
Unresponsive to pain	20. Assesses level of consciousness (AVPU)	** _____		_____
Pupils fixed and dilated	21. Assesses pupils	_____		_____
No rashes noted, no lesions, no bruising	22. Removes all clothing	_____		_____
Rectal temperature 36.1°C (97°F)	23. Measures rectal temperature	_____		_____
	24. Provides psychosocial support to the family and facilitates family presence	_____		_____
	25. States need to obtain a history using CIAMPEDS	_____		_____
Instructor response: "The physician is considering discontinuing resuscitation. What components of the assessment must be re-evaluated prior to discontinuing resuscitation?"				
	26. States need to re-evaluate primary assessment	_____		_____
Instructor response: "Patient remains asystolic, no palpable pulses, no respiratory effort, unresponsive. Pupils fixed and dilated. Patient is pronounced dead."				

Note to instructor: Discuss with the learners the process following the death of a child in the emergency department. Refer to Chapter 13, "Crisis Intervention," for additional information. In the event that a child dies in the emergency department, the following should be considered:

- Provide emotional support to the family and staff.

- Facilitate the family's participation in postmortem care.

- Provide adequate time for the family to complete closure of the resuscitation event.

- Recognize the diversity of grieving among families.

- Provide written bereavement information, including support groups and telephone numbers to contact staff with questions.

- Offer mementos (lock of hair).

- Consider requesting tissue donation.

- Collect and protect forensic evidence for legal authorities.

- Notify legal authorities of incident as appropriate.

SKILL: PEDIATRIC RESUSCITATION

Teaching Case D

An unresponsive 3-year-old boy is brought to the emergency department by his caregivers after choking on a piece of hot dog. The hot dog was dislodged and he vomited. The Pediatric Assessment Triangle reveals that he is unresponsive, apneic, and pale. The child's weight is 15 kg. A support person responds to the resuscitation room to provide support to the family. Please proceed with your primary and secondary assessments and appropriate interventions.

Instructor Responses	Skill Steps	Demonstrated		
		Yes		No
	1. Positions the child AND demonstrates manually opening the airway	_____		_____
	2. Assesses airway patency (at least three of the following):	**_____		_____
No vocalization	• Vocalization			
Unable to visualize tongue because of vomitus	• Tongue obstruction			
No loose teeth or foreign objects; vomitus noted	• Loose teeth or foreign objects			
Vomitus noted	• Vomitus or other secretions			
No edema	• Edema			
Limp, supine on stretcher	• Preferred posture			
Copious secretions and vomitus in the mouth	• Drooling			
Unresponsive	• Dysphagia			
No snoring or stridor	• Abnormal airway sounds			
	3. Demonstrates suctioning the airway	**_____		_____
Instructor response: "The airway is now patent."				

Instructor Responses	Skill Steps	Demonstrated		
		Yes		No
Note to instructor: If the learners identify that there are no respirations, they can move to the intervention without obtaining information about three indicators of breathing effectiveness.	**4. Assesses breathing effectiveness (at least three of the following):**	** _____		_____
Unresponsive	• **Level of consciousness**			
	• **Spontaneous respirations**			
Apneic	• **Rate and depth of respirations**			
	• **Symmetric chest rise and fall**			
Apneic				
Absent	• **Presence and quality of breath sounds**			
Apneic; indicators of work of breathing absent	• **Work of breathing (at least three of the following):**			
	▪ **Nasal flaring**			
	▪ **Retractions**			
	▪ **Head bobbing**			
	▪ **Expiratory grunting**			
Apneic	▪ **Accessory muscle use**			
No jugular vein distention; trachea midline	• **Jugular vein distention and tracheal position**			
	5. Demonstrates bag-valve-mask ventilation with 100% oxygen	_____		_____
	6. Assesses effectiveness of assisted ventilations:	** _____		_____
Symmetric and adequate chest rise with assisted ventilations	• **Chest rise and fall**			
Bilateral breath sounds present	• **Presence of breath sounds**			
	7. States the need to intubate patient	_____		_____
Instructor response: "The team is preparing the equipment for intubation. Proceed with your assessment."				
	8. Assesses perfusion status (at least two of the following):	** _____		_____
Central pulse rate 120 beats/ minute; peripheral pulses present	• **Central AND peripheral pulse rate and quality**			
Skin pale and cool	• **Skin color AND temperature**			
Capillary refill <2 seconds	• **Capillary refill**			
Instructor response: "The child is now intubated. Demonstrate and describe your immediate evaluation of endotracheal tube placement."				

Instructor Responses	Skill Steps	Demonstrated		
		Yes		No
Symmetric chest rise and fall Equal bilateral breath sounds; epigastric sounds absent End-tidal CO_2 device placed; reading indicates positive placement	9. **Demonstrates and describes assessment of endotracheal tube placement (at least two of the following):** ● **Observes chest rise and fall** ● **Listens for breath sounds in the axillary areas AND over epigastric area** ● **Assesses end-tidal CO_2 via monitor or device (if available)**	** _____		_____
	10. **Inserts gastric tube**	_____		_____
Peripheral access obtained	11. **States need to obtain vascular access and infuse maintenance fluids**	** _____		_____
Unresponsive	12. **Assesses level of consciousness (AVPU)**	** _____		_____
Slightly dilated and sluggish to light	13. **Assesses pupils**	_____		_____
	Secondary Assessment			
No additional signs of illness	14. **Removes all clothing**	_____		_____
	15. **States one measure to prevent heat loss:** ● **Warm blankets** ● **Overhead warming lights or other warming device** ● **Warm ambient environment** ● **Warm intravenous fluids** ● **Warm humidified oxygen**	* _____		_____
BP = 94/64 mm Hg Rectal T = 36.2°C (97°F) P = 120 beats/minute R = assisted ventilations at 24 breaths/minute Weight = 15 kg	16. **States need to get a complete set of vital signs**	_____		_____
Electrocardiogram = sinus tachycardia without ectopy	17. **Places cardiac monitor leads on patient**	_____		_____
Oxygen saturation = 98% with assisted ventilations	18. **Places pulse oximeter on patient** .	_____		_____
No evidence of pain or discomfort	19. **Assesses patient for presence of pain or discomfort**	_____		_____

Instructor response: "Normally, you would now conduct a head-to-toe assessment. It has been done. There are no significant findings."

Instructor Responses	Skill Steps	Demonstrated		
		Yes		No
Mother states he was eating a hot dog at the park. Several minutes later, mother noted he had slumped to the ground. She performed Heimlich maneuver, which dislodged the piece of hot dog. He was blue. No allergies or medications. Previously healthy. Immunizations current.	20. States need to obtain a history using **CIAMPEDS**	_____		_____
Instructor response: "What additional diagnostic studies or interventions might be completed?" Note to instructor: If the learner has previously identified any of the appropriate diagnostic studies or interventions listed, include the diagnostic study or intervention in the total of five.				
	21. Identifies appropriate diagnostic studies or interventions (at least five of the following): • **Arterial blood gas** • **Bedside glucose test** • **Chest radiograph** • **End-tidal CO_2 monitor** • **Laboratory studies** • **Prepare for admission or transfer** • **Psychosocial support** • **Urinary catheter**	*_____		_____
Instructor response: "What is the evaluation and ongoing assessment of this patient?"				
	22. States need to re-evaluate primary assessment	_____		_____
	23. States need to re-evaluate vital signs	_____		_____

SKILL: PEDIATRIC RESUSCITATION

Teaching Case E

An 18-month-old toddler is brought to the emergency department by her caregivers because she is not "acting right." Her mother reports that she has had a fever and her heart seems to be beating too fast. The Pediatric Assessment Triangle reveals that she is alert, her respirations are unlabored, and her color is normal. The child's weight is 15 kg. A support person responds to the resuscitation room to provide support to the family. Please proceed with your primary and secondary assessments and appropriate interventions.

Instructor Responses	Skill Steps	Demonstrated		
		Yes		No
	1. **Assesses airway patency (at least three of the following):**	** _____		_____
Talking to mother	● **Vocalization**			
No obstruction	● **Tongue obstruction**			
No loose teeth or foreign objects	● **Loose teeth or foreign objects**			
No vomitus or other secretions	● **Vomitus or other secretions**			
No edema	● **Edema**			
Sitting on mother's lap	● **Preferred posture**			
No drooling	● **Drooling**			
No dysphagia	● **Dysphagia**			
No abnormal airway sounds	● **Abnormal airway sounds (stridor, snoring)**			
Instructor response: "The airway is patent."				
	2. **Assesses breathing effectiveness (at least three of the following):**	** _____		_____
Alert; talking with mother	● **Level of consciousness**			
Spontaneous respirations	● **Spontaneous respirations**			
Respiratory rate 40 breaths/minute; adequate depth	● **Rate and depth of respirations**			
Symmetric chest rise and fall	● **Symmetric chest rise and fall**			
Breath sounds clear and equal	● **Presence and quality of breath sounds**			
No increased work of breathing	● **Work of breathing (at least three of the following):**			
	▪ **Nasal flaring**			
	▪ **Retractions**			
	▪ **Head bobbing**			
	▪ **Expiratory grunting**			
No accessory muscle use	▪ **Accessory muscle use**			
No jugular vein distention; trachea midline	● **Jugular vein distention and tracheal position**			

Instructor Responses	Skill Steps	Demonstrated		
		Yes		No
	3. Assesses peripheral perfusion status (at least two of the following):	**_____		_____
Central and peripheral pulses strong but too rapid to count	• **Central AND peripheral pulse rate and quality**			
Skin pale and warm	• **Skin color AND temperature**			
Capillary refill 2 seconds	• **Capillary refill**			
Electrocardiogram = supraventricular tachycardia that is too rapid to count	4. **Places cardiac monitor leads on patient**	_____		_____
Patient tolerates mask	5. **Applies oxygen via nonrebreather mask**	**_____		_____
Unable to obtain vascular access after three attempts	6. **States need to obtain vascular access**	**_____		_____
Instructor response: "The patient's condition has changed. She is now responding only to verbal stimuli and is restless and agitated. Her skin is mottled, peripheral pulses are faint and capillary refill is 3 seconds. Her heart rate remains at 260 beats/minute. The airway remains patent; respiratory rate and effort have not changed."				
Patient is synchronized cardioverted at 0.5 J/kg (6 J)	7. **States the need to synchronize cardiovert the patient**	**_____		_____
Electrocardiogram = sinus tachycardia	8. **Reassesses cardiac rhythm**	_____		_____
	9. **Reassesses perfusion status (at least two of the following):**	_____		_____
Central and peripheral pulses strong; rate of 140 beats/minute	• **Central AND peripheral pulse rate and quality**			
Skin normal color; temperature warm	• **Skin color AND temperature**			
Capillary refill 2 seconds	• **Capillary refill**			
Alert, looking at her mother	10. **Reassesses level of consciousness (AVPU)**	**_____		_____
Secondary Assessment				
No additional signs of illness	11. **Removes all clothing**	_____		_____
	12. **States one measure to prevent heat loss:**	*_____		_____
	• **Warm blankets**			
	• **Overhead warming lights or other warming device**			
	• **Warm ambient environment**			
	• **Warm intravenous fluids**			
	• **Warm humidified oxygen**			
BP = 92/60 mm Hg P = 140 beats/minute R = 28 breaths/minute Rectal T = 38.6°C (101.4°F) Weight = 15 kg	13. **States need to get a complete set of vital signs**	_____		_____

Instructor Responses	Skill Steps	Demonstrated		
		Yes		No
Oxygen saturation = 96%	14. Places pulse oximeter on patient	_____		_____
Patient is alert, resting comfortably on the stretcher with mother at her bedside, interactive, not demonstrating any signs of discomfort.	15. Evaluates patient's level of pain or discomfort	_____		_____
Instructor response: "Normally, you would now conduct a head-to-toe assessment. It has been done. There are no significant findings."				
Fever started this morning. While rocking the child, the mother felt the child's heart was beating really fast. She called the pediatrician, who told her to bring her to the emergency department. No allergies or medications Has not received immunizations since 6-month checkup	16. States need to obtain a history using CIAMPEDS	_____		_____
Instructor response: "What additional diagnostic studies or interventions may be completed?" Note to instructor: If the learner has previously identified any of the appropriate diagnostic studies or interventions listed, include the diagnostic study or intervention in the total of five.				
	17. Identifies appropriate diagnostic studies or interventions (at least five of the following): ● 12-lead electrocardiogram ● Administer medications ● Bedside glucose test ● Chest radiograph ● Consider pediatric cardiology consult ● Continue psychosocial support ● Prepare for admission or transfer	*_____		_____
Instructor response: "What is the evaluation and ongoing assessment of this patient?"				
	18. States need to re-evaluate primary assessment	_____		_____
	19. States need to re-evaluate vital signs	_____		_____

Instructor discussion: Other therapies used for supraventricular tachycardia include the administration of adenosine intravenously. Because of the patient's deterioration (poor perfusion status), continued intravenous access attempts were stopped and cardioversion was performed immediately. In cases where intravenous access is available and cardioversion is indicated, consider the administration of an analgesic or sedative prior to cardioversion.

SKILL: PEDIATRIC RESUSCITATION

Teaching Case F

A 2-year-old girl is brought to the emergency department by her father. He says that she has been having a "hard time breathing." She also has had a cold and fever. The Pediatric Assessment Triangle reveals that she is crying, her respirations are rapid, and her color is pale. The child's weight is 12 kg. A support person responds to the resuscitation room to provide support. Please proceed with your primary and secondary assessments and appropriate interventions.

Instructor Responses	Skill Steps	Demonstrated		
		Yes		No
	1. Assesses airway patency (at least three of the following):	** _____		_____
Crying	• **Vocalization**			
No visible obstruction	• **Tongue obstruction**			
No loose teeth or foreign objects	• **Loose teeth or foreign objects**			
No vomitus or other secretions	• **Vomitus or other secretions**			
No edema	• **Edema**			
Sitting up in father's lap	• **Preferred posture**			
No drooling	• **Drooling**			
No dysphagia	• **Dysphagia**			
No abnormal airway sounds	• **Abnormal airway sounds**			
	2. Assesses breathing effectiveness (at least three of the following):	** _____		_____
Awake; can be consoled by her father	• **Level of consciousness**			
Present	• **Spontaneous respirations**			
Rate 60 breaths/minute; adequate depth	• **Rate and depth of respirations**			
Symmetric chest rise	• **Symmetric chest rise and fall**			
Decreased breath sounds on right	• **Presence and quality of breath sounds**			
	• **Work of breathing (at least three of the following):**			
Nasal flaring present	▪ **Nasal flaring**			
Substernal and intercostal retractions	▪ **Retractions**			
No head bobbing	▪ **Head bobbing**			
Expiratory grunting	▪ **Expiratory grunting**			
Using accessory muscles	▪ **Accessory muscle use**			
No jugular vein distention; trachea midline	• **Jugular vein distention or tracheal deviation**			

Instructor Responses	Skill Steps	Demonstrated		
		Yes		No
Head of bed elevated; father at bedside	3. Places the child in a position of comfort	_____		_____
Child tolerates mask	4. Applies oxygen via nonrebreather mask	** _____		_____
Central pulse rapid and strong with weak peripheral pulses. Heart rate 180 beats/minute. Skin tones dark; mucous membranes pale; extremities cool; trunk warm Capillary refill greater than 3 seconds	5. Assesses perfusion status (at least two of the following): • Central AND peripheral pulse rate and quality • Skin color AND temperature • Capillary refill	** _____		_____
Vascular access obtained in her right hand	6. States need to obtain vascular access	** _____		_____
Fluid bolus administered	7. States need to administer a 20-ml/kg fluid bolus	** _____		_____
Central pulses strong; peripheral pulses stronger at 166 beats/minute Mucous membranes pale; extremities cool; trunk warm Capillary refill 3 seconds	8. Reassesses perfusion status (at least two of the following): • Central AND peripheral pulse rate and quality • Skin color AND temperature • Capillary refill	_____		_____
Repeat fluid bolus administered	9. States need to administer a repeat 20-ml/kg fluid bolus	_____		_____
Central pulses strong; peripheral pulses strong at 150 beats/minute Mucous membranes pale; extremities and trunk warm Capillary refill 2 seconds	10. Reassesses perfusion status (at least two of the following): • Central AND peripheral pulse rate and quality • Skin color AND temperature • Capillary refill	_____		_____
Opens eyes or cries to verbal stimuli, otherwise keeps eyes closed	11. Assesses level of consciousness (AVPU)	_____ **		_____
Pupils equal and reactive	12. Assesses pupils	_____		_____
	Secondary Assessment			
No additional signs of illness	13. Removes all clothing	_____		_____

Instructor Responses	Skill Steps	Demonstrated		
		Yes		**No**
	14. **States one measure to prevent heat loss:**	* _____		_____
	• **Warm blankets**			
	• **Overhead warming lights or other warming device**			
	• **Warm ambient environment**			
	• **Warm intravenous fluids**			
	• **Warm humidified oxygen**			
BP = 92/56 mm Hg P = 130 beats/minute R = 40 breaths/minute Axillary T = 39.4°C (103°F) Weight = 12 kg	15. **States need to get a complete set of vital signs**	_____		_____
Electrocardiogram = sinus tachycardia without ectopy	16. **Places cardiac monitor leads on patient**	_____		_____
Oxygen saturation = 96% with supplemental oxygen	17. **Places pulse oximeter on patient**	_____		_____
Child is restless; occasional facial grimace; crying intermittently	18. **Assesses patient for presence of pain or discomfort**	_____		_____
Instructor response: "Normally, you would now conduct a head-to-toe assessment. It has been done. There are no significant findings."				
Child has had cold symptoms for past week; fever today with cough and difficulty breathing. No allergies and no medications. No past medical history.	19. **States need to obtain a history using CIAMPEDS**	_____		_____
Instructor response: "What additional diagnostic studies or interventions may be completed?"				
Note to instructor: If the learner has previously identified any of the appropriate diagnostic studies or interventions listed, include the diagnostic study or intervention in the total of five.				
	20. **Identifies appropriate diagnostic studies or interventions (at least five of the following):**	* _____		_____
	• **Arterial blood gas**			
	• **Bedside glucose test**			
	• **Chest radiograph**			
	• **Consider sepsis workup**			
	• **Consider urinary catheter**			
	• **Continue psychosocial support of family**			
	• **Laboratory studies**			
	• **Medications**			
	• **Prepare for admission or transfer**			
	• **Respiratory isolation**			
Instructor response: "What is the evaluation and ongoing assessment of this patient?"				
	21. **States need to re-evaluate primary assessment**	_____		_____
	22. **States need to re-evaluate vital signs**	_____		_____

Appendix A

INJURY PREVENTION RESOURCES

- **National Center for Injury Prevention and Control**
  Centers for Disease Control (CDC)
  Program Development and Implementation
  1600 Clifton Road NE, MS:F-41
  Atlanta, GA 30333
  Telephone: (404) 639-3311

  This is the national coordination and funding source for the major injury control programs in the United States. Staff will direct the caller to resources that might be available through their injury prevention centers. The centers marked with an asterisk (*) are CDC injury prevention centers.

- **Harborview Injury Prevention Research Center***
  University of Washington
  325 Ninth Avenue, Box 359960
  Seattle, WA 98104
  Telephone: (206) 521-1520
  Website: www.weber.u.washington.edu\~hiprc

  ALL AGE GROUPS

  This center provides all types of injury prevention information, literature, and data for all age groups. Contact Frederick Rivaro, MD, MPH, for further information.

- **University of Iowa Injury Prevention Research Center***
  Department of Preventive Medicine and Environmental Health
  126 IREH, Oakdale Campus
  Iowa City, IA 52242
  Telephone: (319) 335-9627
  Website: www.pmeh.uiowa.edu

  ALL AGE GROUPS

  The focus of this organization is mainly on rural injury prevention materials, programs, and research for all age groups.

- **University of North Carolina Injury Prevention Research Center***
  Rosenau Hall, CB #7400
  Chapel Hill, NC 27599
  Telephone: (919) 966-3916
  Website: www.sph.unc.edu\iprc
  Internet E-mail: unciprc@unc.edu

  ALL AGE GROUPS

  This research center has a library of resources and program materials especially related to automobiles, safety restraints, and crashes.

- **The Johns Hopkins Center for Injury, Research and Policy***
  The School of Hygiene and Public Health
  624 North Broadway
  Baltimore, MD 21205
  Telephone: (410) 955-2636
  Website: www.sph.jhu.edu\research\centers\cirp

  ALL AGE GROUPS

  This center provides injury prevention materials and information about injury prevention community programs. They are also currently developing a specialized database on childhood injuries.

- **The American Trauma Society**
  8903 Presidential Parkway
  Suite 512
  Upper Marlboro, MD 20772
  Telephone: (800) 556-7890
  Website: www.amtrauma.org
  Internet E-mail: atstrauma@aol.com

  ALL AGE GROUPS

  Program materials on injury prevention are available.

- **National Resource Center**
  Emergency Medicine Services for Children (EMS-C)
  111 Michigan Avenue, NW
  Washington, DC 20010
  Telephone: (202) 884-4927
  Website: emsc.com/nera
  Internet E-mail: info@emscnrc.com

  CHILDREN ONLY

  This is the clearing house and resource center for all Emergency Medical Services for Children (EMS-C) activities. Literature, curricula, and other resources are available.

- **CSN National Injury and Violence Prevention Resource Center – Georgetown University**
  National Center for Education in Maternal and Child Health
  2000 15th Street North
  Suite 701
  Arlington, VA 22201
  Telephone: (703) 524-7802
  Website: www.ncemch.org
  Internet E-mail: info@ncemch.org

  CHILDREN ONLY

  This is a resource center for program materials.

- **Farm Safety for Kids**
  110 South Chestnut Avenue
  Earlham, IA 50072
  Telephone: (515) 758-2827
  Website: www.fs4jk.org
  Internet E-mail: fs4jk@netins.net

  CHILDREN ONLY

  This is an excellent resource for injury prevention materials related to rural and farm injuries.

- **National Safe Kids Campaign**
  1300 Pennsylvania Avenue, NW
  Suite 1000
  Washington, DC 20004
  Telephone: (202) 662-0600
  Website: www.safekids.org

  CHILDREN ONLY

  This is a national program of the Children's National Medical Center in Washington, DC. Resource materials and program ideas are available. There are also chapters at the state and local levels. Contact the regional, state, or local health department or local children's hospital.

- **National Parent Teachers Association**
  330 North Wabash
  Suite 2100
  Chicago, IL 60611
  Telephone: (312) 670-6782
  Website: www.pta.org
  Internet E-mail: info@pta.org

  This organization has taken a strong position regarding childhood injury prevention and has information and materials related to the topic.

- **US Consumer Product Safety Commission**
  National Injury Information Clearinghouse
  Washington, DC 20207
  Telephone: (800) 638-2772

  ALL AGE GROUPS

  This agency provides injury information related to products on the market, including toys and baby equipment.

- **National Safety Council**
  1121 Spring Lake Drive
  Itasca, IL 60143
  Telephone: (800) 621-7619
  Website: www.nsc.org
  Internet E-mail: customerservice.nsc.org

  ALL AGE GROUPS

  This organization has many materials available regarding injury prevention and occupational injury prevention.

- **Emergency Nurses CARE**
  205 South Whiting Street
  Suite 403
  Alexandria, VA 22304
  Telephone: (800) 942-0011
  Contact: Barbara A. Foley, RN, BS
  Associate Executive Director

Appendix B

CHILDHOOD DEVELOPMENT (INFANT TO ADOLESCENT)

PHYSICAL AND MOTOR DEVELOPMENT	PSYCHOSOCIAL DEVELOPMENT	INTELLECTUAL/ LANGUAGE DEVELOPMENT	PAIN	DEATH
Infant Development (1 Month to 1 Year)				
GROWTH • Period of most rapid growth • Infant weight gain – 1 oz/day • Weight doubles by age 6 months; triples by 1 year	Trust versus Mistrust (Erikson) • When physical needs are consistently met, infants learn to trust self and environment Common Fears (after 6 months) • Separation • Strangers	Sensorimotor Period (Piaget) • Infants learn by the use of their senses and activities	• Infants do experience pain • Degree of pain perceived is unknown	• Infants do not understand the meaning of death • The developing sense of separation serves as a basis for a beginning understanding of the meaning of death
Toddler Development (1 to 2 Years)				
GROWTH • Rate significantly slows down, accompanied by a tremendous decrease in appetite GENERAL APPEARANCE • Potbellied • Exaggerated lumbar curve • Wide-based gait INCREASED MOBILITY • Hallmark of physical development in the toddler	Autonomy versus Shame and Doubt (Erikson) • Increasing independence and self-care activities • Expanding the world with which the toddler interacts • Need to experience joy of exploring and exerting some control over body functions and activity, while maintaining support of "anchor" (i.e., primary caregiver) Common Fears • Separation • Loss of control • Altered rituals • Pain	Sensorimotor Period (Piaget) • Cognition and language not yet sophisticated enough for children to learn through thought processes and communication	• No formal concept of pain, related to immature thought process and poorly developed body image • React as intensely to painless procedures as to ones that hurt, especially when restrained • Intrusive procedures, such as taking temperatures, are very distressing • React to pain with physical resistance, aggression, negativism, and regression • Rare for toddlers to fake pain • Verbal responses concerning pain are unreliable	• Understanding of death still very limited • Belief that loss of significant others is temporary; reinforced by: 　■ Developing sense of object permanence (i.e., objects continue to exist even if cannot be seen) 　■ Repeated experiences of separations and reunions 　■ Magical thinking 　■ TV shows (e.g., cartoon characters)

Appendix B (continued)

PHYSICAL AND MOTOR DEVELOPMENT	PSYCHOSOCIAL DEVELOPMENT	INTELLECTUAL/ LANGUAGE DEVELOPMENT	PAIN	DEATH
		Preschool Development (3 to 5 Years)		
GROWTH • Weight gain – 2 kg/year • Height gain – 6 to 8 cm/year • Usually are half adult height by 2 years of age GENERAL APPEARANCE • "Baby fat" and protuberant abdomen disappear	Initiative versus Guilt (Erikson) • Greater autonomy and independence • Still intense need for caregivers when under stress • Initiate activities, rather than just imitating others • Age of discovery, curiosity, and developing social behavior • Sense of self as individual Common Fears • Mutilation • Loss of control • Death • Dark • Ghosts	Preoperational (Piaget) • Time of trial/error learning • Egocentric – view experiences from own perspective • Understand explanations only in terms of real events or what their senses tell them • No logical or abstract thought; coincidence confused with causation • Magical thinking continues • Difficulty distinguishing between reality and fantasy • May see illness or injury as punishment for "bad" thoughts or behavior • Imaginary friends; fascination with superheros and monsters	• Pain perceived as punishment for bad thoughts or behavior • Difficulty understanding that painful procedures help them get well • Cannot differentiate between "good" pain (as a result of treatment) and "bad" pain (resulting from injury or illness) • React to painful procedures with aggression and verbal reprimands (e.g., "I hate you"; "You're mean")	• Incomplete understanding of death fosters anxiety because of fear of death • Death is seen as an altered state of consciousness in which a person cannot perform normal activities, such as eating or walking • Perceive immobility, sleep, and other alterations in consciousness as death-like states; associate words and phrases (e.g., "put to sleep") with death • Death is seen as reversible; reinforced by TV and cartoons • Unable to perceive inevitability of death due to limited time concept • View death as punishment

Appendix B (continued)

PHYSICAL AND MOTOR DEVELOPMENT	PSYCHOSOCIAL DEVELOPMENT	INTELLECTUAL/ LANGUAGE DEVELOPMENT	PAIN	DEATH
		School-Aged Children (6 to 10 Years)		
GROWTH • Relatively latent period	Industry versus Inferiority (Erikson) • Age of accomplishment, increasing competence, and mastery of new skills • Successes contribute to positive self-esteem and a sense of control • Need parental support in times of stress; may be unwilling or unable to ask Common Fears • Separation from friends • Loss of control • Physical disability	Concrete Operations (Piaget) • Beginning of logical thought • Deductive reasoning develops • Improved concept of time; awareness of possible long-term consequences of illness • More sophisticated understanding of causality • Still interpret phrases and idioms at face value	• Reaction to pain affected by past experiences, parental response, and the meaning attached to it. • Better able to localize and describe pain accurately • Pain can be exaggerated because of heightened fears of bodily injury, pain, and death.	• Concept of death more logically based • Understand death as the irreversible cessation of life • View death as a tragedy that happens to others, not themselves • When death is actual threat, may feel responsible for death and experience guilt

Appendix B (continued)

PHYSICAL AND MOTOR DEVELOPMENT	PSYCHOSOCIAL DEVELOPMENT	INTELLECTUAL/ LANGUAGE DEVELOPMENT	PAIN	DEATH
		Adolescent Development (11 to 18 Years)		
GROWTH • Females – growth spurt begins at age 9 1/2 years • Males – growth spurt begins at age 10 1/2 years PUBERTY • Secondary sex characteristics begin to develop between the ages of 8 and 13 years for females; 10 and 14 years for males	Identity versus Role Confusion (Erikson) • Transition from childhood to adulthood • Quest for independence often leads to family dissention • Major concerns: establishing identity and developing mature sexual orientation • Risk-taking behaviors – feel that nothing bad can happen to them Common Fears • Changes in appearance or functioning • Dependency • Loss of control	Concrete to Formal Operations (Piaget) • Memory fully developed • Concept of time well understood • Adolescents can project to the future and imagine potential consequences of actions and illnesses • Some adolescents do not achieve formal operations	• Can locate and quantify pain accurately and thoroughly • Often hyperresponsive to pain; reacts to fear of changes in appearance or function • In general, highly controlled in responding to pain and painful procedures	• Understanding of death similar to that of adults • Intellectually believe that death can happen to them, but avoid realistic thoughts of death • Many adolescents defy the possibility of death through reckless behavior, substance abuse, or daring sports activities

Appendix C

CONSIDERATIONS IN CHOOSING LANGUAGE

Words that have different meanings can be confusing. If it is likely that the child will hear the standard medical expressions used, these words should be explained or defined. Ideally the child should be asked if he or she knows what nurses and physicians mean when they say these words. Compare, for example, the phrases in the left column with the suggested alternatives in the right.

Potentially Ambiguous	Clearer
Dressing; dressing change *Why are they going to undress me?* *Do I have to change my clothes?* *Will I be naked?*	Bandages; clean, new bandages.
Stool collection *Why do they want to collect little chairs?*	Use child's familiar term, such as "poop" or "BM" or "doody."
Urine *You're in?*	Use child's familiar term, such as "pee."
Shot *Are they mad at me? When people get shot, they're really badly hurt. Are they trying to hurt me?*	Medicine through a (small, tiny) needle.
CT Scan *Will there be cats? Or something that scratches?*	Describe in simple terms, and explain what the letters of the common name stand for.
PICU *Pick you?*	Explain, as above.
ICU *I see you?*	Explain, as above.
IV *Ivy?*	Explain, as above.
Move you to the floor *Why are they going to put me on the ground?*	Unit; ward. (Explain why the child is being transferred and where.)
Take a picture (x-rays, computerized tomography scan, and MRI machines are far larger than a familiar camera, move differently, and don't yield a familiar end product).	A picture of the inside of you. Describe appearance, sounds, and movement of the equipment.

Appendix C (continued)

Words can be experienced as "hard" or "soft," according to how much they increase the perceived threat of a situation. For example, consider the following word choices.

Hard	Soft
This part will hurt.	It (you) may feel (or feel very): sore, achy, scratchy, tight, snug, full, or . . . (other manageable, descriptive term). (Words such as "scratch," "poke," or "sting" might be familiar for some children and frightening to others.)
The medicine will burn.	Some children say they feel a very warm feeling.
The medicine will taste (or smell) bad.	The medicine may taste (or smell) different than anything you have tasted before. After you take it, will you tell me how it was for you?
As big as . . . (e.g., size of an incision or of a catheter)	Smaller than . . .
As long as . . . (e.g., for a duration of a procedure)	For less time that it takes you to . . .

Note: Words or phrases that are helpful to one child may be threatening for another. Health care providers must listen carefully and be sensitive to the child's use and response to language.

Potentially Unfamiliar	Concrete Explanation
Take your vitals (or your vital signs)	Measure your temperature; see how warm your body is; see how fast and strongly your heart is working.
Electrodes, leads	Sticky like a bandage, with a small, wet spot in the center, and small strings that attach to the snap (monitor electrodes); Paste like wet sand, with strings and tiny metal cups that stick to the paste (EEG electrodes). The paste washes off easily afterward; the strings go into a box that will make a picture of how your heart (or brain) is working. (Show the child electrodes and leads before using. Let the child handle them and apply them to a doll or to self.)
Intravenous, IV	Medicine that works best when it goes right **Into a Vein** (**IntraVenous**). It's the quickest way to help you get better. (First ask the child if he or she knows what a vein is, and why some medicine is OK to take by mouth and others work best into a vein. Explain the concept of initials if the child is old enough.)

Hang your (IV) medication	Bring new medicine in a bag, and attach it to the little tube already in your arm. The needle goes into the tube, not into your arm, so you won't feel it.
NPO	Nothing to eat. Your stomach needs to be empty. (Explain why.)
Anesthesia	The physician will give you medicine – you may hear it called "anesthesia." It will help you go into a very deep sleep. You will not feel anything at all. The physicians know just the right amount of medicine to give you so that you will stay asleep through your *whole* operation. When the operation is over, the physician stops giving you that medicine and helps you wake up. (Avoid saying, "They're going to put you to sleep." Children relate being put to sleep with an animal being put to sleep.)
Incision	Small opening. (Follow with discussion of how cuts and scrapes received while playing have healed in the past.)

Adapted from Gaynard L, Wolfer J, Goldberger J, Thompson RH, Redburn L, Laidley L. *Psychosocial Care of Children in Hospitals: A Clinical Practice Manual from the ACCH Child Life Research Project.* Bethesda, Md: Association for the Care of Children's Health; 1990:62-64. Used with permission.

Appendix D

ANATOMIC AND PHYSIOLOGIC DIFFERENCES

AIRWAY	
Differences	**Clinical Significance**
• Infants have smaller upper and lower airways. The tracheal diameter of infants approximates the diameter of the little finger of the infant.	• Small amounts of mucous, edema, or a small foreign body can obstruct the airway and markedly increase airway resistance.
• Infants are obligate nose breathers for the first several months of life.	• Nasal passages must be kept clear of secretions to prevent respiratory distress.
• The tongue is larger in proportion to the mouth.	• The airway can easily become obstructed by the tongue, especially when there is an altered level of consciousness. Repositioning is often all that is needed to open the airway.
• The cartilage of the larynx is softer.	• Any hyperextension or hyperflexion can compress the airway.
• There is increased proportion of soft tissue in the pediatric airway.	• Infants have an increased susceptibility to airway obstruction from edema.
• The larynx is positioned more anteriorly and cephalad.	• There is an increased risk of obstruction by aspiration.
• The epiglottis is floppy, the trachea is shorter, and airway malformations are more common.	• Intubation and maintenance of correct endotracheal tube position are more difficult in infants. Right mainstem intubation is common.
• The cricoid cartilage is the narrowest part of larynx, as opposed to the vocal cords in adults.	• This provides a natural seal for the endotracheal tube. Use uncuffed tubes in children younger than 8 years of age. Cuffed tubes in younger children may be damaging to the airway.

Appendix D (continued)

By about 8 years of age, children's respiratory anatomy and physiology approximate those of adults.

Differences	Clinical Significance
• Because of their size and immaturity, children have less compensatory reserve than adults.	• The younger the child, the more susceptible to respiratory distress and failure. Children tire easily.
• Children have cartilaginous sternum and ribs; the chest wall is softer and more compliant.	• Retractions are common when children experience respiratory distress. Severe retractions compromise the ability to generate adequate tidal volume.
• Intercostal muscles are poorly developed.	• Infants rely primarily on the diaphragm for breathing. Keeping children in respiratory distress upright helps support diaphragmatic function.
• Infants breathe predominately using abdominal muscles.	• Any pressure on the diaphragm from above (e.g., asthma) or below (e.g., abdominal distention) can impede respiratory effort.
• Ribs are more horizontally oriented.	• Chest expansion is decreased during breathing.
• There are fewer and smaller alveoli.	• There is less surface area for gas exchange.
• Collateral pathways of ventilation are incompletely developed.	• Any airway obstruction compromises gas exchange to a greater extent in children.
• Less elastic and collagen tissue is present in the lungs.	• Elastic tissue helps support alveoli and keeps them open at the end of expiration. Having less elastic and collagen tissue increases the lung's susceptibility to air leaks and edema.
• The metabolic rate in infants is approximately two times the adult rate.	• This factor increases the need for oxygen. Hypoxia occurs more rapidly in respiratory distress. Anything that increases the metabolic rate (e.g., fever) contributes to respiratory demands.
• The chest wall is thin.	• Breath sounds are easily transmitted and may be misleading (e.g., breath sounds may be heard over a pneumothorax).

Appendix D (continued)

CIRCULATION

Differences	Clinical Significance
• The myocardium is less compliant (myocardial fibers are shorter and less elastic), contractile mass is less, and stroke volume is limited (1.5 ml/kg/beat/minute compared to 75 to 90 ml/beat in an adult).	• Heart rate rather than stroke volume increases to maintain cardiac output, which falls precipitously with sustained bradycardia or heart rates exceeding 200 beats/minute.
• Infants have a higher cardiac output (200 ml/kg/minute versus 100 ml/kg/minute in an adult).	• This higher output provides for increased oxygen needs, but leaves little cardiac output reserve. Any stresses, such as hypothermia or sepsis, can lead to acute deterioration.
• The circulating blood volume is less than in adults (infant: 90 ml/kg; child: 80 ml/kg; adult: 70 ml/kg).	• Small blood losses can cause circulatory compromise.
• Children are capable of maintaining adequate cardiac output for long periods because of strong compensatory mechanisms. Rapid deterioration can occur when compensatory mechanisms are exhausted.	• Hypotension is late sign of circulatory decompensation. Children may remain normotensive until 25% of their blood volume is lost. Assess capillary refill as an indicator of peripheral circulatory status (capillary refill should be less than 2 seconds).
• A greater percent of total body weight is water. Daily water turnover involves more than half of the extracellular fluid. In the adult, one fifth of the extracellular fluid is exchanged daily.	• There is greater potential for dehydration.
• Infants in the first few months have a decreased ability to concentrate urine (normal urine output – infant: 2 ml/kg/hour; child: 1 ml/kg/hour; adult: 0.5 ml/kg/hour).	• The kidneys cannot efficiently adjust to fluid changes.
• Neonates have an incompletely developed sympathetic nervous system.	• Neonates are particularly sensitive to parasympathetic stimulation (e.g., suctioning, defecating).

Appendix D (continued)

NEUROLOGIC (DISABILITY)

Differences	Clinical Significance
• All primary structures of the brain are present at birth, but additional growth occurs over the first few years of life. The brain is 25% of its mature adult weight at birth, 75% by 2 1/2 years, and 90% by 6 years of age.	• When a neurologic insult occurs in young children, it is difficult to predict the degree of recovery because of continuing brain growth. The outcome may include complete recovery, severe permanent sequelae, or evidence of learning disabilities as they mature.
• The cranial nerves are intact from birth. Immature reflexes (e.g., Moro) and protective reflexes (e.g., gag) are present from birth.	• The presence or absence of the immature reflexes varies with age and can be used to assess the neurologic status of infants.
• Babinski's reflex is normally present until children start walking.	• After children are 2 years of age, Babinski's reflex is an abnormal neurologic finding.
• In infants, the autonomic nervous system is not fully developed.	• The ability to control body temperature in response to environmental changes is limited.
• Infants' posture is predominately one of flexion.	• This is an important indicator of normal neurologic status.
• The cranial sutures in infants are not fused until approximately 16 to 18 months of age.	• The head size can expand to accommodate gradual increases in intracranial pressure.

EXPOSURE (ENVIRONMENT)

Differences	Clinical Significance
• Infants and young children have higher body surface area-to-weight ratios. Their proportionally large head accounts for much of the exposed surface area.	• Infants and children can easily become hypothermic because of the increased surface area from which to lose heat. Effects of hypothermia can include central nervous system depression, respiratory depression, bronchorrhea, myocardial irritability, impaired peripheral oxygen delivery, metabolic acidosis, hypoglycemia, and coagulopathy.
• Infants younger than 3 months of age are unable to produce heat through shivering and must burn brown fat for thermogenesis.	• This process increases oxygen consumption and may lead to hypoxia.

Appendix D (continued)

OTHER PEDIATRIC DIFFERENCES	
Differences	**Clinical Significance**
• Infants younger than 2 to 3 months of age have immature immune systems. Some passive immunity is acquired in utero. However, newborns have had no previous exposures to trigger their own antibody response. After 3 months of age, they are able to develop their own protection against infection.	• Young infants cannot efficiently localize an infection. Infants younger than 2 to 3 months of age are at high risk for developing sepsis.
• Significant changes in body weight occur in infancy and childhood. Approximate weight rules by age: 2 times birth weight by 5 months of age; 3 times birth weight by 1 year of age; 7 times birth weight by 7 years of age; 14 times birth weight by 14 years of age. Average birth weight is 3.5 kg. Another weight estimate is 8 + (2 × age in years) = weight in kilograms.	• Estimation of weights is often necessary in life-threatening and trauma situations; accurate estimates are essential for proper pharmacologic and fluid therapy. Commercially available charts and devices have been developed to assist in the estimation of weights in infants and children. For example, there are pediatric resuscitation tapes that give an estimated weight (up to 34 kg) based on the child's measured length. Measured weights should be obtained in the emergency department whenever possible.
• Children metabolize drugs at different rates.	• All drug dosages should be determined based on children's weight in kilograms. Precalculated drug dosage cards or other tools should be available as a reference for medication dosages and fluid replacement therapy.
• Infants and small children have limited glycogen stores.	• Hypoglycemia occurs frequently in ill or injured children.
• Children have a higher metabolic rate and greater insensible losses than adults.	• Children have a greater maintenance fluid requirement per kilogram than adults. However, because children are smaller, the absolute fluid volume administered will be less than that in adults. Maintenance therapy replaces water and electrolytes lost through respiration, evaporation, the gastrointestinal tract, and urine. Maintenance fluids are calculated individually for children by weight, and adjusted in relation to their condition. It is also important to monitor serum electrolyte values and initiate treatment, as ordered.
• Children have a proportionally larger and heavier head in comparison to body size. This also contributes to a higher center of gravity in children. The head often becomes the lead point of the body. Young children tend to pitch head first during a fall.	• Children are at high risk for head injury. Other injuries in which the head is the lead point of the body also occur (e.g., bucket drownings).
• Children have incomplete bone calcification, rendering their bones more flexible.	• The absence of fractures should not rule out injury to underlying structures.
• Children's bones are still growing.	• Fractures heal more rapidly in children, but injuries to growth plates may arrest bone growth.

Appendix E

VARIETY OF AILMENTS

CULTURAL CONSIDERATIONS OF SOUTHEAST ASIAN FOLK HEALING PRACTICES				
Culture	**Practice**	**Ailments**	**Process**	**Appearance**
• Southeast Asian • Middle Eastern • Chinese	Cupping[1,2]	• Fever • Headache • Cold, cough[1,2]	A vacuum is created in a small glass cup by burning rubbing alcohol, a candle, or paper inside it. The cup is quickly inverted and placed on skin of forehead, shoulder, or trunk for up to 30 minutes.[1,2]	Circular ecchymotic area, may be painful to touch. Multiple cups in vertical rows may be present on the trunk.[1,2]
Southeast Asian	Moxi-bustion[1,2]	• Abdominal pain • Abdominal cramps • Diarrhea • Ulcers • Hernias[1,2]	The moxa herb is shaped and slowly smoldered near or on the skin in the periumbilical area, chest, or back. Incense sticks are sometimes used.[1,2]	If the burning herb is in contact with the skin, lesions resemble cigarette burns, usually in a pattern of four, six, or eight marks, pyramid formation.[1,2]
Southeast Asian	Coining Spooning Fingering[1,2]	• Fever • Pain • Cough • Cold • Vomiting • Headache • Muscle cramps[1,2]	Camphorated oil or salve is rubbed on skin, the area firmly stroked downward with the edge of a coin, spoon, or knuckle. Performed on the neck, back, chest, inner upper arm, shoulder, or abdomen[1,2]	Superficial ecchymotic or red linear marks with petechiae. Striped pattern appearance. On the back, parallel linear marks on each side of the spine with linear marks along the rib contour.[1,2]
Southeast Asian	Burning[2]	• Pain • Cough • Diarrhea • Failure to thrive[2]	A weed-like grass is dried and dipped in hot lard or fat, and the tip is ignited and applied to the skin. Last-resort treatment.[2]	Single burn in center of forehead or two vertical rows of burns down the neck and trunk.[2]
Southeast Asian	Pinching[1,2]	• Headache • Cold • Pain • Flu[1,2]	The skin is repeatedly pinched with a snapping motion. Camphorated salve or water may be used to lubricate the skin. Performed between eyebrows, on neck, or chest.[1,2]	Small welts in a regular pattern; may be ecchymotic areas. On the neck, may have pattern of two or three vertical rows on each side of the trachea.[1,2]

References

1. Ratliff SS, Nguyen H. *Southeast Asian Healing Practices, Birthmarks, and Amulets*. Columbus, Ohio: Children's Hospital; 1989. Poster.

2. Schreiner D. *Southeast Asian Healing Practice/Child Abuse?* Presented at the Indochinese Health Care Conference in Eugene, Ore. Portland, Ore: Peck Health Center; 1981.

Appendix F

DISTRACTION/COPING KIT

A distraction or coping kit provides a centralized location to store a variety of items to facilitate the use of distraction techniques. The individual items are placed in a container with a lid for storage for use in treatment or examination rooms.

Distraction kits should provide an array of items appropriate for a variety of age groups. All the items may be stored in one container, or smaller kits for specific ages or developmental levels may also be effective. When age-specific kits are developed, containers can be color coded to facilitate selection of the appropriate kit. Clear plastic containers with colored lids or colored plastic containers work well for storing the items. The advantages of plastic containers are durability and ease of cleaning. Items should be cleaned with an appropriate nontoxic cleaning agent prior to being returned to the kit.

Suggested Distraction Kit Contents

■ Infants, Toddlers, and Preschoolers

- Rattle
- Plastic keys
- Infant toy
- Unbreakable mirror
- Pop-up book
- Infant or toddler picture book (with heavy cardboard pages)
- Finger puppets
- Glitter wand
- Pacifier (for one patient use only)
- Infant music box
- Books with sound effects
- Cassette tape or compact disc of child's story or soothing music if a tape or compact disk player is available
- Videotape (e.g., Barney or other currently recognizable preschool characters) if a videocassette recorder is available
- Soap bubbles
- Pinwheel

■ School-Aged Children and Adolescents

- Pinwheel
- Soap bubbles
- Soft foam "squeeze" ball
- Glitter wand
- Small, erasable dry ink board or doodle board
- Small Etch A Sketch®
- Hand-held electronic game
- Playing cards or game cards (e.g., Uno™)
- Silly Putty™
- Cassette tape or compact disk of soothing music if a tape or compact disk player is available
- Videotape of current family oriented, nonviolent movie if a videocassette recorder is available
- Picture book (e.g., soothing scenery)

Appendix G

NONPHARMACOLOGIC GUIDELINES FOR PAIN MANAGEMENT

GENERAL STRATEGIES

- Form a trusting relationship with child and family:
  - Express concern regarding their reports of pain.
  - Take an active role in seeking effective pain management strategies.
- Use general guidelines to prepare child for procedure.
- Prepare child before potentially painful procedures but avoid "planting" the idea of pain. For example, instead of saying, "This is going to (or may) hurt," say, "Sometimes this feels like pushing, sticking, or pinching, and sometimes it doesn't bother people. Tell me what it feels like to you."
  - Use "nonpain" descriptors when possible (e.g., "It feels like intense heat" rather than "It's a burning pain").
  - This allows for variation in sensory perception, avoids suggesting pain, and gives child control in describing reactions.
- Avoid evaluative statements or descriptions (e.g., "This is a terrible procedure" or "It really will hurt a lot").
- Stay with child during a painful procedure.
  - Encourage parents to stay with child if child and parent desire; encourage parent to talk softly to child and to remain near child's head.
  - Involve parents in learning specific nonpharmacologic strategies and assisting child in their use.
- Educate child about the pain, especially when explanation may lessen anxiety (e.g., that child's pain is expected after surgery and does not indicate something is wrong; reassure that child is not responsible for the pain).
- For long-term pain control, give child a doll, which becomes "the patient," and allow child to do everything to the doll that is done to the child. Pain control can be emphasized through the doll by stating, "Dolly feels better after the medicine."
- Teach procedures to child and family for later use.

SPECIFIC STRATEGIES

Distraction

- Involve parent and child in identifying strong distractors.
- Involve child in play; use radio, tape recorder, record player; have child sing or use rhythmic breathing.
- Have child take a deep breath and blow it out until told to stop.
- Have child blow bubbles to "blow the hurt away."
- Have child concentrate on yelling or saying "ouch" by focusing on "yelling loud or soft as you feel it hurt; that way I know what's happening."

Appendix G (continued)

- Have child look through kaleidoscope (type with glitter suspended in fluid-filled tube) and encourage to concentrate by asking, "Do you see the different designs?"

- Use humor, such as watching cartoons, telling jokes or funny stories, or acting silly with child.

- Have child read, play games, or visit with friends.

Relaxation

- With an infant or young child:

  - Hold in a comfortable, well-supported position, such as vertically against the chest and shoulder.

  - Rock in a wide, rhythmic arc in a rocking chair or sway back and forth, rather than bouncing child.

  - Repeat one or two words softly, such as "Mommy's here."

- With a slightly older child:

  - Ask child to take a deep breath and "go limp as a rag doll" while exhaling slowly, then ask child to yawn (demonstrate if needed).

  - Help child assume a comfortable position (e.g., pillow under neck and knees).

  - Begin progressive relaxation: Starting with the toes, systematically instruct child to let each body part "go limp" or "feel heavy"; if child has difficulty relaxing, instruct child to tense or tighten each body part and then relax it.

  - Allow child to keep eyes open, since children may respond better if eyes are open rather than closed during relaxation.

Guided Imagery

- Have child identify some highly pleasurable real or pretend experiences.

- Have child describe details of the event, including as many senses as possible (e.g., "feel the cool breezes," "see the beautiful colors," "hear the pleasant music").

- Have child write down or record story.

- Encourage child to concentrate only on the pleasurable event during the painful time; enhance the image by recalling specific details, such as reading the story or playing the record.

- Combine with relaxation.

Positive Self-Talk

- Teach child positive statements to say when in pain (e.g., "I will be feeling better soon," "When I go home, I will feel better and we will eat ice cream").

Appendix G (continued)

Thought Stopping

- Identify positive facts about the painful event (e.g., "It does not last long").

- Identify reassuring information (e.g., "If I think about something else, it does not hurt as much").

- Condense positive and reassuring facts into a set of brief statements, and have child memorize them (e.g., "Short procedures, good veins, little hurt, nice nurse, go home").

- Have child repeat the memorized statements whenever thinking about or experiencing the painful event.

CUTANEOUS STIMULATION

- Include simple rhythmic rubbing; use of pressure, electric vibrator, massage with hand lotion, powder, or menthol cream; application of heat or cold, such as an ice cube on the site before giving injection or application of ice to the site opposite the painful area (e.g., if right knee hurts, place ice on left knee).

- A more sophisticated method is transcutaneous electrical nerve stimulation (TENS) (use of controlled low-voltage electricity to the body via electrodes placed on the skin).

Behavior Contracting

- Informal – may be used with children as young as 4 or 5 years of age:

  - Use stars or tokens as rewards.

  - Give uncooperative or procrastinating children (during a procedure) a limited time (measured by a visible timer) to complete the procedure.

  - Proceed as needed if child is unable to comply.

  - Reinforce cooperation with a reward if the procedure is accomplished within specified time.

- Formal – use written contract, which includes the following:

  - Realistic (seems possible) goals or desired behavior.

  - Measurable behavior (e.g., agrees not to hit anyone during procedures).

  - Contract written, dated, and signed by all persons involved in any of the agreements.

  - Identified rewards or consequences are reinforced.

  - Goals can be evaluated.

  - Required commitment and compromise from both parties (e.g., while time is used, nurse will not nag or prod child to complete procedure).

Adapted from Wong DL. Family-Centered Care of the Child During Illness and Hospitalization. In: Wong DL, ed. *Whaley and Wong's Nursing Care of Infants and Children.* 6th ed. St. Louis, Mo: Mosby-Year Book; 1997:1090. Used with permission.

Appendix H

PAIN RATING SCALES FOR CHILDREN

Oucher scale[2] – This tool uses six pictures of a child's face representing from "no hurt" to "biggest hurt ever." It also includes a vertical scale with numbers from zero to 100 to use with older children. The child is asked to choose the face that best describes his or her pain. This scale can be used for children 3 to 13 years of age. The numeric scale can be used if the child can count to 100.

Poker chip tool – This tool uses four red poker chips placed in front of the child. The chips are placed horizontally and the child is told that "these are pieces of hurt." Explain to the child that each chip represent a piece of hurt. Ask him or her how many pieces of hurt they have right now. Record the number of chips the child selected. This tool can be used for children over 3 years of age once they can count and understand numbers.

Faces scale[1] – This tool consists of six cartoon faces ranging from a smiling face for "no pain" to a tearful face for "worst pain." Explain to the child that each face is for a person who feels happy because there is no pain or sad because there is some or a lot of hurt. Ask the child to pick the face that best describes his or her pain. This scale can be used for children as young as 3 years of age.

Numeric scale[1] – This scale uses a straight line with end points that are labeled as "no pain" and "worst pain." Divisions with corresponding numbers from 0 to 10 are marked along the line. The child is asked to choose the number that best describes his or her pain. This scale can be used on children over 4 years of age once that can count and understand numbers.

No pain   Worst pain

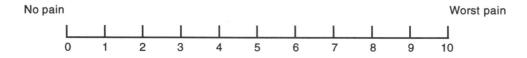

0   1   2   3   4   5   6   7   8   9   10

Visual analogue scale – This scale uses a 10 cm horizontal line with end points marked "no pain" and "worst pain." The child is asked to place a mark on the line that best describes the amount of his or her pain. Measure the distance with a ruler from the "no pain" end and record the measurement as the pain score. This scale can be used on children over 4 1/2 years of age.

Word-graphic rating scale – This scale uses descriptive words to describe varying intensities of pain. Examples of the words along the scale may include "no pain," "little pain," "medium pain," "large pain," and "worst possible pain." The child is asked to mark along the line the words that best describe his or her pain. Measure the distance with a ruler from the "no pain" end to the mark and record the measurement as the pain score. This scale can be used for children 5 years of age and over however they made need explanation of the words.

References

1. Beyer JE. *The Oucher: A User's Manual and Technical Report.* Denver, Colo: University of Colorado; 1989. Reprinted with permission.
2. Wong DL. In: Wong DL, ed. *Whaley & Wong's Essentials of Pediatric Nursing.* 5th ed. St. Louis, Mo: Mosby-Year Book; 1997:624-626. Reprinted with permission.

Appendix I

GUIDELINES FOR USING EUTECTIC MIXTURE OF LOCAL ANESTHETICS (EMLA)[1] (lidocaine hydrochloride 2.5% and prilocaine 2.5%)

1. Explain to the child the EMLA is like a "magic cream that takes hurt away." Tap or lightly scratch the site of the procedure to show the child that the "skin is now awake."

2. Apply a thick layer (dollop) of EMLA over normal, intact skin to anesthetize the site (about half of a 5-gram tube; can use one third of the tube if the puncture site is localized and superficial (e.g., intradermal injection of heel or finger puncture).

3. For venous access, apply to two sites. Place enough cream on the antecubital fossa to cover medial and lateral veins. Do not rub.

4. Place transparent occlusive dressing over EMLA. Make sure the cream remains a dollop. A piece of plastic film (c.g., food wrap) with tape to seal the edges can be used. Use only as much adhesive as needed to prevent leakage.

5. To make the dressing less accessible, cover it with a self-adhering bandage, such as Coban®, or an intravenous catheter protector, such as I.V. House®. Label the dressing with "EMLA applied," the date, and the time, to distinguish it from other types of dressings. Instruct older children not to disturb the dressing. (Covering the dressing with an opaque material may reduce the attraction and discourage "fingering.") Supervise younger or cognitively compromised children throughout the application time.

6. Leave EMLA on the skin for at least 60 minutes for superficial puncture and 120 minutes for deep penetration (e.g., intramuscular injection, biopsy). Alternatively, EMLA may be applied at home. It may need to be kept on longer in persons with dark and/or thicker skin. Anesthesia may last up to 3 hours after EMLA is removed.

7. Remove the dressing before the procedure and wipe the cream from the skin. With transparent adhesive, grasp opposite sides and, while holding the dressing parallel to the skin, pull the sides away from each other to stretch and loosen the dressing. An adhesive remover may be used.

8. Observe the skin reaction. It should either be blanched or reddened. If there is no obvious skin reaction, EMLA may not have penetrated adequately; test skin sensitivity and, if needed, reapply.

9. Repeat tapping or light scratching of the skin to show the child that the "skin is asleep" so that "it cannot feel a needle either."

10. After the procedure, assess the child's behavioral response. If the child was upset, use a pain scale to help the child distinguish between pain and fear.

Appendix I (continued)

11. In the United States, EMLA is not approved for use in infants younger than 1 month of age. In Canada, it is not approved for use in infants younger than 6 months of age. It should not be used in those rare patients with congenital or idiopathic methemoglobinemia or in infants younger than 1 year of age who are receiving treatment with methemoglobin-inducing agents (e.g., sulfonamides, phenytoin sodium, phenobarbital sodium, and acetaminophen).

12. EMLA is contraindicated in anyone with a known history of sensitivity or allergy to amide-type local anesthetics (lidocaine hydrochloride, prilocaine, mepivocaine hydrochloride, bupivacaine, or etidocaine hydrochloride) or to any other component of the product.

13. Maximum recommended application area of EMLA cream to intact skin for infants and children:

Body Weight (kg)	Maximum Application Area (cm^2)
Up to 10 kg	100
10 to 20 kg	600
Greater than 20 kg	2,000

These are broad guidelines for avoiding systemic toxicity in applying EMLA to patients with normal, intact skin and with normal renal function and hepatic function.

14. For more individualized calculation of how much lidocaine hydrochloride and prilocaine may be absorbed, practitioners can use the following estimates of lidocaine hydrochloride and prilocaine absorption for children and adults:

The estimated mean (+SD) absorption of lidocaine hydrochloride is 0.045 (+0.016) $mg/cm^2/hour$.
The estimated mean (+SD) absorption of prilocaine is 0.077 (+0.036) $mg/cm^2/hour$.

Reference

1. Wong DL. Family-centered care of the child during illness and hospitalization. In: Wong DL, ed. *Whaley & Wong's Essentials of Pediatric Nursing*. 5th ed. St. Louis, Mo: Mosby-Year Book; 1997:641. Reprinted with permission.

Appendix J

BLOOD PRESSURE LISTING BY AGE

DEFINITIONS	
Term	**Definition**
Normal blood pressure	Systolic and diastolic blood pressures <90th percentile for age and sex
High normal blood pressure*	Average systolic and/or average diastolic blood pressure between 90th and 95th percentiles for age and sex
High blood pressure (hypertension)	Average systolic and/or average diastolic blood pressure ≥95th percentile for age and sex with measurements obtained on at least three occasions

*If the blood pressure reading is high normal for age, but can be accounted for by excess height for age or excess lean body mass for age, such children are considered to have a normal blood pressure.

CLASSIFICATION OF HYPERTENSION BY AGE GROUP		
Age Group	**Significant Hypertension (mm Hg)**	**Severe Hypertension (mm Hg)**
Newborn 7 days 8 to 30 days	Systolic BP ≥96 Systolic BP ≥104	Systolic BP ≥106 Systolic BP ≥110
Infant (<3 years)	Systolic BP ≥112 Diastolic BP ≥74	Systolic BP ≥118 Diastolic BP ≥82
Children (3 to 5 years)	Systolic BP ≥116 Diastolic BP ≥76	Systolic BP ≥124 Diastolic BP ≥84
Children (6 to 9 years)	Systolic BP ≥122 Diastolic BP ≥78	Systolic BP ≥130 Diastolic BP ≥86
Children (10 to 12 years)	Systolic BP ≥126 Diastolic BP ≥82	Systolic BP ≥134 Diastolic BP ≥90
Adolescents (13 to 15 years)	Systolic BP ≥136 Diastolic BP ≥86	Systolic BP ≥144 Diastolic BP ≥92
Adolescents (16 to 18 years)	Systolic BP ≥142 Diastolic BP ≥92	Systolic BP ≥150 Diastolic BP ≥98

Adapted from Task Force on Blood Pressure Control in Children. Report of the Second Task Force on Blood Pressure Control in Children. *Pediatrics.* 1997;79:1-25. Used with permission.

Appendix K

CONVERSIONS AND ESTIMATES

TEMPERATURE

To convert centigrade to Fahrenheit (9/5 × temperature) + 32

To convert Fahrenheit to centigrade (temperature − 32) × 5/9

CENTIGRADE (CELSIUS)	FAHRENHEIT	CENTIGRADE (CELSIUS)	FAHRENHEIT
34.2	93.6	38.6	101.5
34.6	94.3	39.0	102.2
35.0	95.0	39.4	102.9
35.4	95.7	39.8	103.6
35.8	96.4	40.2	104.4
36.2	97.2	40.6	105.2
36.6	97.9	41.0	105.9
37.0	98.6	41.4	106.5
37.4	99.3	41.8	107.2
37.8	100.0	42.2	108.0
38.2	100.8	42.6	108.7

Adapted from Barkin R, Rosen P, eds. *Emergency Pediatrics*. St. Louis, Mo: Mosby-Year Book.; 1994:778. Used with permission.

Appendix L

QUICK REFERENCE TO PEDIATRIC EMERGENCY EQUIPMENT*

EQUIPMENT	Premature	Neonate	6 Months	1 Year	2 Years	3 Years	4 Years	5 Years	6 Years	7 Years	8 Years	9 Years	10 Years	11-18 Years
Airway Oral airway[1] (size)	Infant	Infant/Small	Small	Small	Small	Small	Med	Med	Med	Med	Med/Lg	Med/Lg	Med/Lg	Large
Endotracheal tube[2] (mm)	2.5-3.0	3.0-3.5	3.5-4.0	4.0-4.5	4.0-4.5	4.0-4.5	5.0-5.5	5.0-5.5	5.5-6.0	5.5-6.0	6.0*-6.5*	6.0*-6.5*	6.0*-6.5*	7.0*-8.0*
Laryngoscope blade[1] s = straight c = curved	0 s	1 s	1 s	1 s	1 s	1 s	2 s/c	2 s/c	2 s/c	2 s/c	2-3 s/c.	2-3 s/c	2-3 s/c	3 s/c
Suction catheter[2] (French)	5	6	6	8	8	8	10	10	10	10	10	10	10	12
Breathing Face mask[1] (size)	Preemie NB	NB	NB	Ped	Ped	Ped	Ped	Ped	Ped	Ped	Ad	Ad	Ad	Ad
Bag-valve device[1] (size)	Inf	Inf	Inf	Ped	Ped	Ped	Ped	Ped	Ped	Ped/Ad	Ad	Ad	Ad	Ad
Chest tube[1] (French)	10-14	12-18	14-20	14-24	14-24	14-24	20-32	20-32	20-32	20-32	28-38	28-38	28-38	28-38
Circulation Over-the-needle catheter[3] (gauge)	22-24	22-24	22-24	20-22	20-22	20-22	20-22	18-22	18-20	18-20	16-20	16-20	16-20	14-18
Intraosseous device (gauge)	18	15	15	15	15	15	15	15	-	-	-	-	-	-
Gastrointestinal Nasogastric tube[4] (French)	5	5	8	8	10	10	10	10	10	12	12	12	12	14-16
Urinary catheter[1] (French)	5 feeding tube	5-8 feeding tube	8	10	10	10	10-12	10-12	10-12	10-12	12	12	12	12-18

[1] American College of Surgeons, Committee on Trauma. *Advanced Trauma Life Support Manual.* Chicago, Ill: Author; 1989.

[2] Motoyama E. Endotracheal intubation. In: Motoyama E, Davis P, eds. *Smith's Anesthesia for Infants and Children.* St. Louis, Mo: Mosby; 1990.

[3] Chameides L, ed. *Textbook of Pediatric Advanced Life Support.* Dallas, Tex: American Heart Association; 1938.

[4] Skale N. *Manual of Pediatric Nursing Procedures.* Philadelphia, Pa: JB Lippincott; 1992.

*This reference demonstrates suggested sizes only. Always consider each child's size and health condition when selecting appropriate equipment for procedures.

Adapted from Bernardo LM, Bove MA, eds. *Pediatric Emergency Nursing Procedures.* Boston, Mass: Jones & Bartlett; 1993. Used with permission.

Appendix M

PEDIATRIC COMA SCALE

		EYE OPENING		
Score	*>1 Year*			*<1 Year*
4	Spontaneously			Spontaneously
3	To verbal command			To shout
2	To pain			To pain
1	No response			No response

		BEST MOTOR RESPONSE		
Score	*>1 Year*			*<1 Year*
6	Obeys			Spontaneous
5	Localizes pain			Localizes pain
4	Flexion-withdrawal			Flexion-withdrawal
3	Flexion-abnormal (decorticate rigidity)			Flexion-abnormal (decorticate rigidity)
2	Extension (decerebrate rigidity)			Extension (decerebrate rigidity)
1	No response			No response

	BEST VERBAL RESPONSE		
Score	*>5 Years*	*2 to 5 Years*	*0 to 23 Months*
5	Oriented and converses	Appropriate words/phrases	Smiles and coos appropriately
4	Disoriented and converses	Inappropriate words	Cries and is consolable
3	Inappropriate words	Persistent cries and/screams	Persistent, inappropriate crying and/or screaming
2	Incomprehensible sounds	Grunts	Grunts, agitated, and restless
1	No response	No response	No response

TOTAL = 3 to 15

Adapted from Simon J, Goldberg A. *Prehospital Pediatric Life Support.* St. Louis, Mo: Mosby-Year Book; 1989:11. Used with permission.

Appendix N

PEDIATRIC TRAUMA SCORE

The Pediatric Trauma Scale score is the only trauma score available with the special needs of children in mind. It functions as a useful triage tool to identify life-threatening injuries and accurately predict the severity of injuries.

PEDIATRIC TRAUMA SCORE			
Severity	**+ 2**	**+ 1**	**− 1**
Weight	>44 lb (>20 kg)	22 to 44 lb (10 to 20 kg)	<22 lb (10 kg)
Airway	Normal	Oral or nasal airway	Invasive: Intubation cricothyrotomy
Blood pressure*	>90 mm Hg	50 to 90 mm Hg	<50 mm Hg
Level of consciousness	Awake Alert	Obtunded Any loss of consciousness	Comatose
Open wound	None	Minor	Major or penetrating
Fractures	None	Single Simple	Open or multiple

*An assessment of pulse can be used in place of the blood pressure. Scoring is as follows:
Radial: + 2; Femoral: + 1; Absent: − 1

Adapted from Tepas JJ III, Mollitt DL, Talbert JL, Bryant M. Pediatric trauma score as a prediction of injury severity in the injured child. *J Pediatr Surg*. 1987;22:14. Used with permission.

Appendix O

CRANIAL NERVE ASSESSMENT

A gross evaluation of cranial nerve function can be completed relatively quickly. However, the child's condition and developmental level may preclude evaluation of all cranial nerves. Basic cranial nerve evaluation should include eye movement and function, gag reflex, and facial symmetry.

Evaluation of Eye Movement and Function (Cranial Nerves II, III, IV, and VI)[1,2]

- In the conscious child, evaluation of eye movement and function includes an assessment of extraocular movements and gross visual acuity. However, complete evaluation of all extraocular movements may not be possible in children younger than 2 to 3 years of age. The assessment includes evaluation for the presence of:

    - Equal rise of eyelids.

    - Equality of pupil size and reactivity to light and accommodation.

    - Ability to see and track an object.

    - Ability to identify color.

    - Ability to follow an object through the six fields of gaze.

- In conscious infants younger than 3 months of age, the assessment includes evaluation for the presence of:

    - Equal rise of eyelids.

    - Equality of pupil size and reactivity to light and accommodation.

    - Blinking in response to a bright light.

    - Ability to follow or track a dangling object, or moving the head to follow an object.[3]

- In infants and children with an altered level of consciousness, the position of the eyes at rest and the presence of abnormal spontaneous eye movement should also be noted.[4] The assessment includes evaluation for the presence of:

    - Equal rise of eyelids (if eye opening response present).

    - Equality of pupil size and reactivity to light and accommodation.

    - Abnormal eye position:

        - Deviation of the eyes toward one field of gaze.

        - Dysconjugate gaze.

    - Abnormal movement (nystagmus).

Appendix O (continued)

Evaluation of Reflex Responses (Cranial Nerves IX and X [Gag, Cough, and Swallowing]; Cranial Nerves V and VII [Corneal Reflex]; Cranial Nerves III, VI, and VIII [Oculocephalic and Oculovestibular])[2,5,6]

- The assessment of reflex response includes evaluation for the function of:

    - Cranial nerves IX and X:

        - Ability to swallow.

        - Ability to cough.

        - Presence of gag reflex.

        - Presence of clear speech or alterations in speech pattern.

    - Cranial nerves V and VII:

        - Spontaneous blinking.

        - Blinking in response to corneal stimulus.

    - Cranial nerves III, VI, and VIII: Oculocephalic and oculovestibular responses are only tested for the evaluation of severe brain stem dysfunction in the unresponsive infant or child. This assessment includes evaluation for the presence of:

        - Doll's eyes is when the head is turned but the eyes move in the opposite direction. If the eyes move in the same direction the head is turned, doll's eyes are considered absent, and this is an abnormal finding.

        - Nystagmus in response to ice water caloric test. No eye movement or asymmetric eye movement in response to the ice water caloric test is considered an abnormal response.

Evaluation of Facial Movement and Expression (Cranial Nerves V and VII)[2,5,6]

- The assessment of facial movement and expression includes evaluation for the presence of:

    - Facial symmetry with movement or during crying and sucking in infants.

    - Ability to raise eyebrows, smile, clench teeth, and chew.

    - Tears with crying.

    - Sucking reflex and strength of reflex in infants.

Evaluation of Motor and Muscular Function (Cranial Nerves XI and XII)[2,5,6]

- The assessment of motor and muscular function related to the cranial nerves includes observing for the presence of the child's ability to:

    - Shrug shoulders.

    - Turn head and move upper extremities.

    - Stick out tongue. In infants, the position of the tongue when crying is observed; the midline position is the norm.

Appendix O (continued)

Basic Evaluation of Hearing (Cranial Nerve VIII)[3,6]

- The assessment of hearing function includes observing for the presence of the child's ability to:

  - Respond to verbal commands and answer questions.

  - Repeat words.

- In infants younger than 3 months of age, the following behaviors are observed:

  - Spontaneous movements and/or sucking stop in response to voice or sounds. The infant should then resume the activity.

  - Quieting to the sound of voice or soothing sounds.

  - Turning of head or eyes toward the sound.

  - Vocalization in response to sounds or voice.

References

1. Hector JE. Neurologic evaluation and support in the child with an acute brain insult. *Pediatr Ann.* 1986;15:16-22.

2. Hazinski MF. Neurologic disorders. In: Hazinski MF, ed. *Nursing Care of the Critically Ill Child.* St. Louis, Mo: Mosby-Year Book; 1992:521-628.

3. Gordon N. The neurologic examination. In: Gordon N, ed. *Neurologic Problems in Childhood.* Boston, Mass: Butterworth-Heinemann; 1993:1-24.

4. Dolan M. Head trauma. In: Barkin RM, ed. *Pediatric Emergency Medicine: Concepts and Clinical Practice.* St. Louis, Mo: Mosby-Year Book; 1992:184-198.

5. Emergency Nurses Association. Consciousness. In: *Course in Advanced Trauma Nursing: A Conceptual Approach.* Park Ridge, Ill: Author; 1995:287-331.

6. Brucker JM. Neurologic disorders. In: Brucker JM, Wallin KD, eds. *Manual of Pediatric Nursing.* Boston, Mass: Little, Brown and Company; 1996:251-297.

Appendix P

PEDIATRIC BASIC LIFE-SUPPORT GUIDELINES

COMPONENTS	INFANT (YOUNGER THAN 1 YEAR)	CHILD (1 TO 8 YEARS)
Airway	• Head tilt-chin lift • Jaw thrust (trauma)	• Head tilt-chin lift • Jaw thrust (trauma)
Breathing Initial Subsequent	• Two breaths at 1.0 to 1.5 sec/breath • 20 breaths/minute	• Two breaths at 1.0 to 1.5 sec/breath • 20 breaths/minute
Circulation Pulse check Compression area Compression: Depth Rate Compression-ventilation ratio	• Brachial/femoral • Lower third of sternum with two to three fingers • 0.5 to 1.0 inch • At least 100/minute • 5:1 (pause for ventilation) Neonates 3:1 with interposed compressions and ventilation	• Carotid • Lower third of sternum with heel of one hand • 1.0 to 1.5 inches • 100/minute • 5:1 (pause for ventilation)
Foreign-body airway obstruction	• Back blows (up to five) then chest thrusts (up to five)	• Heimlich maneuver up to five times

Adapted from Emergency Cardiac Care Committee and Subcommittees, American Heart Association. Guidelines for cardiopulmonary resuscitation and emergency cardiac care. *JAMA.* 1992;268:2259. Used with permission.

Appendix Q

DRUGS USED IN PEDIATRIC RESUSCITATION

DRUG	DOSE	REMARKS
• Adenosine	• 0.1 to 0.2 mg/kg Maximum single dose: 12 mg	• Rapid intravenous (IV) bolus
• Atropine sulfate	• 0.02 mg/kg per dose	• Minimum dose: 0.1 mg • Maximum single dose: 0.5 mg in child 1.0 in adolescent
• Bretylium tosylate	• 5 mg/kg: may be increased to 10 mg/kg	• Rapid IV bolus
• Calcium chloride 10%	• 20 mg/kg per dose	• Give slowly
• Dopamine hydrochloride	• 2 to 20 mcg/kg/minute	• a–Adrenergic action dominates at $\geq$15 to 20 mcg/kg/minute
• Dobutamine hydrochloride	• 2 to 20 mcg/kg/minute	• Titrate to desired effect
• Epinephrine hydrochloride (for bradycardia)	• IV or IO: 0.01 mg/kg (1:10,000) ET: 0.1 mg/kg (1:1,000)	• Be aware of effective dose of preservatives administered (if preservatives are present in epinephrine preparation) when high doses are used
• Epinephrine hydrochloride (asystole or pulseless arrest)	• First dose: IV or IO: 0.01 mg/kg (1:10,000) ET: 0.1 mg/kg (1:1,000) Doses as high as 0.2 mg/kg may be effective • Subsequent doses: IV, IO, or ET: 0.1 mg/kg (1:1,000) Doses as high as 0.2 mg/kg may be effective	• Be aware of effective dose of preservatives administered (if preservatives present in epinephrine preparation) when high doses are used
• Epinephrine hydrochloride infusion	• Initially at 0.1 mcg/kg/minute • Higher infusion dose if asystole present	• Titrate to desired effect (0.1 to 1.0 mcg/kg/minute)
• Lidocaine hydrochloride	• 1 mg/kg per dose	
• Lidocaine hydrochloride infusion	• 20 to 50 mcg/kg/minute	
• Sodium bicarbonate	• 1 mEq/kg per dose or 0.3 mEq × kg × base deficit	• Infuse slowly and only if ventilation is adequate

Adapted from Emergency Cardiac Care Committee and Subcommittees, American Heart Association. Guidelines for cardiopulmonary resuscitation and emergency cardiac care. *JAMA*. 1992;268:2262-2275. Used with permission.

Appendix R

PREPARATION OF INFUSIONS

DRUG	PREPARATION*	DOSE
● Epinephrine hydrochloride	0.6 × body weight (kg) equals milligrams added to diluent† to make 100 ml	Then 1 ml/hour delivers 0.1 mcg/kg/minute; titrate to effect
● Dopamine hydro-chloride, dobutamine hydrochloride	6 × body weight (kg) equals milligrams added to diluent to make 100 ml	Then 1 ml/hour delivers 1.0 mcg/kg/minute; titrate to effect
● Lidocaine hydrochloride	120 mg of 40 mg/ml solution added to 97 ml of 5% dextrose in water, yielding 1,200 mcg/ml solution	Then 1 ml/kg/hour delivers 20 mcg/kg/minute

* Standard concentration may be used to provide more dilute or more concentrated drug solution, but then individual dose must be calculated for each patient and each infusion rate.
† Diluent may be 5% dextrose in water, 5% dextrose in one half normal saline, normal saline, or lactated Ringer's solution.

Adapted from Chameides L, Hazinski MF, eds. *Textbook of Pediatric Advanced Life Support*. Dallas, Tex: American Heart Association; 1988:56. Used with permission.

Appendix S

SUGGESTED TREATMENT FOR ASYSTOLE AND PULSELESS ARREST

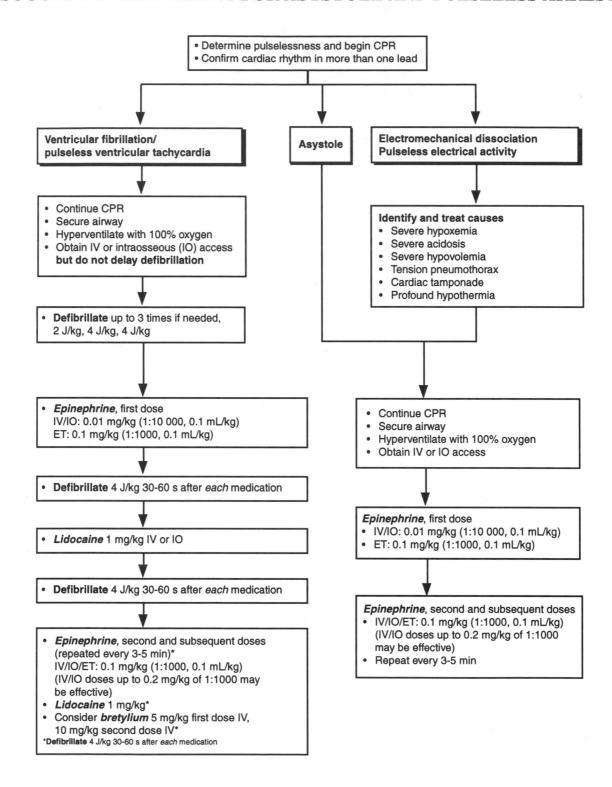

From Chameides L, Hazinski MF, eds. *Pediatric Advanced Life Support*. Dallas, Tex: American Heart Association; 1997:7-11. Reprinted with permission.

Appendix T

SUGGESTED TREATMENT FOR BRADYCARDIA

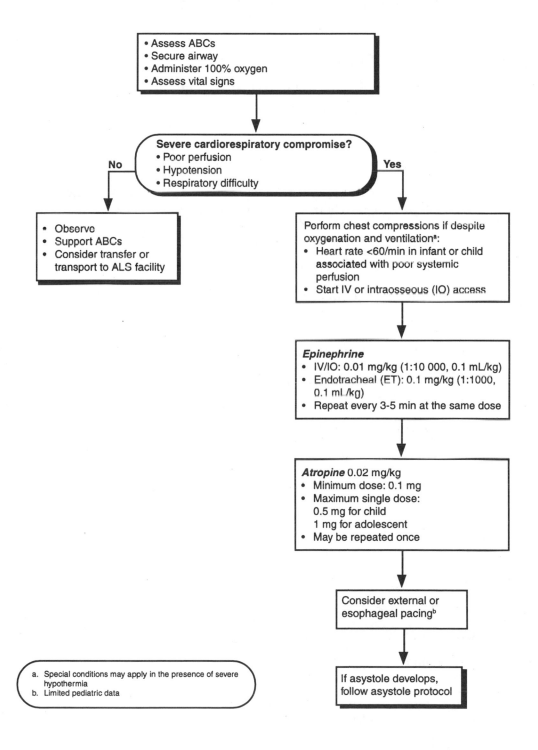

- Assess ABCs
- Secure airway
- Administer 100% oxygen
- Assess vital signs

Severe cardiorespiratory compromise?
- Poor perfusion
- Hypotension
- Respiratory difficulty

No

Yes

- Observe
- Support ABCs
- Consider transfer or transport to ALS facility

Perform chest compressions if despite oxygenation and ventilation[a]:
- Heart rate <60/min in infant or child associated with poor systemic perfusion
- Start IV or intraosseous (IO) access

Epinephrine
- IV/IO: 0.01 mg/kg (1:10 000, 0.1 mL/kg)
- Endotracheal (ET): 0.1 mg/kg (1:1000, 0.1 mL/kg)
- Repeat every 3-5 min at the same dose

Atropine 0.02 mg/kg
- Minimum dose: 0.1 mg
- Maximum single dose:
  0.5 mg for child
  1 mg for adolescent
- May be repeated once

Consider external or esophageal pacing[b]

If asystole develops, follow asystole protocol

a. Special conditions may apply in the presence of severe hypothermia
b. Limited pediatric data

From Chameides L, Hazinski MF, eds. *Pediatric Advanced Life Support*. Dallas, Tex: American Heart Association; 1997:7-9. Reprinted with permission.

Appendix U

CARE OF THE SEXUALLY ABUSED CHILD
IN THE EMERGENCY DEPARTMENT

Interviewing the Sexually Abused Child

The following techniques are used during the ED interview of a child who has been sexually abused:

- Interview the verbal child alone:
    - Interviewing the child alone may provide an opportunity for him or her to make verbal statements regarding the possible sexual abuse.
    - Even if the caregiver accompanying the child is not a suspect, the child may be reluctant to disclose the abuse, especially if the abuser is a relative or friend of the family.
- Never interview the child in the presence of the possible abuser.
- Use a quiet, private room for the interview.
- Establish trust and rapport with the child; convey interest, sincerity, and respect.
- Use clear, simple language.
- Determine and use the child's own terminology for describing body parts.
- Use age-appropriate media including anatomic drawings and anatomically correct dolls to facilitate verbal communication.
- Limit the interview to 1 hour or less.
- Avoid multiple interviews by the emergency health care workers and others.
- Do not make promises you cannot keep or have no control over.

History

- The history may include a report of the following characteristic behaviors:
    - Sexual acting out with siblings, peers, or adults.
    - Preoccupation with sexual matters.
    - Excessive masturbation.
    - Regressive behavior.
    - Enuresis or encopresis.
    - Sleep disorders or nightmares.
    - Excessive fears.
    - Refusal to sleep alone at night.
    - Fatigue.

- ■ Depression.

- ■ Suicidal ideation or gestures.

- ■ Substance abuse.

- ■ Runaway behavior.

- ■ School problems.

- ● History of the sexual abuse incidents:

  - ■ Location of incidents.

  - ■ Dates and times of incidents.

  - ■ Name of the offender if known by the child.

  - ■ Statements made by offender or child during the incidents.

  - ■ Occurrence of threats, bribes, intimidation, physical force, or other violent activity.

  - ■ Involvement of other children or adults.

  - ■ Knowledge of photographs or movies taken of the child.

  - ■ Use of any pornography.

Diagnostic Procedures

Laboratory Studies

- ● Vaginal, cervical, or rectal cultures for chlamydia and gonorrhea.

- ● Vaginal and rectal fluids for spermatozoa and prostatic acid phosphatase.

- ● Pregnancy test.

- ● Saliva for ABO-antigen typing.

- ● Hair specimen.

- ● Blood for human immunodeficiency virus antibodies or sexually transmitted diseases.

Appendix V

ASSESSMENT FINDINGS IN THE NEONATE AND POTENTIAL CAUSES

Assessment Findings	Potential Causes

Cyanosis of the mucous membranes or trunk	• Hypoxia
	• Respiratory distress or failure
	• Congenital heart disease
	  ■ Congestive heart failure, causing impaired alveolar ventilation
	  ■ Right-to-left shunting resulting from cardiac lesion
	• Infection or sepsis
	• Poor perfusion, shock
	• Acidosis
	• Polycythemia
	• Methemoglobinemia
	• Central nervous system injury, malformation, or disease causing a diminished respiratory drive

Mottling of skin	• Hypothermia or cold stress (vascular instability) • Poor perfusion from hypovolemia • Infection or sepsis • Hypoxia • Congenital heart disease
Pallor of the soles of feet, palms of hands, nailbeds, or mucous membranes	• Poor perfusion • Poor oxygenation • Low hemoglobin • Infection or sepsis • Hypothermia • Shock • Hypoxia • Congenital heart disease
Jaundice	• Hyperbilirubinemia secondary to blood group incompatibilities • Primary liver disease • Extrahepatic obstruction, such as biliary atresia • Infection or sepsis • Hemolysis reaction secondary to bruising during delivery • Physiologic jaundice • Breast milk jaundice • Genetic and metabolic disorders
Lethargy, hypotonia. Decreased muscle tone, poor feeding or lack of interest in feeding, difficult to arouse or elicit a response to stimuli, increased sleeping times, decreased reflexes (suck, grasp, startle, rooting).	• Sepsis • Hypoxia • Respiratory distress or failure • Dehydration • Shock • Hypoglycemia

Assessment Findings	Potential Causes
Irritability: Increased activity level, poor sleep patterns or decreased sleeping times, inconsolability	• Infection • Pain or discomfort • Colic • Withdrawal from maternal substance abuse • Hypoglycemia • Feeding intolerance • Overstimulation
Hypertonia: Arms and hands tightly flexed, arching of back and neck, legs stiff and extended, startles easily	• Meningitis • Neurologic injury or dysfunction

Jitteriness or seizure activity: Lip smacking, eye fluttering or repeated eye movements, bicycling movements of legs, shaking of one or more extremities	• Hypoglycemia
	• Hypocalcemia
	• Sepsis
	• Seizure disorder
	• Electrolyte disturbance
	  ■ Secondary to diarrhea and vomiting
	  ■ Secondary to error in formula preparation
	• Meningitis
	• Increased intracranial pressure
	• Neurologic injury or dysfunction

Hypothermia • Axillary temperature <36.5°C (97.7°F) • Rectal temperature <36°C (96.8°F)	• Sepsis • Cold ambient environment • Neurologic dysfunction
Hyperthermia • Axillary temperature >37.5°C (99.5°F) • Rectal temperature >38°C (100.4°F)	• Sepsis • Warm ambient environment • Bundled heavily in clothing and blankets in warm environment
Apnea	• Airway obstruction from congenital deformity, swelling, secretions, positioning • Sepsis • Respiratory infection • Gastroesophageal reflux • Hypoglycemia • Seizures
Bradypnea	• Respiratory failure • Cardiopulmonary failure • Neurologic compromise

Assessment Findings	Potential Causes
Tachypnea: Consistent respiratory rate >60 breaths/minute after 6 to 8 hours of age	<ul><li>Respiratory infection; pneumonia</li><li>Hypoxia</li><li>Sepsis</li><li>Hyperthermia</li><li>Congenital heart disease; congestive heart failure</li><li>Hypoglycemia</li><li>Acidosis</li><li>Dehydration</li><li>Shock</li><li>Pain or discomfort</li></ul>
Bradycardia: Heart rate <100 beats/minute	<ul><li>Late response to hypoxia</li><li>Late response to shock</li><li>Apnea</li><li>Sepsis</li><li>Hypothermia</li><li>Neurologic compromise</li></ul>
Tachycardia: Sustained heart rate >180 beats/minute	<ul><li>Dehydration</li><li>Shock</li><li>Hypotension</li><li>Acidosis</li><li>Sepsis</li><li>Respiratory distress</li><li>Hypoxia</li><li>Congenital heart disease</li><li>Hyperthermia</li><li>Crying</li></ul>
Depressed or sunken anterior fontanelle	<ul><li>Dehydration</li></ul>
Bulging anterior fontanelle: Assessed with the infant in an upright position and quiet	<ul><li>Hydrocephalus</li><li>Increased intracranial pressure</li></ul>
Diarrhea: Increased number of stools with an increased water content	<ul><li>Viral infection</li><li>Bacterial infection</li><li>Toxic reaction to food or other poison</li><li>Formula intolerance</li><li>Antibiotic therapy side effect</li></ul>

Assessment Findings	Potential Causes
Constipation: First newborn stool should be passed by 36 hours of age	• Infrequent passage of stool • May be accompanied by abdominal distention and discomfort • Stool may be hard • Stool may be blood-streaked • Formula incompatibility (change of formula) • Meconium plug • Meconium ileus (early sign of cystic fibrosis) • Congenital intestinal obstruction, atresia, or stenosis • Malrotation • Hirschsprung's disease
Vomiting: Forceful ejection of the gastric contents, may be present with abdominal distention	• Infection • Pyloric stenosis • Bowel obstruction, atresia, or stenosis • Malrotation • Gastroesophageal reflux • Necrotizing enterocolitis

References

1. Nelson W, ed. *Nelson Textbook of Pediatrics.* 15th ed. Philadelphia, Pa: WB Saunders; 1996:452.

2. Wong DL, ed. *Whaley & Wong's Essentials of Pediatric Nursing.* 5th ed. St. Louis, Mo: Mosby-Year Book; 1997.

3. Cloherty JP, Stark AR, eds. *Manual of Neonatal Care.* 3rd ed. Boston, Mass: Little, Brown and Company; 1992.

4. Bailey C, Boyle R, Kattwinkel J, Ferguson J. *Outpatient Perinatal Education Program, Book Two: The Infant At Risk After Discharge.* Charlottesville, Va: Division of Neonatal Medicine, University of Virginia Health Sciences Center; 1997.

Appendix W

THE PREMATURE INFANT

Premature infants will generally be discharged to home when the following criteria are met:

- Weight around 1,800 gm (about 4 lbs) with a steady weight gain of 20 to 30 gm/kg/day.

- Able to maintain temperature when bundled in an open crib.

- Able to tolerate feedings (either oral or tube).

Considerations in the Assessment and Care of the Preterm Infant in the Emergency Department

- The premature infant is:

  - More prone to hypothermia and cold stress.

  - More prone to hypoglycemia if stressed.

  - More prone to dehydration and shock if vomiting and diarrhea occur.

  - More prone to bruising due to fragile skin and capillaries.

  - Less able to tolerate periods without fluids and nutrients.

- Delays in all areas of development may be seen in the premature infant. The delays may be secondary to the prematurity itself, to complications of prematurity, or to an extended time spent on ventilatory support and medications.

- Development should be assessed by using a one-half correction for gestational age:

  - Determine the number of weeks premature at delivery.

  - Divide the number of weeks premature by 2.

- Subtract this number from the current chronologic age.

- Neurologic abnormalities may be present; these may be related to a delay in maturation of the central nervous system or secondary to neurologic damage:

  - Increased or decreased muscle tone.

  - Abnormal posture.

  - Increased or decreased deep tendon reflexes.

  - Clonus.

  - Persistence of primitive reflexes.

- Abdominal musculature and structures close late in fetal development. Problems related to abdominal wall development are common in both male and female preterm infants:

  - Undescended testes in preterm males.

  - Inguinal hernias.

  - Umbilical hernias.

- Complications of prematurity:

  - Bronchopulmonary dysplasia.

  - Vision loss secondary to retinopathy of prematurity. This occurs from the effects of hyperoxia, hypoxia, acidosis, and hypercarbia on the poorly vascularized retina.

  - Hearing loss may be present as the result of infection, ototoxic drugs, or hypoxemia causing injury to the auditory pathways of the brain.

Appendix X

RECOMMENDED EQUIPMENT LIST FOR DELIVERY OF AN INFANT

■ **OBSTETRIC PACK (EQUIPMENT FOR A NORMAL DELIVERY)**

- Sterile towels for drying the baby
- Bulb syringe for suctioning the mouth and nose
- Cord clamps for the umbilical cord
- Scalpel or scissors
- Identification bands for mother and infant
- May have a footprint kit

■ **HEAT SOURCE**

- Ideally, a heated radiant warmer. A prewarmed isolette is useful for keeping a stable baby warm, but it cannot be easily used during resuscitative efforts
- Heat lamps
- Warmed blankets
- Crushable hot packs – wrap in a cloth diaper or a towel, before placing around the baby, to prevent burns

■ **RESUSCITATION MASKS**

- Infant, newborn, and premature

■ **RESUSCITATION BAG**

- Self-inflating bag (500 ml) with oxygen reservoir
- Anesthesia bag

■ **MECHANICAL SUCTION WITH PRESSURE REGULATOR**

- Negative pressure should not exceed 100 mm Hg (suctioning can usually be done with 80 to 100 mm Hg)

■ **LARYNGOSCOPE HANDLE AND BLADES**

- 0 straight
- 1 straight

■ **ENDOTRACHEAL TUBES**

- 2.5-mm, 3.0-mm, 3.5-mm, 4.0-mm
- Endotracheal tube stylet (small)

■ **SUCTION CATHETERS**

- 5-French to 6-French (for 2.5 endotracheal tube)
- 8-French (for larger endotracheal tube)
- 8-French to 14-French (for suctioning the mouth)

■ **GASTRIC OR FEEDING TUBES**

- 5-French, 8-French, 10-French

■ **SYRINGES**

- 1-ml, 3-ml, 10-ml

■ **MISCELLANEOUS**

- Umbilical catheters (3.5-French and 5-French) with stopcock
- Meconium aspirator
- Medications
- Gloves (and other protective devices as desired)

Appendix Y

MEDICATIONS FOR NEONATAL RESUSCITATION

MEDICATION	CONCENTRATION TO ADMINISTER	DOSAGE/ROUTE*	RATE/PRECAUTIONS
Epinephrine hydrochloride	1:10,000	0.01 to 0.03 mg/kg (0.1 to 0.3 ml/kg) IV, IO, or ET	Give rapidly, may dilute with normal saline to 1 to 2 ml if giving ET
Volume expanders	Blood, 5% albumin, normal saline, lactated Ringer's solution	10 ml/kg IV or IO	Give over 5 to 10 minutes
Sodium bicarbonate	0.5 mEq/ml (4.2% solution) 8.4% solution must be diluted 1:1 to 4.2% solution	2 mEq/kg IV	Give *slowly,* over at least 2 minutes. Give only if the infant is being effectively ventilated.
Naloxone hydrochloride	0.4 mg/ml	0.1 mg/kg (0.25 ml/kg) IV, ET, IM, SQ	Give rapidly IV, ET preferred; IM, SQ acceptable
	1.0 mg/ml	0.1 mg/kg (0.1 ml/kg) IV, ET, IM, SQ	
*IM = Intramuscular; ET = Endotracheal; IV = Intravenous; SQ = Subcutaneous; IO = Intraosseous			

Adapted from *Textbook of Neonatal Resuscitation.* Elk Grove Village, Ill: American Academy of Pediatrics; 1994:6-51. Used with permission.

Appendix Z

NEONATAL RESUSCITATION GUIDELINES FOR CPR

- **AIRWAY**
  - "Sniffing" or neutral position
  - Endotracheal intubation as needed

- **VENTILATION**
  - Oxygen
    - Preferred method: simple face mask held firmly on face using 5 to 10 liters/minute flow
    - May use standard oxygen tubing and a flow rate of 5 to 10 liters/minute to direct blow-by oxygen toward the neonate's nares
  - Bag-valve-mask ventilation
    - Rate: 40 to 60 breaths/minute
    - Adequate ventilation is assessed by chest wall movement and auscultation of bilateral breath sounds
    - Bag-valve volume for full-term neonate: at least 450 to 750 ml

- **COMPRESSIONS**
  - Acceptable methods in newborns
    - Thumb technique (preferred method): two thumbs on the lower third of sternum with hands encircling the body and fingers supporting the back
    - Two-finger technique: two fingers, using the tips of the fingers to compress the lower third of sternum and the other hand to support the back (unless on a firm surface)
  - Compression-ventilation ratio
    - 3:1 ratio (three compressions to one ventilation)
    - Results in 90 compressions and 30 ventilations/minute
    - Important to allow for adequate ventilation between compressions
  - Compression depth: depress the sternum 0.50 to 0.75 inch

Adapted from Emergency Cardiac Care Committee and Subcommittees, American Heart Association. Guidelines for cardiopulmonary resuscitation and emergency cardiac care. *JAMA*. 1992;268:2276-2281. Used with permission.

Appendix AA

CLASS OF CHILD BASED ON BLOOD LEAD CONCENTRATIONS

	CLASS OF CHILD BASED ON BLOOD LEAD CONCENTRATIONS	
Class	**Blood Lead Concentration (mcg/dL)**	**Comment**
I	≤9	A child in Class I is not considered to be lead poisoned.
IIA	10 to 14	The incidence of many children (or a large proportion of children) with blood lead levels in this range should trigger community-wide childhood lead poisoning prevention activities. Children in this range may need to be rescreened more frequently.
IIB	15 to 19	A child in Class IIB should receive nutritional and educational interventions and more frequent screening. If the blood lead level persists in this range, environmental investigation and intervention should be done.
III	20 to 44	A child in Class III should receive environmental evaluation and remediation and a medical evaluation. Such a child may need pharmacologic treatment of lead poisoning.
IV	45 to 69	A child in Class IV will need both medical and environmental interventions, including chelation therapy.
V	≥70	A child with Class V lead poisoning is a medical emergency. Medical and environmental management must begin immediately.

Adapted from *Preventing Lead Poisoning in Young Children*. Atlanta, Ga: Centers for Disease Control; 1991. US Dept of Health, Education, and Welfare Publication. chronological. Used with permission.

Appendix BB

GENERAL INDICATIONS FOR ANTIVENOM ADMINISTRATION FOR VENOMOUS SNAKE BITES IN AUSTRALIA

Indications for Antivenom

- Muscle weakness:
  - Respiratory and ocular muscles are particularly sensitive to snake neurotoxins.
  - Generalized muscle weakness may result in poor respiratory effort.
  - Changes in predicted peak flow measurement can be an early indicator of envenomation.
- Presence of coagulation disturbance.
- Headache (early sign).
- Evidence of systemic involvement.
- Tender or enlarged lymph nodes (not conclusive).

Administration of Antivenom (Australia)

The use of antivenom carries a high risk of anaphylaxis. Previous administration of antivenom must be determined. Children who have received antivenom for previous bites have a greater risk for anaphylaxis with subsequent doses.

ANAPHYLAXIS PROPHYLAXIS

- Epinephrine hydrochloride 0.01 ml/kg, intramuscularly (never intravenously).
- Promethazine hydrochloride, 0.5 to 1.0 mg/kg, intravenously.
- Hydrocortisone acetate, 2.0 mg/kg, intravenously.

ANTIVENOM ADMINISTRATION

- Assure correct antivenom is used:
  - If the snake cannot be positively identified, then polyvalent antivenom is appropriate.
  - Wound swabs as well as a urine sample can assist in the identification process with the use of a venom detection kit.
- The dosage for children and adults is the same. The amount required is the amount of antivenom necessary to relieve the presenting signs and symptoms and alleviate pain.
- Dilute antivenom to a concentration of 1:10.
- Commence slowly, at a rate of 1.0 ml/minute for 5 minutes, with close observation of airway, breathing, and circulatory status.
- Observe for signs of anaphylactic reaction:
  - If no reaction is noted, continue infusion over next 30 minutes.
  - Observe closely throughout infusion.
  - Administer medications for anaphylaxis if reaction occurs.
- Serum sickness may be prevented with a short follow-up course of oral steroids.

GENERAL INDICATIONS FOR ANTIVENOM ADMINISTRATION FOR VENOMOUS SNAKE BITES IN AUSTRALIA

Appendix CC

LEGAL CONSIDERATIONS

Children have health care rights, such as the right to privacy and the right to confidentiality. The emergency care team has the legal responsibility to provide prudent, competent care to infants, children, and adolescents who come to the emergency department for treatment. Six acts that violate the legal rights of children are negligence, assault, battery, abandonment, breach of confidentiality, and breach of duty to report. A definition and example of each act is listed in the following table:

ACTS THAT VIOLATE THE RIGHTS OF THE PEDIATRIC PATIENT		
Act	*Definition*	*Example*
Negligence	Deviation from accepted standards of care.[1]	Not obtaining frequent vital signs in a trauma patient whose condition subsequently deteriorates.
Assault	Intentionally threatening to harm an individual, coupled with the immediate ability to carry out the threat.[2]	Threatening to slap a child who is uncooperative.
Battery	Unconsented touching of another person that results in injury or offensive touching.[2]	Slapping a child who is uncooperative.
Abandonment	Unilateral termination of a nurse (physician)-patient relationship by the nurse (physician).[1]	Refusal to care for a child in the emergency department who is HIV positive.
Breach of Confidentiality	Child's rights to privacy about his or her health condition are violated.	Giving out information about a child's condition to the news media without the consent of the child or caregiver; talking about a child's condition to another family member without the child's or caregiver's consent.
Breach of Duty to Report	Information required by state law is not reported to the proper authorities. Such information may include animal bites, sexual assault, child maltreatment, gunshot or stab wounds, children who are dead on arrival, and communicable diseases (measles, sexually transmitted diseases).	Suspected child maltreatment is not reported to the proper authorities, as required by state law.

Appendix CC (continued)

Informed consent, assent, and permission for treatment must also be considered when treating children presenting to the emergency department. These terms are described in the following table:

Term	Description
Informed consent from the child	Informed consent must be obtained from children who have reached the statutory age of majority as well as mature or emancipated minors. To obtain informed consent for treatment, the following information must be provided to the patient: ● The diagnosis or description of the health problem. ● The recommended treatment and its chances for success. ● The risk and benefits involved in the treatment. ● The risk and benefits of alternative or no treatment.
Assent from the child	Assent means agreement or acceptance. When a child assents to treatment, the child agrees or complies with the treatment plan. Attempt to obtain assent from children as young as 7 or 8 years of age in addition to the caregiver's permission. Assent means that the child has: ● A developmentally appropriate understanding of the health problem. ● Been informed of the treatment method and what will happen during that treatment. ● Demonstrated willingness to receive the treatment.
Informed permission from the caregiver	Informed permission is obtained from the caregiver of infants and children. *Informed permission* means that the caregiver understands the same bulleted information described in "Informed consent from the child."

References

1. Korin JB. Legal aspects of emergency department pediatrics. In: Fleisher GR, Ludwig, S, eds. *Textbook of Pediatric Emergency Medicine.* 2nd ed. Baltimore, Md: Williams & Wilkins; 1988:1230-1245.

2. *Black's Law Dictionary.* 6th ed. St. Paul, Minn: West Publishing; 1990.

Glossary

Acyanotic heart lesion – lesions that produce a left-to-right shunt. Typically, these defects do not produce cyanosis because there is sufficient oxygenated blood in the circulation. This type of shunt produces increased pulmonary blood flow and increased workload on the heart. Examples of this type of lesion include patent ductus arteriosus and ventricular septal defect.

Antegrade amnesia – the inability to recall events that occur after the onset of amnesia; the inability to form new memories.

Babinski's reflex - first described by Joseph Babinski, a French neurologist. Stroking the outer sole of the foot upward from the heel across the ball of the foot causes the big toe to dorsiflex and the other toes to hyperextend. The reflex is normal in newborns (disappears after 1 year of age), and abnormal in children and adults.

Bag-valve-mask device – self-inflating device, consisting of a manually compressible bag with a port for room air or supplemental oxygen and a mask that fits over the mouth and nose of the patient. The device delivers room air at 21% oxygen unless supplemental oxygen is provided. To deliver a consistently higher oxygen concentration, a bag-valve-mask device should be equipped with an oxygen reservoir.

Barrier protection – barrier methods of contraception, such as the condom or cervical diaphragm, that prevent passage of spermatozoa into the uterus.

Battle's sign – ecchymosis behind the ear over the mastoid process; may indicate basilar skull fracture of the posterior fossa; first described by W. Battle (1855-1936), an English surgeon who was the surgical advisor to *Lancet* and was known for his work in obstetrics as well as surgery.

Bezoar – a hard ball of hair or vegetable fiber that may develop within the stomach of humans. A ball of pill fragments or tablets may develop after large ingestions and may remain lodged in the intestinal tract. This is also referred to as a *bezoar*.

Broselow tape™ – commercially available resuscitation measuring tape. This length-based resuscitation tape provides a measurement that corresponds with critical resuscitation information such as drug dosages, approximate weight, predicted normal vital signs, and other information. Measurement also corresponds with color coding that can be correlated with commercially packaged pediatric resuscitation equipment.

Brudzinski's sign – involuntary flexion of the knees and hips following flexion of the neck while supine. This is a manifestation of meningeal irritation. In some children, particularly in those younger than 12 to 18 months of age, this sign may not be evident.

Caregiver – parent, guardian, or any individual responsible for the child.

Cephalopelvic disproportion (CPD) – obstetric condition in which a baby's head is too large or a mother's birth canal is too small to permit normal labor or birth.

Cervical spine stabilization – whenever head or neck injury is suspected, the cervical spine must be stabilized. Cervical spine stabilization is the manual technique of ensuring that the neck is maintained in neutral alignment.

Chain of evidence – documentation of all persons handling evidence.

Glossary (continued)

Clubbing – abnormal enlargement of the distal phalanges. In children, it usually is associated with cyanotic heart disease. The mechanism that diminishes oxygen tension in the blood, causing clubbing, is not understood. Clubbing is present if the transverse diameter of the base of the fingernail is greater than the transverse diameter of the most distal joint of the digit.

Cold stress – neonate or young infant's response to a cool ambient environment, which results in physiologic stress because of the infant's limited ability to maintain heat.

Contrecoup injury (brain) – applied force to the brain causes the brain to strike the interior skull on the same side as the applied force (coup); then the brain moves (accelerates) and strikes the opposite side of the skull. The contrecoup injury occurs when the brain strikes the opposite side of the skull.

Costovertebral angle (CVA) tenderness – the CVA is one of two angles that outlines a space over the kidney. CVA tenderness to percussion is often noted with pyelonephritis and other infections of the kidney and adjacent structures.

Coup injury (brain) – applied force to the brain causes the brain to strike the interior skull on the same side as the applied force.

Crisis – state of disequilibrium that occurs when usual coping strategies are inadequate and immediate interventions are required.

Cyanotic heart lesion – lesion with a right-to-left shunt with either reduced or increased pulmonary blood flow. This shunt causes unoxygenated blood to be shunted from the right to the left side of the heart, and then to all parts of the body. Examples of cyanotic heart lesions include pulmonary valve atresia or stenosis, truncus arteriosus, and hypoplastic left heart syndrome.

Defibrillation – untimed depolarization of a critical mass of myocardial cells to allow spontaneous organized myocardial depolarization to resume. Defibrillation is the definitive treatment for ventricular fibrillation or pulseless ventricular tachycardia.

Diastatic fracture – linear fracture that occurs in one of the cranium sutures. This occurs more commonly at the lambdoid suture.

Droplet precautions – droplet transmission occurs when droplets containing microorganisms are transferred from the infected person, usually during sneezing, talking, coughing, or during certain procedures, such as suctioning. The microorganisms are propelled a short distance (usually within 3 feet). Droplet precautions include private room (preferred), closed door, and the use of a mask if within 3 feet of the patient.

Envenomation – injection of snake or insect venom into the body.

Family – persons with an established mutual relationship with a child.

Family-centered care philosophy – philosophy that incorporates the key elements of family-centered care. The philosophy provides the foundation for integrating the psychosocial care of the child and family in the emergency care setting.

Family presence – practice of providing families the option to remain with their child during all phases of treatment or interventions including resuscitation, stabilization, and invasive procedures.

Glossary (continued)

Fever – abnormal elevation of body temperature. Fever results from an imbalance between the elimination and production of heat. No single theory explains the mechanism whereby the temperature is increased. Fever has no recognized function in conditions other than infection.

Fiftieth percentile weight – statistical distribution for ranking children by weight. The standardized 50th percentile weight chart identifies the expected weight for the age group. Approximately 50% of children will be heavier and 50% will be lighter than the specified weight.

Functional asplenia – absence of the immunologic function of the spleen.

Gatekeeper – health care professional, usually a primary care physician or a nurse, who is the patient's first contact with the health care system. The gatekeeper triages the patient's further access to the system.

Glasgow coma scale – scoring system to measure the patient's level of consciousness. Score ranges from 3 to 15; points correspond to responses in three areas: eye opening, verbal response to pain, and motor response to pain. The patient's best responses in each of the three areas are added for a total score; developed by Drs. Jennett and Teasdale who are from Glasgow, Scotland.

Grasp reflex – pathologic reflex induced by stroking the palm or sole, with the result that the fingers or toes flex in a grasping motion. The reflex occurs in diseases of the premotor cortex. In young infants, the tonic grasp reflex is normal. When the examiner strokes the infant's palms, the child grasps the examiner's fingers so firmly that the child can be lifted into the air. The grasp reflex may also be called Darwinian reflex.

Head tilt–chin lift – method of opening the airway. The rescuer uses one hand to tilt the head, extending the neck. The index finger of the rescuer's other hand lifts the mandible outward by lifting on the chin. Head tilt should not be performed if cervical spine injury is suspected.

Hyphema – hemorrhage into the anterior chamber of the eye, usually caused by a blunt injury or trauma.

Immunocompromised – pertaining to an immune response that has been weakened by a disease or an immunosuppressive agent.

Jaw thrust – safest method of opening the airway of the victim with suspected neck or cervical spine injury. The jaw thrust can be accomplished without extension of the neck. Two or three fingers are placed under each side of the lower jaw at its angle and the jaw is lifted upward and outward.

Kernig's sign – diagnostic sign for meningitis, marked by a loss of the ability of a supine patient to completely straighten the leg when it is fully flexed at the knee and hip. Pain in the lower back and resistance to straightening the leg constitute a positive Kernig's sign. Usually the patient can extend the leg completely when the thigh is not flexed on the abdomen.

KPa – measurement to report arterial blood gas values in the United Kingdom. Conversion is the value in mm Hg divided by 7.5.

Kussmaul respirations – abnormally deep, very rapid sighing respirations, characteristics of diabetic ketoacidosis.

Mottling – patchy discoloration of the skin related to peripheral vasoconstriction.

Myolysis – dissolution or liquefaction of muscular tissue, frequently proceeded by degenerative changes, such as atrophy and fatty degeneration.

Glossary (continued)

Neonate – infant from birth to 4 weeks of age. If the infant is preterm, he or she remains a neonate until the expected due date plus 28 days.

Orthostatic vital signs – abnormal vital sign changes that occur when an individual assumes the sitting or standing posture. Abnormally low blood pressure that occurs when standing is called *orthostatic hypotension* or *postural hypotension.*

Overbed radiant warmer – commercially available overbed warming device that emits controlled radiant heat outwardly and downwardly.

Oxygen challenge test – test used to assist in differentiating the cause of cyanosis (respiratory versus cardiac). Arterial blood gases are measured with the neonate on room air and then on 100% oxygen. If the PaO_2 increases by more than 20 torr or is greater than 200 torr on oxygen, the cyanosis is probably respiratory in origin.

Paracetamol – acetaminophen product commercially available outside of the United States, in countries such as Australia, Canada, and Great Britain.

Paradoxical chest wall movement – traditional description for the respiratory effort of a patient with a flail chest. Generally, multiple rib fractures and/or a sternum fracture are present. The continuity of the thorax is destroyed, and the rib cage no longer moves evenly and in unison. The injured parts of the bony thorax do not respond with normal movements of inspiration or expiration. The flail segment appears to move paradoxically.

Paradoxical irritability – when the young child or infant cries with comforting measures and is quiet when left alone. A young child or infant without paradoxical irritability is quieted with comfort measures and cries when left alone.

Pediatric coma scale – scoring system, adapted from the Glasgow Coma Scale, to measure the young child's level of consciousness. The scale incorporates pediatric developmental considerations. The pediatric version of the Glasgow Coma Scale includes assessment of eye opening, best motor response, and best verbal response. Response in each category is rated on a scale of 1 to 5. The highest possible score is 15; a score of 8 or less is indicative of coma.

Pediatrics – branch of medicine concerned with the development and care of infants, children, and adolescents (birth through 21 years of age).

Pericardiocentsis – emergency procedure to relieve a pericardial tamponade; blood in the pleural sac is removed via an over-the-needle catheter inserted into the sac.

Permanent tooth bud – during embryonic life, a tooth-forming organ develops in the dental lamina for each permanent tooth that will be needed after the deciduous teeth are gone. These tooth-producing organs slowly form the permanent teeth throughout the first 6 to 20 years of life. When each permanent tooth becomes fully formed, it pushes upward through the bone of the jaw. This erodes the root of the deciduous tooth and eventually causes it to loosen and fall out. The permanent tooth bud is the evolving tooth behind the deciduous tooth.

Persistent pulmonary hypertension of the newborn – syndrome characterized by pulmonary hypertension that results in severe hypoxemia secondary to right-to-left shunting through persisting fetal channels (foramen ovale and ductus arteriosis) in the absence of structural heart disease.

Petechiae – small (under 3 mm in diameter), reddish, purple, macular lesions. They are a result of tiny hemorrhages within the dermal or submucosal layers.

Plantar reflex – normal response elicited by firmly stroking the outer surface of the sole from heel to toes, characterized by flexion of the toes.

Poisoning – condition or physical state produced by the ingestion of, injection of, inhalation of, or exposure to a poisonous substance or product in doses sufficient to cause poisoning.

Preventive services – procedure, measure, substance, or program designed to prevent a disease from occurring or a mild disorder from becoming more severe. Services focus on disease prevention and health maintenance.

Protective (reverse) isolation – isolation process used to protect the immunocompromised patient from exposure to harmful microorganisms.

Prudent layperson – any health care consumer.

Purpura – ecchymotic areas reflecting blood in the skin or mucosal membranes. This may occur with several different bleeding disorders, meningococcemia, or sepsis.

Raccoon's eyes – ecchymosis around the eyes; may indicate basilar skull fracture of the anterior fossa.

Rapid sequence induction (RSI) – anesthesiology term relating to the use of certain drugs to induce anesthesia; induction relates to Stage 1 (analgesia and consciousness) and Stage 2 (unconscious yet no skeletal muscle relaxation); RSI is a method to facilitate the insertion of an endotracheal tube in a trauma patient or responsive child.

Respiratory distress – compensated state in which normal gas exchange is maintained at the expense of an increased work of breathing.

Respiratory failure – failure of the physiologic process of oxygen transport to cells and the removal of carbon dioxide from cells. Clinically, respiratory failure is characterized by inadequate ventilation or oxygenation.

Reticular activating system (RAS) – functional system in the brain, essential to wakefulness, attention, concentration, and introspection. A network of nerve fibers in the thalamus, hypothalamus, brain stem, and cerebral cortex contribute to the system.

Retrograde amnesia – loss of memory for events occurring before a particular time in a person's life, usually before the event that precipitated the amnesia.

Rooting reflex – normal response in newborns, when the cheek is touched or stroked along the side of the mouth, to turn the head toward the stimulated side and begin to suck. The reflex disappears by 3 to 4 months of age but in some infants may persist until 1 year of age.

Sexual contact – legal definitions for sexual contact varies by state and country. The National Center on Child Abuse and Neglect defines sexual contact as:
- The offender touches the child's intimate parts.
- The offender induces the child to touch his or her intimate parts.
- Frottage (the offender rubs genitals against the victim's body or clothing).

Shaken impact syndrome – one of several terms ascribed to the range of craniospinal injuries sustained by infants and young children as a consequence of violent physical actions of a caregiver. Shaken impact syndrome is also referred to as *nonaccidental head injury, shaken baby syndrome,* and *shaken infant syndrome.*

Glossary (continued)

Special needs – any type of condition with the potential to interfere with normal growth and development.

Spinal cord injury without radiographic abnormality (SCIWORA) – phenomenon in children in which the child sustains a spinal cord injury from hyperextension, flexion, or traction without an associated vertebral fracture.

Spinal immobilization – immobilization of the vertebral column includes the application of cervical collar, towel rolls, or lateral stabilization device, and straps, or commercially available immobilization devices. The purpose of spinal immobilization is to prevent the occurrence or exacerbation of spinal cord injury in the child with a potentially unstable spinal injury.

Startle reflex – reflex response to a sudden, unexpected stimulus. The reaction may be accompanied by flexion of the trunk muscles and is rapid, pervasive, and uncontrollable, regardless of the unexpected stimulus.

Stress – relationship between a person and the environment that is appraised by the person as taxing or exceeding his or her resources and endangering his or her well-being.

Sucking reflex – involuntary sucking movements of the circumoral area in newborns in response to stimulation. Persists throughout infancy, even without stimulation, such as during sleep.

Synchronized cardioversion – restoration of the heart's normal rhythm by delivery of a synchronized electric shock through two paddles, which are attached to an appropriate delivery device. Synchronized cardioversion provides depolarization that is timed or synchronous with the patient's intrinsic electrical activity.

Syndrome of inappropriate antidiuretic hormone (SIADH) – abnormal condition characterized by the excessive release of antidiuretic hormone (ADH) that alters the body's fluid and electrolyte balance. It results from various malfunctions, such as the inability to produce and secrete dilute urine, water retention, increased extracellular fluid volume, and hyponatremia. SIADH develops in association with diseases that affect the osmoreceptors of the hypothalamus.

Tanner staging – may also be referred to as *sexual maturity rating*. A system for objectively determining sexual maturity, correlating chronologic age with a group of anatomic parameters, or determining the degree of adolescent maturation. In females, five stages of maturation are recorded for pubic hair and breast development; in males, five stages are recorded for pubic hair, growth of the penis, and growth of the testicles. The most commonly used system was described by Tanner.

Triage – process used to determine the urgency of need for emergency care based on assessment findings. The word *triage* means to sort or choose.

Triage decision – decision resulting from a process in which a group of patients are sorted according to their need for care. Triage decisions may be classified as emergent, urgent, or nonurgent.

Widening pulse pressure – pulse pressure is determined by systolic pressure minus diastolic pressure. A widening pulse pressure is determined by trending the changes in blood pressure that reflect elevation of systolic reading, decreases in diastolic reading, or both.

Wolff-Parkinson-White syndrome – a disorder of atrioventricular conduction, characterized by two AV conduction pathways. This syndrome is often identified by a characteristic delta wave seen on an electrocardiogram at the beginning of the QRS complex.